Antisense Technology in the Central Nervous System

Antisense Technology in the Central Nervous System

Edited by

RONALD A. LESLIE
SmithKline Beecham Pharmaceuticals, Harlow, Essex

A. JACKIE HUNTER
SmithKline Beecham Pharmaceuticals, Harlow, Essex

and

HAROLD A. ROBERTSON
Department of Pharmacology, Dalhousie University, Halifax, Nova Scotia, Canada

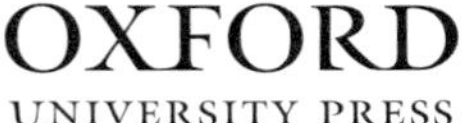

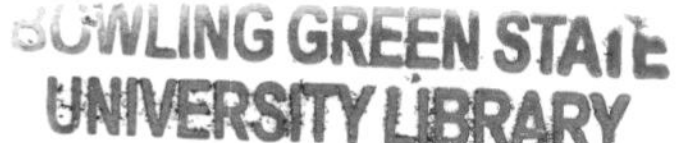

OXFORD
UNIVERSITY PRESS

Great Clarendon Street, Oxford OX2 6DP

Oxford University Press is a department of the University of Oxford and furthers the University's aim of excellence in research, scholarship, and education by publishing worldwide in

Oxford New York

Athens Auckland Bangkok Bogotá Buenos Aires Calcutta Cape Town Chennai Dar es Salaam Delhi Florence Hong Kong Istanbul Karachi Kuala Lumpur Madrid Melbourne Mexico City Mumbai Nairobi Paris São Paulo Singapore Taipei Tokyo Toronto Warsaw

and associated companies in Berlin Ibadan

Oxford is a registered trade mark of Oxford University Press in the UK and in certain other countries

Published in the United States by Oxford University Press Inc., New York

First published 1999

A catalogue record for this book is available from the British Library

Library of Congress Cataloging in Publication Data

Antisense technology in the central nervous system/edited by Ron A. Leslie, J. Hunter, H. Robertson.
Includes bibliographical references and index.
1. Neurogenetics. 2. Antisense nucleic acids. 3. Genetic regulation. I. Leslie, Ron A. II. Hunter, Jackie, 1956– III. Robertson, H. (Harry A.)
QP356.22.A58 1999 573.8′6–dc21 99–16187

ISBN 0 19 850316 4 (Hbk)
0 19 850538 8 (Pbk)

Typeset by Footnote Graphics, Warminster, Wilts
Printed in Great Britain on acid-free paper by Bookcraft (Bath) Ltd, Midsomer Norton, Avon

Foreword

by Prof. Claude Hélène, Museum National d'Histoire Naturelle, Laboratoire de Biophysique, Paris

The avalanche of information arising from sequencing the genomes of different organisms, including the human genome, is stimulating the development of new tools to investigate gene function. Functional genomics is now at the centre stage of research activities aimed at understanding the physiology of living organisms. How information derived from such studies can be exploited to develop new treatments for human disorders is, of course, the focus of intensive research in the pharmaceutical industry, in biotech companies, and in public research laboratories. Most clinically active drugs that are presently available target proteins—the products of gene expression. One noticeable exception is represented by drugs that target DNA, but in general these act by non-sequence-specific mechanisms. The idea of developing novel strategies to target specific sequences of nucleic acids is not new. However it is only recently that several concepts have emerged with the ambitious goal of inhibiting a single gene in a living cell. The simplest way to recognise a nucleic acid is to use nucleic acids themselves. In the antisense approach, an oligonucleotide binds to its complementary sequence on a messenger RNA. In the antigene strategy an oligonucleotide is designed to bind a target sequence on the double helix of DNA, forming a local triple helix. The oligonucleotide inhibits either the translation of the mRNA (antisense) or the transcription of the gene itself (antigene) in a sequence-specific manner.

Antisense oligonucleotides provide interesting tools to investigate gene function. Intravenous injection of oligonucleotides incorporating phosphorothioate backbones has demonstrated that they distribute in all tissues except brain because they do not cross the blood–brain barrier, as would be expected for such polyanionic molecules. Therefore the utilisation of antisense oligonucleotides to investigate gene function in the brain requires a direct administration by either intracerebroventricular infusion or intracerebral injection. Antisense oligonucleotides with a phosphodiester or a phosphorothioate backbone inhibit messenger RNA translation by directing a sequence-specific cleavage of the mRNA by endogenous RNase H. This enzyme is involved, during normal cell life, in removing RNA primers after DNA replication and before cell division. Therefore RNase H activity might be a limiting factor in an approach targeting cells that do not divide, such as mature neurons. However several reports have described a decrease in mRNA levels after oligonucleotide administration to the brain, an observation which suggests that even non-dividing cells might contain enough RNase H activity to sustain an antisense effect. In any case, brain tissue might represent a good opportunity to investigate oligonucleotide analogues that do not reduce RNase H cleavage but exhibit an antisense activity by a different mechanism.

The different chapters of this book address some of the basic questions raised by antisense technologies and their applications to brain studies. There are strategies other than antisense technology which can be used to obtain information on gene function through sequence-specific inhibition of protein synthesis, for instance ribozymes which are described in Chapter 14. More recent technologies that have not yet been applied to brain research (or not yet described) would be worth testing by local administration techniques. Antigene oligonucleotides with high affinity and sequence specificity are now available to control the transcription of specific genes; they may either compete with transcription factor binding or arrest the transcription machinery during the elongation process. Other DNA ligands, apart from oligonucleotides, such as minor groove-binding polyamides could also be used to modulate gene transcription in a sequence-selective manner. Transcription can also be modulated by double-stranded oligonucleotides that act as decoys for transcription factors. Since a given transcription factor is involved in the regulation of several genes, the decoy strategy is not expected to be specific for a single gene. Chimeric DNA/RNA oligonucleotides have been described as inducing targeted mutations and could be used to change gene expression. More recently double-stranded RNAs have been shown to interfere with gene expression in a sequence-specific manner, at least in organisms such as *Caenohabditis elegans*, *Drosophila*, and trypanosomes.

Furthermore, instead of targeting DNA or mRNAs, oligonucleotides can be selected to bind proteins and inhibit their activity. These 'aptamers' are described in Chapter 13. All the technologies mentioned above would certainly be worth investigating as tools to decipher gene function in the brain. Forthcoming studies will certainly tell us how far these approaches will be exploited in order to understand brain organisation and function and to provide a basis for the indentification of new therapeutic targets and/or new strategies to fight brain diseases.

Acknowledgments

The editors wish to thank Marion Leslie for help with the design and artwork on the front cover.

Contents

3. The design of appropriate control experiments to ensure specificity in antisense oligonucleotide function 21

Wolfgang Brysch

4. Modulation of gene expression in the CNS as a tool in behavioral pharmacology 42

Wolfgang Sommer and Markus Heilig

Contributors

SUDHIR AGRAWAL
Hybridon, Inc., 155 Fortune Blvd., Milford, MA 01757, USA.

DAVID L. BECKER
Department of Anatomy and Developmental Biology, University College London , Gower Street, London WC1E 6BT, UK.

WOLFGANG BRYSCH
Biognostik GmbH, Gerhard-Gerdes-Str. 19, 37079 Göttingen, Germany.

RICHARD C. CONRAD
Eli Lilly & Co., Lilly Research Labs, Lilly Corporate Center, Indianapolis IN 46285, USA.

IAN CREESE
Center for Molecular and Behavioral Neuroscience, Rutgers, The State University of New Jersey, 197 University Avenue, Newark, NJ 07102, USA.

EMMANUEL CULETTO
Laboratory of Molecular Signalling, Department of Zoology, University of Cambridge, Downing Street, Cambridge CB2 3EJ, UK.

COLIN R. GREEN
Department of Anatomy with Radiology, School of Medicine, University of Auckland, Private bag 92019, Auckland, New Zealand.

PAUL R. HARTIG
CNS Department, DuPont Pharmaceuticals Research Laboratories, P.O. Box 80400 Experimental Station E400, Wilmington, DE 19880-0400, USA.

MARKUS A. HEILIG
Addiction Center South, Huddinge University Hospital, M67 Karolinska Institutet, S-14186 Huddinge, Sweden.

SIEW PENG HO
CNS Department, DuPont Pharmaceuticals Research Laboratories, P.O. Box 80400 Experimental Station E400, Wilmington, DE 19880-0400, USA.

A. J. HUNTER
SmithKline Beecham Pharmaceuticals, New Frontiers Science Park North, Third Avenue, Harlow, Essex CM19 5AW.

EKAMBAR R. KANDIMALLA
Hybridon, Inc., 155 Fortune Blvd., Milford, MA 01757, USA.

SIMRANJIT KAUR
Center for Molecular and Behavioral Neuroscience, Rutgers, The State University of New Jersey, 197 University Avenue, Newark, NJ 07102, USA.

RAI KNEE
Department of Physiology and Biophysics, Faculty of Medicine, Dalhousie University, Halifax, Nova Scotia, Canada.

R. LANDGRAF
Max Planck Institute of Psychiatry, Kraepelinstrasse 10, 80804 Munich, Germany.

MARC B. LEE
Department of Human Anatomy and Genetics, Oxford University, South Parks Road, Oxford OX1 3QX, UK.

R. A. LESLIE
SmithKline Beecham Pharmaceuticals, New Frontiers Science Park North, Third Avenue, Harlow, Essex CM19 5AW.

AUDREY W. LI
Department of Physiology and Biophysics, Faculty of Medicine, Dalhousie University, Halifax, Nova Scotia, Canada.

JUN SHENG LIN
Department of Anatomy with Radiology, School of Medicine, University of Auckland, Private bag 92019, Auckland, New Zealand.

DAGMARA MOHUCZY
Department of Physiology, University of Florida College of Medicine, P.O. Box 100274, Gainesville FL 32610, USA.

PAUL R. MURPHY
Department of Physiology and Biophysics, Faculty of Medicine, Dalhousie University, Halifax, Nova Scotia, Canada.

GAVRIL W. PASTERNAK
Department of Neurology, Memorial Sloan Kettering Cancer Center, 1275 York Avenue, NY 10021, USA.

M. IAN PHILLIPS
Department of Physiology, University of Florida College of Medicine, P.O. Box 100274, Gainesville FL 32610, USA.

LEONIDAS A. PHYLACTOU
The Cyprus Institute of Neurology and Genetics, 6 International Airport Avenue, P.O. Box 23462, 1683 Nicosia, Cyprus.

DENNIS W. RICKMAN
Department of Ophthalmology and Visual Sciences, University of Iowa, 200 Hawkins Drive, Iowa City IA 52242, USA.

H. A. ROBERTSON
Department of Pharmacology, Dalhousie University, Sir Charles Tupper Medical Building, Halifax, Nova Scotia B3H 4H7, Canada.

DAVID B. SATTELLE
Laboratory of Molecular Signalling, Department of Zoology, University of Cambridge, Downing Street, Cambridge CB2 3EJ, UK.

WOLFGANG SOMMER
Addiction Center South, Huddinge University Hospital, M67 Karolinska Institutet, S-14186 Huddinge, Sweden.

XIAOPING TANG
Department of Physiology, University of Florida College of Medicine, P.O. Box 100274, Gainesville FL 32610, USA.

JAMES M. TEPPER
Center for Molecular and Behavioral Neuroscience, Rutgers, The State University of New Jersey, 197 University Avenue, Newark, NJ 07102, USA.

MATTHEW J. A. WOOD
Department of Human Anatomy and Genetics, Oxford University, South Parks Road, Oxford OX1 3QX, UK.

Abbreviations

AAV	adeno-associated virus
ACh	acetylcholine
AChE	acetylcholinesterase
ALT	alanine aminotransferase
AP-1	activator protein-1
β-APP	amyloid peptide precursor
APS	ammonium persulfate
AST	aspartate aminotransferase
AVP	arginine vasopressin
BDNF	brain-derived neurotrophic factor
CGE	capillary gel electrophoresis
CMV	cytomegalovirus
CNS	central nervous system
CREB	cAMP response element binding [protein]
CRH	corticotropin-releasing hormone
DEB	diepoxybutane
DMT	dimethoxytrityl
DOR	delta opioid receptor
DPDPE	[D-Pen^{2},D-Pen^{5}]enkephalin
DRADA	double-stranded RNA-specific adenosine deaminase
dsRNAi	double-stranded RNA interference
EMS	ethyl methanesulfonate
FES	filter elution solution
FGF-2	basic fibroblast growth factor
FITC	fluorescein isothiocyanate
FNM	fluphenazine-*N*-mustard
GABA	γ-aminobutyric acid
GCL	ganglion cell layer
GFAP	glial fibrillary acidic protein
GFP	green fluorescent protein
GnRH	gonadotropin releasing hormone
HDV	hepatitis delta virus
HPLC	high performance liquid chromatography
i.c.v.	intracerebroventricular
IEG	immediate–early gene
IGF-II	insulin-like growth factor II
INL	inner nuclear layer
IPL	inner plexiform layer
LTR	long terminal repeat
MBO	mixed-backbone oligonucleotide

M6G	morphine-6β-glucuronide
MOI	multiplicity of infection
MOR	mu opioid receptor
nAChR	nicotinic acetylcholine receptor
NO	nitric oxide
NOS	nitric oxide synthase
NPY	neuropeptide Y
NT-4	neurotrophin-4
ODN	oligodeoxynucleotide
6-OHDA	6-hydroxydopamine
ORF	open reading frame
PAGE	polyacrylamide gel electrophoresis
PBMC	peripheral blood mononuclear cell
PBS	phosphate-buffered saline
PCNA	proliferating cell nuclear antigen
PNA	peptide nucleic acid
PND	postnatal day
PO-ON	phosphodiester oligonucleotide
PS-ON	phosphorothioate oligonucleotide
aPTT	activated partial thromboplastin time
RT-PCR	reverse transcription–polymerase chain reaction
SHR	spontaneously hypertensive rat
SNAP	synaptosome-associated protein
TH	tyrosine hydroxylase
TMP-UV	trimethylpsoralen–ultraviolet light
TR	thyroid hormone receptor
UTR	untranslated region
VTA	ventral tegmental area
YAC	yeast artificial chromosomes
YC	yellow crescent

1

Antisense oligonucleotide regulation of gene expression in the CNS: an overview

R. A. LESLIE, A. J. HUNTER AND H. A. ROBERTSON

1. Introduction

As more and more genes are sequenced and mapped by the human genome project, the determination of the function of novel genes becomes of increasing importance. Transgenic animals have usually been used to study the effects of either overexpression, or abolition of expression, of individual genes. The process for producing such transgenic animals is, however, very time consuming (taking up to a year in some cases) and is complicated by possible variations in gene expression in different strains of mouse and compensatory mechanisms that occur during pre- and post-embryonic development. These considerations have driven the development of novel technologies to allow the modulation of expression of genes that alter the production of specific proteins—the building blocks of the cell. These technologies make it increasingly possible to manipulate gene expression in order to study normal or pathological cellular metabolic processes, often with the aim of alleviating or curing disease.

Specifically designed antisense oligodeoxynucleotides (ODNs) have effectively been used to 'knock down' expression of specific genes in living tissues and cells in order to study the function of their protein products. Experimental or therapeutic antisense ODNs are short lengths of man-made genetic material, designed according to known gene sequence information, to lessen or prevent the production of the protein encoded by the gene. These engineered molecules interfere with one or more stages in the process of protein formation, and the cell ends up manufacturing less of the particular encoded product. Studies on the cells or tissues, now rendered deficient in the particular protein, may shed light on the function of that protein. Alternatively, if the function of the protein is already known, and it is determined that a disease process results from a particular tissue containing too much of the protein, the method could in theory correct the problem and effect a cure for the disorder (1, 2, 3).

The technology is still at an early stage of development and the many technical problems experienced by the pioneers of the methods are only now beginning to be understood and circumvented. Some of these are unique to the use of antisense knockdown approaches in the nervous system. For example, problems of design and synthesis of antisense molecules, administration of them to the brain, and prevention of their destruction by metabolic processes once they have been introduced, are still under active study. Furthermore, the newly introduced genetic fragments can be toxic to healthy brain tissue and cause irreparable damage. These problems and others have caused (and continue to cause) many investigators to worry about the usefulness of this approach for biological studies or for potential therapeutic use (4). None the less, successes that have been achieved to date by use of these methods strongly suggest that these problems will be solved and that the technique will become much more routine and trustworthy, at least for some types of investigations and/or therapies.

This book summarizes the background to the technology of antisense ODN knockdowns, explains its potential for central nervous system (CNS) research and therapy, and discusses the problems associated with its use, particularly in the nervous system. Emphasis is given to practical ways in which these problems can and should be addressed. The advantages and disadvantages of the technique, as compared with alternatives such as the use of transgenic mice with specific gene knockouts, are explained. The future of antisense knockdown in research and therapeutics as well as aspects of developing alternative technologies (such as aptamers and ribozymes) are also discussed.

2. The theory of antisense gene knockdown and design of synthetic antisense molecules

The most efficient way to approach antisense ODN gene knockdown in practice is still under development. One theoretical strategy of the antisense ODN approach is to cause the formation of a short triple-helical structure in the genetic material of a cell by the binding of a synthetic ODN designed to hybridize in an antisense manner to a portion of the DNA molecule during transcription. Thus the process of coding for a new mRNA molecule is inhibited. Another strategy would target mRNA after the transcription process has taken place and inhibit its translation into protein. Cleavage of mRNA by endogenous RNase H activity has been shown to be involved in some cases of inhibition of gene expression by the action of antisense ODNs (see Chapter 2).

The design of synthetic ODNs for antisense gene knockdown is critical. For example, the size of the molecule is important: in some instances at least, little leeway is tolerable in this. Unfortunately there is no hard-and-fast rule that will always work to yield an optimally sized ODN and it is probable that the molecules that will provide the best knockdown in a given situation will have to be determined by empirical means. For example, some ODNs as short as 12 nucleotides have been found to provide good discrimination amongst different gene sequences, but in other cases ODNs 16 bases long provide no selectivity. If an ODN is too short it will not be selective at all, but if it is too long it will not be accessible to the tissue and will be difficult to work with in an experimental or therapeutic situation (and may not even be selective).

Similarly, there are issues about longevity of synthetic ODNs once they have been administered to cells and tissues. Endogenous RNases presumably work quickly to break the molecules down and it appears to be often necessary to protect against this in order for the ODNs to have a practical antisense effect. Factors such as the frequency of turnover of the proteins in question as well as the biological environment of the cells will all play a role in this process. Phosphorothioate 'protection' of ODNs is often designed into their manufacture to minimize their breakdown by RNase activity and this in turn affects their optimum size: the addition of the sulfur groups requires that such ODNs be longer than 'unprotected' ODNs in order to 'work'.

Some investigators have spent considerable effort in experimenting with strategies to optimize the design of antisense ODNs. One procedure for rational design of ODNs is discussed in Chapter 2. The efficacy of antisense ODNs is unpredictable, in part due to the presence of secondary and tertiary structures within mRNA molecules that hinder access of antisense ODNs. The RNA mapping described here uses a library of semi-random ODNs that are allowed to hybridize to the target RNA. The binding regions are identified with RNase H, which cleaves RNA only at sites where RNA–DNA hybrids occur. The cleaved RNA fragments are sequenced and those areas of the mRNA accessible to antisense ODNs are identified. In studies using such an approach, targeting the start codon sequence with phosphorothioated ODNs was no more successful than targeting other regions of the target gene. The thioprotected ODNs appeared to exert their effects via induction of RNase H activity, while another type of oligonucleotide, using 2-methoxyribonucleotide sequences, was effective only when it was designed to recognize the start codon, suggesting that it caused arrest of translation.

3. Advantages and disadvantages of the technique—comparison with transgenics

A popular research technique in current use is the construction of transgenic animals to study the effect of a single gene on a biological system. This technique involves genetic manipulation of experimental mice to generate animals that either do not express a gene of interest throughout development or overexpress the gene. While antisense ODNs cannot be used for overexpression studies, they do have some advantages over transgenic animals for gene underexpression studies. Such advantages include effectiveness in any species, not just mice, reversibility of the underexpression, relative low cost, potential for therapeutic use, and the knockdown of as many genes as desired. However, there are disadvantages as well, which include incomplete knockdown of target, sequence-independent effects, narrow window of effect and CNS administration problems. Another practical disadvantage is the often-experienced toxicity associated with the administration of antisense ODNs, particularly those that have been designed with phosphorothioate protection against RNase degradation. A detailed discussion of ODN design is given in Chapter 8.

4. Uptake of antisense ODNs by experimental cells and tissues and the issue of controls

Obviously, for the antisense inhibition approach to work, *in vitro* or *in vivo*, for either research or therapeutic purposes, the molecules used must not only be efficacious in knocking down gene expression but they must also be specific to the gene in question. To address the issue of efficacy, studies have been done using fluorescent markers to monitor the uptake of antisense ODNs into tissues and cells. An interesting finding was that uptake into primary cultured cells can be good in some situations whereas poor uptake into cloned cell lines has often proved to be a problem; this phenomenon may explain why some laboratories have experienced a lack of effect of their ODNs in established cell lines. Thus the strategy of using cloned cells to determine whether an antisense technique will work (which is often used by laboratories newly interested in the antisense ODN technique) may not be a sensible one.

Control experiments are essential for any studies using antisense ODNs. Much of the scepticism that surrounds antisense oligonucleotide knockdown as a strategy results from studies that have been reported that have not included appropriate controls. There are many possible types of control experiment that can be used (see Chapter 3). One common type is the use of 'mismatch ODNs', which are scrambled antisense sequences, having the advantage of automatically keeping the same GC content as the specific ODN. Another is the use of 'sense' control ODNs, but this can result in very confusing results for sound biological reasons (see below). Other types of control experiments involve 'randomized' control ODNs and 'reverse' controls. A great advantage can be the inclusion of a positive control in an experimental protocol. A good illustration of this is given in Chapter 4, where it can be seen that specific antisense ODNs can be effective against an immediate early gene product (such as Fos, the transcription factor encoded by c-*fos*) but not against related targets (such as the protein target coded by c-*jun*). Thus the experimenter can convince him/herself that the antisense ODN 'works' and is selective.

The issue of use of a sense probe as a control for the effects of an antisense

ODN is a complex one which has implications for antisense gene knockdown as well as any other technique using antisense technology (such as *in situ* hybridization histochemistry using oligoprobes). Any studies using sense ODNs as control must be interpreted with great caution, because it is becoming increasingly apparent that some cells can produce naturally occurring antisense molecules that can obscure the effects in these cells of synthetic sense molecules. Naturally occurring antisense is involved in gene regulation by a number of mechanisms, including transcriptional termination, RNA processing, transcript stability, ribosome binding and translation. A growing number of eukaryotic genes are known to be bidirectionally transcribed, and one of these, *FGF-2*, is discussed in detail in Chapter 12. *FGF-2* sense and antisense transcripts have been reported to form double-stranded RNA duplexes *in vivo*, which are targeted for post-transcriptional modification by a double-stranded RNA specific adenosine deaminase. Expression of the antisense RNA in *Xenopus* oocytes is associated with decreased *FGF-2* mRNA stability, suggesting that *FGF-2* may be regulated by its natural antisense. In situations like this, then, the introduction of a sense ODN as a control will provide misleading results, because the sense ODN will have biological activity and produce physiological effects of its own. Hence the commonly-used sense sequence control molecules in antisense ODN experiments probably are best avoided in all cases.

5. Antisense oligodeoxynucleotide delivery systems

Antisense ODNs can be administered to cells or tissues in several different ways. For example, cells *in vitro* can be incubated in solutions containing the synthetic ODNs, or the ODN solutions can be injected directly into individual cells. This is, of course, impractical in most situations where one desires to effect gene knockdown in many or all cells in a population. Especially in intact tissues and organs, such as the brain, it is necessary to devise some technique to introduce antisense molecules to all the cells of interest. Direct parenchymal injections or intracerebrovascular injections have both been used with some success.

The use of molecular biological approaches for delivery of antisense ODNs, such as adeno-associated viral (AAV) vectors, is becoming popular as it is realized that such delivery systems can provide more efficacious and targeted delivery, especially in CNS tissues (see Chapter 11). Access to the mammalian CNS is more problematic than to peripheral tissues because of the existence of the blood–brain diffusion barrier ('blood–brain barrier'). AAV is a 'dependent' virus which requires adenovirus to replicate and therefore is safe to use *in vivo*; it has a number of advantages over other viral vectors in that it does not cause an inflammatory or immune response. AAV enters non-dividing cells and integrates into their chromosomes. Recombinant AAV can be prepared with added cytomegalovirus (CMV) promoters, and cDNA for the gene of interest can be inserted in the antisense direction. Stable cell lines can be transfected with the vector contents for *in vitro* studies, or *in vivo* experiments can use injections of the constructs into CNS areas. Reporter genes such as *lacZ* can be included in the construct to give a preliminary indication of the success and extent of the transfection of injections, and such studies have been used to produce long-lasting antisense inhibition in some systems without any apparent toxicity.

Other innovative ways of maximizing the efficient delivery of ODNs to tissues are being explored and developed. One of these involves the use of pluronic gels as matrices for ODNs; this technique is explained in Chapter 10. Another approach that has been tried with some success *in vitro* is to conjugate the ODNs to cell-penetrant peptides such as penetratin. These peptides are short fragments derived from the homeodomain of antennapedia, a *Drosophila* transcription factor. They appear to interact with phospholipids and cholesterol-rich domains in the plasma membrane and are internalized via a non-endocytotic process. ODNs can be linked by disulfide bonds which are rapidly reduced inside the cell, leading to the dissociation of the ODN from its carrier peptide.

6. Alternative gene knockdown technologies

Molecules similar to, but somewhat more complex than antisense ODNs have been used for gene knockdown studies and have been suggested as being more efficaceous and reliable. These molecules, called 'hammerhead ribozymes', offer two theoretical advantages over antisense ODNs:

- they catalytically cleave the mRNA and positively halt the translation process
- they may have greater specificity than'regular' antisense ODNs because they have two separate mRNA-binding regions.

Chemical modifications of ribozyme structure do not appear to exert non-specific effects. As for antisense ODNs, ribozymes can be expressed from a variety of viral vectors to cause long-term effects. Ribozymes can be constructed and then selected based upon their secondary structure, mRNA target sequence accessibility and, if appropriate, cross-species homology. Ribozymes appear to be taken up readily *in vivo*, but require help *in vitro* (see Chapter 14). In some studies, ribozymes have been delivered to target tissues by adenoviral vectors and head-to-head comparisons of ribozymes with 15- and 20-mer phosphorothioated antisense ODNs have indicated that the ribozymes gave superior gene knockdown.

Several other approaches have been put forward as alternatives to antisense ODNs for gene knockdown. Aptamers are small nucleic acids (DNA, RNA or modified molecules) that bind with high specificity to targets ranging from organic molecules to protein assemblies. The term 'aptamer' is derived from the Latin, *aptare*, which means 'to fit' or 'to accommodate'. Aptamers can act as inhibitors of protein function and are selected from a pool of random nucleotide sequences produced for the purpose. The process has been termed 'selective enrichment of ligands through exponential enrichment' (SELEX), and is described in Chapter 13. Target molecules are immobilized in a column or matrix and ODNs that bind to them are extracted and amplified by PCR. Chosen sequences are cloned to produce aptamers with high affinity and selectivity, and that can inhibit target nucleic acid function to produce a gene knockdown. Although theoretically this appears to be a sound strategy for gene knockdown, no information is yet available on entry of aptamers into cells, and little is yet known about the possible selectivity of aptamers in binding to molecules other than their targets.

Yet another similar strategy that has been proposed for gene knockdown involves a new class of molecules termed 'peptide nucleic acids' (PNAs; see Chapter 8). These DNA-mimetic molecules have the deoxyribose phosphodiester nucleic acid backbone replaced by a novel type of molecular building block, *N*-(2-aminoethyl)glycine. Molecules of this nature have been demonstrated to act as near-perfect mimics of DNA, being able to form the familiar double-helical complex using normal Watson–Crick base pairing. PNAs can also complex with single-stranded DNA in the normal base-pairing fashion, and Hoogsteen base pairing can form triple-stranded complexes in purine-rich sequences. All these attributes would theoretically allow PNAs to be used to modulate gene expression and cause gene knockdown. PNAs would have several practical advantages over oligonucleotides as experimental or therapeutic molecules: they are non-chiral, uncharged, and are more stable and are less dependent upon the ionic strength of the medium in which they are prepared. Furthermore, PNA–RNA complexes do not form a substrate for RNase H as is the case for 'normal' RNA. PNA molecules most probably depend upon inhibiting the passage of ribosomes along the RNA to inhibit translation, and experiments have shown that they can inhibit RNA function in start-codon regions as well as in downstream areas of the gene. Like some of the other approaches mentioned in this book, PNAs have problems in terms of access to internal cellular compartments. Again, special delivery systems have been tried, and conjugation with cell-penetrant peptides have been shown to enhance penetration across the plasma membrane. Recently, PNAs conjugated to the cell-penetrant peptides transportan or penetratin have been shown to regulate mRNA levels in the spinal cord. (5)

References

1. Zamecnik, P. and Stephenson, M. (1978) *Proc. Natn. Acad. Sci., USA.* **75,** 280–4.
2. Agrawal, S. (1996) *Trends Biotech.* **14,** 376–87.
3. Crooke, S. T. ed. (1998) Antisense research and application. In *Handbook of Pharmacology*, Vol. **131**, Springer-Verlag.
4. Gura, T. (1995) *Science.* **270,** 575–7.
5. Pooga (1998) *Nature Biotech.* **16,** 857–61.

2

Antisense knockdown in the CNS—optimizing the strategy

SIEW PENG HO AND PAUL R. HARTIG

1. Introduction

Application of antisense oligodeoxynucleotides (ODNs) to CNS targets has been a much more difficult task than originally envisioned. Early reports of success have sometimes proven irreproducible in other laboratories or have been confounded by oligonucleotide-induced toxicities at doses only slightly higher than, or overlapping with, effective doses. As experience has grown and more studies on the mechanism, toxicities and desirable control experiments have been published, the success rate has significantly improved. In this chapter, we review many of the experimental approaches and controls that our laboratory and others have found important for reducing the toxic effects, increasing the specificity and improving both the reproducibility and success rate in CNS antisense experiments. In particular, much larger degrees of both protein and mRNA knockdown (over 60%) can be obtained by these approaches than are reported in most published CNS antisense experiments. Additional discussions of CNS antisense methodologies can be found in related chapters of this book, and in recent published reviews (1–3).

2. Selection of potent oligonucleotide sequences for the antisense experiment

The design of antisense oligonucleotides is, in theory, a simple exercise. An antisense sequence is the complementary sequence, based on Watson–Crick base pairing, of the stretch of RNA being targeted. In practice, only 20–30% of antisense sequences selected are sufficiently active to reduce protein levels by 50% (4–6). The region around the start codon is one area that is frequently targeted, but ODNs directed against this site are sometimes of modest activity or even inactive (7–9). The importance of selecting potent sequences should not be underestimated. Large reductions in protein provide important biochemical support for any functional differences observed between treatment groups.

The mRNA target of antisense ODNs has significant secondary structure (double-helical stems, hairpin loops, internal bulges) and tertiary structure which render certain regions in the RNA inaccessible. To identify highly potent sequences, multiple ODNs can be randomly selected and screened (7,9,10). As an example of the variability seen amongst ODN sequences, of 34 antisense sequences targeted against c-Raf kinase mRNA, 45% of the ODNs had little to no antisense effect, whereas four ODNs reduced RNA levels by 70% or more.

Alternatively, to improve upon the selection procedure, a more empirical approach may be adopted. We and others have developed methods whereby ODN or ribozyme libraries consisting of every possible sequence are used to identify RNA sites that are relatively accessible to ODN hybridization (11–16). In our method, RNA sites which bind DNA ODNs are cleaved by ribonuclease H (RNase H) (*Figure 1*). The location of these sites is then determined by sequencing experiments. RNA transcripts subjected to such RNA mapping experiments exhibit specific cleavage sites and not a smear of bands, consistent with the notion that not all regions in RNA molecules are equally accessible to ODN hybridization. In our experiments, ODNs targeted to 80% of the accessible sites were active, producing antisense effects of at least 50% in tissue culture (11,12). ODNs selected by use of this method were also effective in CNS *in vivo* experiments against the angiotensin type-1 receptor (12) and the corticotropin-releasing hormone (CRH) receptors (unpublished data).

3. Tissue culture experiments

Once antisense sequences have been selected, *in vitro* experiments should be performed to demonstrate ODN efficacy, verify sequence specificity (through

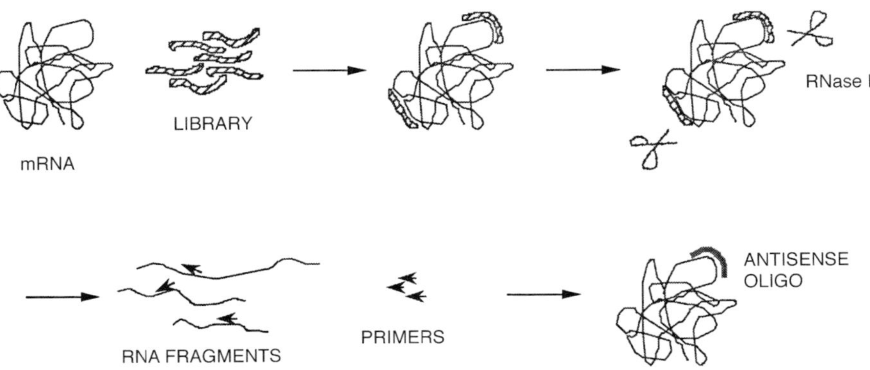

Figure 1. Scheme for antisense sequence selection. A library of ODNs is allowed to hybridize with the RNA molecule of interest. Accessible regions of RNA that are bound by ODN are cleaved with RNase H. Sequencing of RNA fragments generated reveals the location of accessible sites. Antisense ODNs are targeted to these sites.

the use of several different control sequences) and select the best sequences for animal experiments. Optimizing ODNs in tissue culture prior to initiating *in vivo* work can be a time saver in the long run. The success of cell-based experiments often depends upon the efficiency of ODN uptake into cells in culture (4,17). Antisense ODNs are large (typically 6–7 kDa) and highly charged (a 20 nt sequence has 19 negative charges) molecules. These properties impede the effective uptake of ODN in many different cell types, particularly continuous cell lines and some primary cultures (18–21). Therefore, before embarking on cell-based experiments, ODN uptake in the cells of interest should be demonstrated. This can be accomplished through microscopic examination of cells treated with ODNs labeled with fluorophores. Antisense experiments are less likely to succeed if intracellular levels of ODN are not sufficiently high.

If the cells of interest demonstrate poor ODN uptake, an effective way to overcome this problem is by the use of cationic liposomes (22–24). These positively charged lipid reagents form electrostatic complexes with DNA which are taken up by cells primarily through endocytic mechanisms. In the endosomes, fusion of liposomal and endosomal membranes occurs, resulting in release of the ODNs to the cytoplasm and nucleus (25–27). The use of liposomes should be carefully optimized because of their potential cytotoxicity. Liposomes are most effective at mediating uptake when the molar ratio between the positive charges (on the liposome) to the negative charges (on the ODN) is greater than 1 (28). However, increasing the positive-to-negative charge ratio can lead to increasing cytotoxicity. This is monitored through an assay for mitochondrial activity (MTT assay) or by cell counting (24). Fluorescence microscopy of cells treated with fluorescein-labeled ODNs allows successful uptake (nuclear and cytoplasmic localization) to be distinguished from cases where the complex is endocytosed, but where the ODN is still trapped in endosomes. Finally, quantitative fluorescence-activated cell sorting can be used to select the best experimental conditions and the most effective liposome for a particular tissue culture system (24).

As an example of the improvements possible with cationic liposomes (22, 26), oligonucleotides against the angiotensin type-1 receptor mRNA were completely inactive at concentrations up to 15 μM ODN. However, in the presence of the cationic liposome Lipofectin, the ODNs were maximally effective at 0.25 μM (24). In general, potent antisense sequences (in the presence of cationic lipids) should reduce protein levels by 60–80% when administered to cells at concentrations of 150–400 nM.

4. Selecting parameters for the *in vivo* experiment

In contrast to cell culture studies, *in vivo* experiments do not make use of cationic liposomes. However, the presence of the blood–brain barrier requires direct delivery of ODNs to the brain. Several studies describing the tissue penetrance and distribution of intracerebrally administered biotin-, fluorescein- or radiolabeled ODNs have been reported (29–36). Intraventricular delivery is optimal for targeting periventricular brain regions, while intraparenchymal administration is required for more distal brain regions. In either case, penetration of ODN into the brain tissue is somewhat limited, highly dose-dependent, and stable in its extent of penetration by 1 h post-injection. At any given dose, intraparenchymal delivery produces greater tissue penetration than intraventricular administration (*Figure 2*), perhaps at the expense of more significant tissue damage. For instance, ODN penetration extended for 2–3 mm from the injection site following a single striatal injection of 2 nmol of ODN. A similar dose delivered into the lateral ventricle resulted in tissue penetration no greater than 1 mm from that ventricle (29).

A zone of tissue damage, extending up to 200 μm from the needle track, invariably occurs following intracerebral injections. This zone is characterized by a reduction in the number of neurons and by intense nuclear and cytoplasmic ODN-labeling of the remaining cells. While ODN diffusion extended for 1–2 mm from the injection site following an intrastriatal injection of 0.2 nmol of ODN, penetrance of ODN did not extend beyond the zone of damage with a 0.02 nmol injection (29). These observations should be kept in mind when targeting small brain nuclei with low doses of intraparenchymally administered ODN.

ODNs may be administered by repeated bolus injections or continuously infused using osmotic mini-pumps. There are few direct comparions between the two routes of administration in antisense experiments (37). In general, larger quantities of ODN are delivered per day via the continuous infusion route. These large doses can, however, produce significant toxic effects in the animals (35).

Before initiating an *in vivo* study, it is important to ensure that ODN dosage and route of administration will produce adequate ODN penetration to the brain region of interest. Our recent dose–response studies can serve as a guide (29), or ODN tracers may be used to demonstrate penetration to the target area. Although there is good overlap between the extent of ODN penetrance and the area of brain tissue exhibiting antisense effects (29,38), presence of ODN by itself is not sufficient to guarantee antisense effects. Many other factors, such as ODN potency, stability and intracellular distribution, will determine antisense efficacy. In addition, microscopic examination of brain tissue following antisense experiments should be performed to rule out tissue damage or infection as a cause of protein or mRNA down-regulation or behavioral changes.

5. Cellular localization of ODNs *in vivo*

A recent study in our group has examined this issue in detail. One hour and 6 h following ODN administration, large reservoirs of fluorescein-labeled ODN

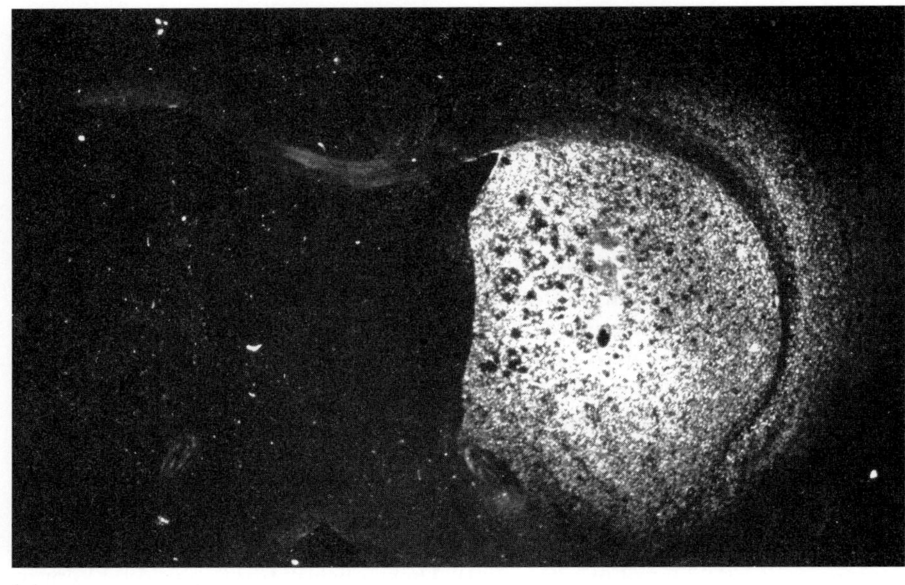

(a)

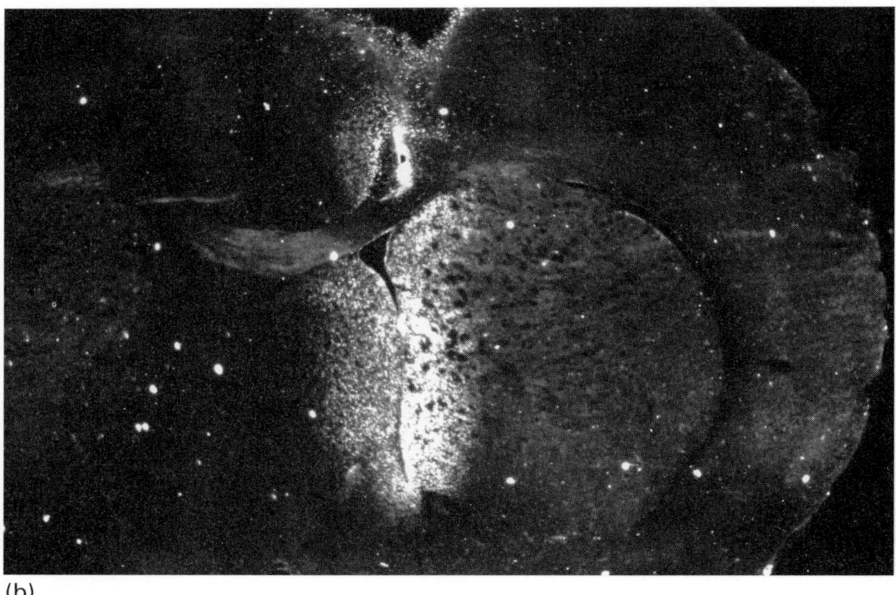

(b)

Figure 2. Dark-field photomicrographs of transverse sections through the striatum 24 h following intracerebral delivery of 2 nmol of biotin-labeled ODN. (a) Intracerebroventricular delivery of ODN; (b) intrastriatal delivery of ODN. The extent of penetration is significantly greater with intraparenchymal delivery.

were present in the extracellular space. In addition, ODN could be detected in the nucleus by confocal microscopy. By 16 h post-injection, the ODN was primarily sequestered in cytoplasmic vesicles. This change in the intracellular distribution of fluorescein-labeled ODN paralleled the temporal loss of activity of a single injection of *c-fos* antisense ODN (29). These data demonstrate that, when ODNs are trapped within cytoplasmic vesicles, they are unable to interact with their mRNA target in the nucleus and cytoplasm and hence are inactive.

When performing these types of experiments, it is important to analyze the tissue immediately after sectioning to avoid artefactual redistribution of ODN. This redistribution has been observed upon tissue storage due to the poor reactivity of ODNs with the aldehyde fixatives used in perfusion fixation (29).

6. Controls

The use of antisense ODNs should be accompanied by the testing of several different control sequences which should have minimal effects on the protein or mRNA of interest. This is addressed in depth in Chapter 3. In addition, wherever possible, antisense effects should be demonstrated using at least two non-contiguous ODN sequences. Sequence specificity can also be demonstrated by studying the antisense effects on closely related gene products (39–41). In experiments against the angiotensin type-1 receptor, ODNs which potently suppressed angiotensin type-1 receptor synthesis had minimal effects on angiotensin type-2 receptor levels (12,42).

7. Mechanisms of antisense knockdown in the brain

There is increasing evidence supporting the involvement of RNase H in cell culture experiments. In this antisense mechanism, the enzyme cleaves the mRNA in the vicinity of the antisense ODN binding site (43,44). Subsequent degradation of the targeted RNA by other ribonucleases leads to reductions in both protein and RNA levels. Some ODNs produce their antisense effects through a translational arrest mechanism. ODNs that work by this mechanism are directed either at the start codon or in the 5′-untranslated region of the RNA (45). ODNs directed downstream of the start codon are considerably less effective at translational arrest (24). Hybridization of antisense ODNs to upstream 5′-sites may interfere with the assembly of the ribosome machinery. When antisense knockdown occurs by this mechanism, protein levels are reduced but RNA levels are unchanged.

A similar situation seems to exist for CNS antisense experiments in animals. In *in vivo* experiments against the corticotropin-releasing hormone type-2 (CRH-2) receptor, ODNs were targeted against a site within the mRNA

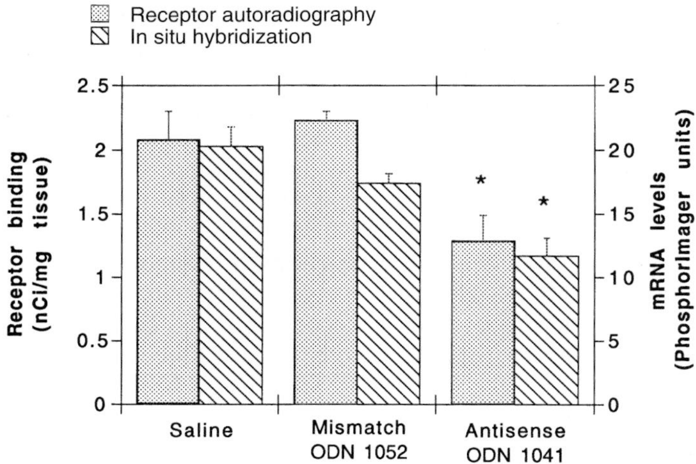

Figure 3. Effect of antisense ODN 1041 and 4-base mismatch ODN 1052 on CRH-2 receptor binding and mRNA levels. $n = 6–8$ rats. ANOVA: $P < 0.0001$ for receptor autoradiography and *in situ* hybridization data. Fisher analysis: $*P < 0.005$ for rats treated with ODN 1041 as compared with those treated with saline or ODN 1052. Reductions in both receptor binding and RNA levels suggests the involvement of RNase H-like enzymes. Antisense ODN 1041 has eight 2′-deoxyribonucleotide phosphorothioate residues at the 5′ portion of the ODN, and twelve 2′-methoxyribonucleotide phosphodiester residues.

coding region. Several ODN analogs that support the activity of RNase H reduced both receptor and RNA levels in the lateral septum (46) (*Figure 3*). In contrast, a 2′-methoxyribonucleotide ODN analog that does not support RNase H had no effect on either protein or RNA levels (46). These data are not consistent with a translational arrest mechanism but point to the involvement of an RNase H-like enzyme. In experiments using ODNs directed against the start codon, others have obtained evidence suggesting a translational arrest mechanism (37,47,48). The emerging picture of antisense mechanisms in the CNS therefore does not seem to be too different from mechanisms in cell culture systems.

The issue of antisense mechanisms is relevant to the selection of appropriate ODN analogs for CNS *in vivo* experiments. Since many phosphorothioate sequences are toxic (see following section), replacing phosphorothioates with other chemical analogs requires some knowledge of the operative antisense mechanism. Numerous ODN chemistries exist which are relatively stable to nuclease degradation but which are not substrates for RNase H cleavage (49–52)—see Chapter 8. To use such analogs, the ODNs should be directed against regions which will support the hybrid arrest mechanism. Conversely, if antisense ODNs are directed at sites within the coding region of the mRNA or at the 3′-untranslated region, they are likely to produce their antisense effects through an RNase H-type mechanism.

A note of caution: when examining effects of antisense ODNs on target mRNA levels, it is important to remember that residual antisense ODN may remain in brain tissue at far higher concentrations than the probes used in the RNA detection experiment (whether by *in situ* hybridization, RT-PCR, RNase protection or other methods). Therefore, care must be exercised in the design and conduct of such studies.

8. Selection of chemical analogs for *in vivo* antisense experiments

Phosphodiester ODNs (*Table 1*) are highly susceptible to celluıar nucleases, with a half-life in serum of about 20 min (53). The CSF and brain, however, have relatively low levels of nuclease activity and phosphodiester ODNs have been successfully applied to CNS experiments (37,54–56). In general, higher doses of these ODNs are required and the ODNs are administered more frequently, e.g. every 8–12 h instead of every 24 h.

Since a major route of ODN degradation is 3′-exonuclease digestion, phosphodiester ODNs may be protected to some extent by introducing one or more phosphorothioate linkages to the ends of the ODNs (end-protected phosphodiester ODNs). Such analogs can be used against targets with a rapid mRNA and protein turnover rate. In experiments targeting the immediate–

Table 1. Chemical structure and antisense-related properties of ODN analogs

Analog	Structure	Stability against nucleases	Hybridization to RNA	Activation of RNase H
2′-Deoxy phosphodiester	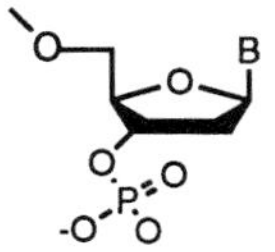 [sugar with B; 3′-O-P(=O)(O)-O⁻]	–	++	++
2′-Deoxy phosphorothioate	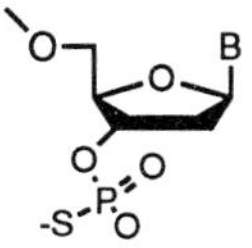 [sugar with B; 3′-O-P(=O)(O)-S⁻]	++	+	+++
2′-Methoxy phosphodiester	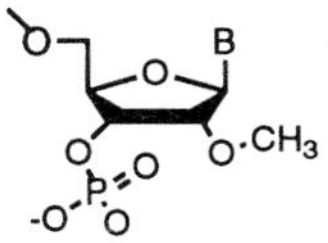 [sugar with B, 2′-O-CH_3; 3′-O-P(=O)(O)-O⁻]	+	+++	–

Key: –, poor; +, fair; ++, good; +++, excellent.

early gene c-*fos*, a phosphodiester antisense ODN was ineffective at suppressing c-*fos* immunoreactivity (57). Suppression could be observed for 2 h, however, using an end-protected phosphodiester ODN of identical sequence (58). The phosphorothioate analog was the most effective, suppressing c-*fos* immunoreactivity for up to 10 h (59).

Phosphorothioate ODNs are used in many CNS antisense experiments because of their relative stability against cellular nucleases. There is increasing evidence, however, that these analogs can be toxic in rodents when administered centrally. Undesired side effects that have been reported include fevers (60), induction of inflammatory mediators (61), general symptoms of ill health (46,62) and weight loss (46,63). When compromising symptoms are present, phosphorothioate ODNs cannot be used without confounding the interpretation of functional data.

Chimeric molecules, consisting of a combination of 2′-methoxyphosphodiester nucleotides and phosphorothioate residues represent a new alternative. These ODNs retained the ability to activate RNase H due to the stretch of eight phosphorothioate residues (46). In these analogs, reduction of the number of phosphorothioate linkages eliminated the toxic symptoms and weight loss (46). An animal's weight gain (or loss) appears to be a very sensitive indicator of toxic side effects. These analogs were almost as potent as phosphorothioate ODNs, reducing CRH-2 receptor levels by about 45% after 5 days of ODN treatment (*Figure 3*).

On a practical note: ODNs for *in vivo* use should be purified by HPLC and extracted with butanol to remove organic impurities. Ammonium salts (ODNs without any purification) and triethyl ammonium salts (ODNs after reversed phase HPLC) of ODNs may cause cellular toxicity (64). ODNs should therefore be converted to their sodium salt form.

9. Biochemical evidence for antisense effects—increasing protein and RNA knockdown

Antisense experiments demonstrating functional effects should be accompanied by biochemical evidence for selective protein and RNA knockdown. Although several examples of robust antisense effects at the protein level have been reported (at least 60% reduction; 12,42,54,65), there are many more examples where protein knockdown is minimal. Although several extensive experimental series convincingly demonstrate antisense effects after relatively small reductions in target protein levels (41,56,66,67), larger reductions of target proteins (at least within the relevant physiological brain regions) would be expected before many biological functions would be affected. For example, human PET scans have demonstrated that 70% or higher occupancy of dopamine D_2 receptors by antipsychotics is required for clinical efficacy (68,69). Furthermore, approximately 80% reductions in striatal dopamine inputs can be tolerated in Parkinsonian patients before movement disorders are triggered (70). Even larger reductions of enzyme protein levels may be necessary in antisense studies since pharmacological blockade of enzyme activity generally requires >90% blockade of an enzyme's active site. Antisense studies showing significantly smaller reductions of receptor or enzyme protein levels should be accompanied by extensive controls and cautious interpretation, especially since different physiological effects may arise as higher levels of protein knockdown are achieved.

Antisense sequences with poor activity (or phosphodiester ODNs dosed once a day) may contribute to low levels of protein reduction. Duration of dosing, in relation to the half-life of the target protein, is probably one of the most important considerations in achieving significant reductions in target mRNA and protein levels. Theoretically, maximal antisense effects are obtained after ODN treatment for three protein half-lives. Substantial antisense effects can be obtained within hours to 1 day in gene targets with short protein and RNA half-lives, such as c-*fos* (38,59). In contrast, seven-transmembrane-domain receptors have much longer protein half-lives, ranging from 2 to 8 days (46). To maximize the antisense knockdown against such targets, animals should be dosed for substantially longer periods of time. Lengthening the *in vivo* dosing period from 5 days to 9 days in the CRH-2 receptor system increased knockdown of that receptor protein from about 50% to 78% (46).

10. Summary

Successful application of antisense ODNs in the living brain is a challenging task, requiring careful consideration of many experimental details. In this review, we addressed eight critical areas in the design and conduct of *in vivo* antisense studies for the mammalian CNS. Attention to these areas greatly lowers the nonspecific actions of ODNs and increases the experimental success rate.

Antisense ODNs of maximum potency can be designed by targeting accessible regions of mRNA. Although random screening for effective ODNs may be used, an RNase H digestion–mapping procedure can efficiently map accessible regions for antisense experiments. Recently, a new generation of chimeric ODNs have been applied to *in vivo* CNS studies. These analogs incorporate a region capable of inducing RNase H cleavage, along with flanking regions of low nuclease sensitivity and low toxicity. These ODNs do not elicit the toxic effects commonly observed with many phosphorothioate sequences. Together, these two approaches provide a rational approach to optimized ODN design.

Cell culture testing of antisense ODNs is an important and efficient means of verifying ODN efficacy and sequence specificity prior to initiating time-consuming *in vivo* studies. The extent of tissue penetrance of ODN following intraparenchymal and intraventricular routes of ODN delivery is highly dose dependent. In general, the zone of spread of ODNs correlates closely with the zone of effective antisense knockdown. Intracellular redistribution of ODNs into large cytoplasmic vesicular compartments occurs 12–16 h after injection and correlates with termination of the antisense effect. Finally, matching the duration of ODN administration to the magnitude of the target protein half-life appears to be one of the more important considerations in achieving >60% reduction of target mRNA and protein levels.

With important experimental factors carefully controlled and optimized, CNS antisense experiments should be more routine and reliable. In the near future, further improvements in the technology may come from the application of ribozyme approaches (see Chapter 14), and from the use of stable, self-replicating antisense plasmid and virus constructs (Chapter 11). Although the development of antisense technologies for *in vivo* CNS applications has proven much more difficult than originally anticipated, its great potential for rapidly evaluating the function of unknown gene products now appears within reach.

References

1. Wahlestedt, C. (1994) *Trends Pharmacol. Sci.*, **15**, 42.
2. Chiasson, B. J., Armstrong, J. N., Hooper, M. L., Murphy P. R. and Robertson, H. A. (1994) *Cell. Mol. Neurobiol.*, **14**, 507.
3. Robinson, E. S. J., Nutt, D. J., Jackson, H. C. and Hudson, A. L (1997) *J. Psychopharmacol.*, **11**, 259.
4. Gewirtz, A. M., Stein, C. A. and Glazer, P. M. (1996) *Proc. Natl Acad. Sci. USA*, **93**, 3161.
5. Branch, A. D. (1998) *Trends Biochem. Sci.*, **23**, 45.
6. Wahlestedt, C. (1996) In: Raffa, R. B. and Porreca, F. (Eds), *Antisense Strategies for the Study of Receptor Mechanisms*, pp. 1–10. R. G. Landes Co., Austin, TX
7. Monia, B. P., Johnston, J. F., Geiger, T., Muller, M. and Fabbro, D. (1996) *Nature Med.* **2**, 668.
8. Schlingensiepen, R. and Schlingensiepen, K.-H. (1997) In: Schlingensiepen, R., Brysch, W. and Schlingensiepen, K.-H. (Eds), *Antisense—from Technology to Therapy*, pp. 3–28. Blackwell Science, Berlin.
9. Peyman, A., Helsberg, M., Kretzschmar, G., Mag, M., Gravley, S. and Uhlmann, E. (1995) *Biological Chemistry (Hoppe-Seyler)*, **376**, 195.
10. Dean, N. M., McKay, R., Condon, T. P. and Bennett, C. F. (1994) *J. Biol. Chem.*, **269**, 16416.
11. Ho, S. P., Britton, D. H. O., Stone, B. A., Behrens, D. L., Leffet, L. M., Hobbs, F. W., Miller, J. A. and Trainor, G. L. (1996) *Nucleic Acids Res.*, **24**, 1901.
12. Ho, S. P., Bao, Y., Lesher, T., Malhotra, R., Ma, L. Y., Fluharty, S. J. and Sakai, R. R. (1998) *Nature Biotechnol.*, **16**, 59.
13. Birikh, K. R., Berlin, Y. A., Soreq, H. and Eckstein, F. (1997) *RNA*, **3**, 429.
14. Lima, W. F., Brown-Driver, V., Fox, M., Hanecak, R. and Bruice, T. W. (1997) *J. Biol. Chem.*, **272**, 626.

15. Milner, N., Mir, K. U. and Southern, E. M. (1997) *Nature Biotechnol.*, **15**, 537.
16. Lieber, A. and Strauss, M. (1995) *Mol. Cell. Biol.*, **15**, 540.
17. Zelphati, O. and Szoka, F. C., Jr (1996) *J. Contr. Release*, **41**, 99.
18. Beltinger, C., Saragove, H. U., Smith, R. M., LeSauteur, L., Shah, N., DeDionisio, L., Christensen, L., Raible, A., Jarett, L. and Gewirtz, A. M. (1995) *J. Clin. Invest.*, **95**, 1814.
19. Marti, G., Egan, W., Noguchi, P., Zon, G., Matsukura, M. and Broder, S. (1992) *Antisense Res. Dev.*, **2**, 27.
20. Noonberg, S. B., Garovoy, M. R. and Hunt, C. A. (1993) *J. Invest. Dermatol.*, **101**, 727.
21. Kreig, A. M., Gmelig-Meyling, F., Gourley, M. F., Kisch, W. J., Chrisey, L. A. and Steinberg, A. D. (1991) *Antisense Res. Dev.*, **1**, 161.
22. Bennett, C. F., Chiang, M.-Y., Chan, H., Shoemaker, J. E. and Mirabelli, C. K. (1992) *Mol. Pharmacol.*, **41**, 1023.
23. Lewis, J. G., Lin, K.-Y., Kothavale, A., Flanagan, W. M., Matteucci, M. D., DePrince, R. B., Mook, R. A., Jr, Hendren, R. W. and Wagner, R. W. (1996) *Proc Natl Acad. Sci. USA*, **93**, 3176.
24. Ho, S. P., Bao Y., Lesher T. and Conklin D. (1999) *Mol. Brain Res.* **65**, 23.
25. Zelphati, O. and Szoka, F. C., Jr (1996) *Proc Natl Acad Sci USA*, **93**, 11493.
26. Zelphati, O. and Szoka, F. C., Jr (1996) *Pharmaceut. Res.*, **13**, 1367.
27. Wrobel, I. and Collins, D. (1995) *Biochim. Biophys. Acta*, **1235**, 296.
28. Gershon, H., Ghirlando, R., Guttman, S. B. and Minsky, A. (1993) *Biochemistry*, **32**, 7143.
29. Grzanna, R., Dubin, J. R., Dent, G. W., Ji, Z., Zhang, W., Ho, S. P. and Hartig, P. R. (1998) *Mol. Brain Res.* **63**, 35.
30. Zhang, S. P., Zhou, L. W., Morabito, M., Lin, R. C. S. and Weiss, B. (1996) *J. Mol. Neurosci.*, **7**, 13.
31. Ogawa, S., Brown, H. E., Okano, H. J. and Pfaff, D. W. (1995) *Regul. Peptides*, **59**, 143.
32. Yaida, Y. and Nowak, T. S., Jr (1995) *Regul. Peptides*, **59**, 193.
33. Szklarczyk, A. and Kaczmarek, L. (1995) *J. Neurosci. Methods*, **60**, 181.
34. Szklarczyk, A. and Kaczmarek, L. (1997) *Neurochem. Intl*, **31**, 413.
35. Whitesell, L., Geselowitz, D., Chavany, C., Fahmy, B., Walbridge, S., Alger, J. R. and Neckers, L. M. (1993) *Proc. Natl Acad. Sci. USA*, **90**, 4665.
36. Yee, F., Ericson, H., Reis, D. J. and Wahlestedt, C. (1994) *Cell. Mol. Neurobiol.*, **14**, 475.
37. Wahlestedt, C., Golanov, E., Yamamoto, S., Yee, F., Ericson, H., Yoo, H., Inturrisi, C. E. and Reis, D. J. (1993) *Nature*, **363**, 260.
38. Sommer, W., Rimondini, R., O'Connor, W., Hansson, A. C., Ungerstedt, U. and Fuxe, K. (1996) *Proc Natl Acad. Sci. USA*, **93**, 14134.
39. Dean, N., McKay, R., Miraglia, L., Howard, R., Cooper, S., Giddings, J., Nicklin, P., Meister, L., Ziel, R., Geiger, T., Muller, M. and Fabbro, D. (1996) *Cancer Res.*, **56**, 3499.
40. Widnell, K. L., Self, D. W., Lane, S. B., Russell, D. S., Vaidya, V. A., Miserendino, M. J. D., Rubin, C. S., Duman, R. S. and Nestler, E. J. (1996) *J. Pharmacol. Exp. Ther.*, **276**, 306.
41. Weiss, B., Zhou, L. W., Zhang, S. P. and Qin, Z. H. (1993) *Neuroscience*, **55**, 607.

42. Sakai, R. R., He, P. F., Yang, X. D., Ma, L. Y., Guo, Y. F., Reilly, J. J., Moga, C. N. and Fluharty, S. J. (1994) *J. Neurochem.*, **62**, 2053.
43. Inoue, H., Hayase, Y., Iwai, S. and Ohtsuka, E. (1987) *FEBS Lett.*, **215**, 327.
44. Crooke, S. T., Lemonidis, K. M., Neilson, L., Griffey, R., Lesnik, E. A. and Monia, B. P. (1995) *Biochem. J.*, **312**, 599.
45. Chiang, M. Y., Chan, H., Zounes, M. A., Freier, S. M., Lima, W. F. and Bennett, C. F. (1991) *J. Biol. Chem.*, **266**, 18162.
46. Ho, S. P., Livanov, V., Zhang, W., Li, J.-H. and Lesher, T. (1998) *Mol. Brain Res.* **62**, 1.
47. Rickman, D. W. and Rickman, C. B. (1996) *Proc. Natl Acad. Sci. USA*, **93**, 12564.
48. Skutella, T., Schwarting, R. K. W., Huston, J. P., Sillaber, I., Probst, J., Holsboer, F. and Spanagel, R. (1997) *Eur. J. Neurosci.*, **9**, 210.
49. Gryaznov, S. M. (1995) *Proc. Natl Acad. Sci. USA*, **92**, 5798.
50. Monia, B. P., Lesnik, E. A., Gonzalez, C., Lima, W. F., McGee, D., Guinosso, C. J., Kawasaki, A. M., Cook, P. D. and Freier, S. M. (1993) *J. Biol. Chem.*, **268**, 14514.
51. Miller, P. S. (1991) *Bio-Technology*, **9**, 358.
52. Jones, R. J., Lin, K. Y., Milligan, J. F., Wadwani, S. and Matteucci, M. D. (1993) *J. Org. Chem.*, **58**, 2983.
53. Sands, H., Gorey-Feret, L. J., Cocuzza, A. J., Hobbs, F. W., Chidester, D. and Trainor, G. L. (1994) *Mol. Pharmacol.*, **45**, 932.
54. Wahlestedt, C., Pich, E. M., Koob, G. F., Yee, F. and Heilig, M. (1993) *Science*, **259**, 528.
55. Akabayashi, A., Wahlestedt, C., Alexander, J. T. and Leibowitz, S. F. (1994) *Mol. Brain Res.*, **21**, 55.
56. Standifer, K. M., Chien, C. C., Wahlestedt, C., Brown, G. P. and Pasternak, G. W. (1994) *Neuron*, **12**, 805.
57. Hooper, M. L., Chiasson, B. J. and Robertson, H. A. (1994) *Neuroscience*, **63**, 917.
58. Hebb, M. O. and Robertson, H. A. (1997) *Mol. Brain Res.*, **47**, 223.
59. Chiasson, B. J., Hooper, M. L., Murphy, P. R. and Robertson, H. A. (1992) *Eur. J. Pharmacol.*, **227**, 451.
60. Schobitz, B., Pezeshki, G., Probst, J. C., Reul, J. M., Skutella, T., Stohr, T., Holsboer, F. and Spanagel, R. (1997) *Eur. J. Pharmacol.*, **331**, 97.
61. Pezeshki, G., Schobitz, B., Pohl, T. and Reul, J. M. (1996) *Neurosci. Lett.*, **217**, 97.
62. Skutella, T., Stohr, T., Probst, J. C., Ramalho-Ortigao, F. J., Holsboer, F. and Jirikowski, G. F. (1994) *Hormones Metab. Res.*, **26**, 460.
63. Heinrichs, S. C., Lapsansky, J., Lovenberg, T. W., Souza, E. B. D. and Chalmers, D. T. (1997) *Regul. Peptides*, **71**, 15.
64. Brysch, W., Rifai, A., Tischmeyer, W. and Schlingensiepen, K.-H. (1996) In: Agrawal, S. (Ed.), *Antisense Therapeutics*, p. 159. Humana Press, Totowa, NJ.
65. Zhang, M. and Creese, I. (1993) *Neurosci. Lett.*, **161**, 223.
66. Zhou, L. W., Zhang, S. P., Qin, Z. H. and Weiss, B. (1994) *J. Pharmacol. Exp. Ther.*, **268**, 1015.
67. Standifer, K. M., Jenab, S., Su, W., Chien, C. C., Pan, Y. X., Inturrisi, C. E. and Pasternak, G. W. (1995) *J. Neurochem.*, **65**, 1981.
68. Seeman, P. (1992) *Neuropsychopharmacology*, **7**, 261.
69. Seeman, P. (1995) *Int. Clin. Psychopharm.*, **10**, *Suppl. 3*, 5.
70. Langston, J. W. (1985) *Trends Neurosci.*, **8**, 79.

3

The design of appropriate control experiments to ensure specificity in antisense oligonucleotide function

WOLFGANG BRYSCH

1. Introduction

Synthetic oligodeoxynucleotides (ODNs) used for antisense gene knockdown can cause a number of different and often unexpected biological effects in neuronal cell cultures, organotypic cultures like brain slices, and live animals. The researcher working with antisense ODNs in such biological systems faces the difficult task of differentiating between those effects which are due to the desired sequence-specific inhibition of the targeted mRNA and the undesired sequence-related and non-sequence-related effects that many antisense ODNs can cause.

The following section will describe some of these specific and non-specific effects. A good understanding of these effects will help the experimenter to choose and design appropriate control ODNs as described in the second section of this chapter. The third section reviews some of the more popular assays used to measure and evaluate the effect of antisense ODNs as well as the advantages and disadvantages of each assay with respect to specificity and validity. This chapter focuses exclusively on antisense ODNs targeted against cellular mRNA; not all of the approaches described here will be appropriate for alternative approaches such as triple-helical or transfected antisense RNA.

2. Effects of antisense oligodeoxynucleotides

2.1 Sequence-specific effects

Sequence-specific effects are due to the hybridization of antisense ODNs with the targeted cellular mRNA (or viral DNA/RNA) in a sequence-dependent complementary fashion. Binding is exclusively via hydrogen bonds where A–T (A–U) base pairs form two hydrogen bonds and C–G base pairs form three hydrogen bonds. Only those effects which are the result of such sequence-specific binding are regarded as true 'antisense' effects.

2.2 Sequence-related side effects

Sequence-related side effects result from the particular sequence of an ODN but are not caused by its hybridization to the desired target mRNA. Sequence-related side effect may have different causes including:

1. *Sequence homologies*: the commonest cause of sequence-related side effects is the partial or total homology of the mRNA target sequence with other mRNA sequences in related, or even completely unrelated genes. Such homologies may result in the total or partial suppression of other genes and lead to a misinterpretation of the observed biological effects (1). Sequences with a high G–C content are especially prone to form stable hybrids with unrelated genes. A perfect match of as little as eight to ten bases of a G–C rich sequence may be sufficient to cause an inhibitory effect.
2. *Sequence motifs*: certain short sequence motifs can cause unwanted side effects in most cell types. One of the best known motifs is the G-quartet, i.e. four G-bases in a row (2,3); also two or more G-triplets within one ODN often result in non-specific effects. Other motifs only seem to play a role in certain cell types under certain conditions such as the stimulatory effect of the CpG motif on immune cells (4,5). If non-specific effects due to certain motifs are suspected, control ODNs which bear this motif in different sequence contexts can be used to clarify this point (see Section 3.3, below).
3. *Higher-order structures*: depending on their sequence, ODNs—especially longer ones—can form secondary structures which may bind to various proteins. This phenomenon is exploited in the so-called aptamer approach (6; see Chapter 13) for the design of novel agonist/antagonist compounds. With antisense ODNs the formation of secondary or higher-order structures always bears the risk of unwanted protein binding (7,8) (*Figure 1a*). The G-quartet and G-triples mentioned in the previous paragraph foster the formation of ODN quadruplex structures. Four identical ODNs with these motifs can form a quadruplet in a parallel/antiparallel fashion. These quadruplets can have pronounced biological effects by binding to proteins (*Figure 1b*). Palindromic motifs within the ODN may lead to dimerization and the formation of double-stranded pieces of DNA, which can serve as potential binding sites for transcription factors. Again, this phenomenon has been exploited to design novel competitive blocking agents for transcription factors (9), but in ODNs which are designed as antisense reagents such double-stranded binding sites should be avoided (*Figure 1c*).

The effects described above are often classified as non-sequence-specific. In

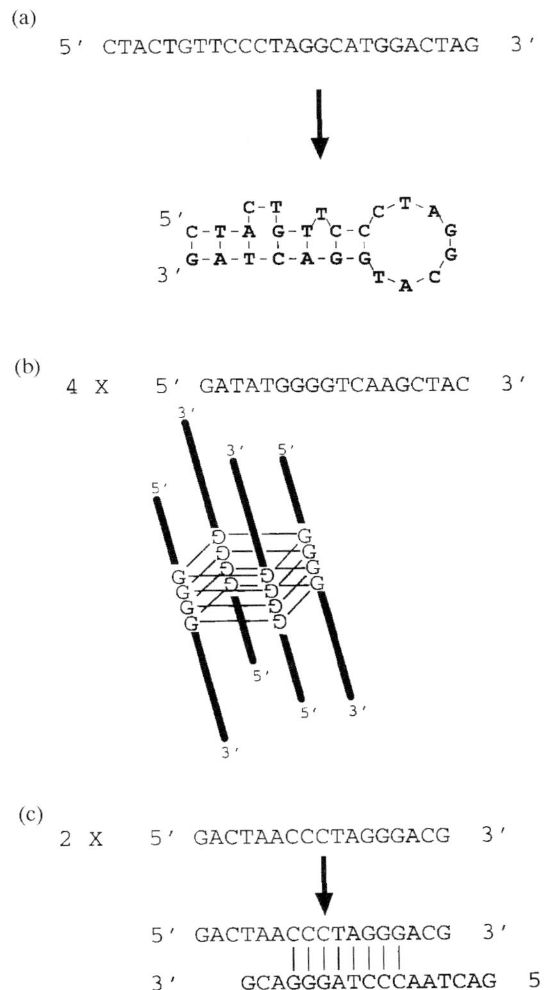

Figure 1. Higher-order structures of oligodeoxynucleotides (ODNs) that can lead to protein binding. (a) Formation of a secondary structure within a self-complementary ODN. (b) Formation of a quadruplex structure from four identical ODNs which contain a GGGG motif. (c) Formation of a dimer through a palindromic motif.

my view, this is a misnomer. Even though these effects are not caused by Watson–Crick type base pairing with a target mRNA, the effects are the result of the specific sequence of ODNs. Every ODN has a sequence and the fact that this sequence may not 'make sense' to the researcher does not mean that the effects of this ODN are not sequence-specific. Thus we usually refer to such effects as 'sequence-related'.

2.3 Substance-related effects

Antisense ODNs are macromolecules, usually between 14 and 25 bases in length. Depending on their size, sequence and chemical modification and on the ancillary chemical groups coupled to the ODN, these molecules may have a number of desired and undesired biological effects which result from the gross chemical properties of the compound, irrespective of the individual base sequence. Those effects that are due to the chemical substance 'oligonucleotide' should be differentiated from effects that are related to the sequence of the individual ODN. Negative controls as described below are usually employed to demonstrate that a biological effect is not caused by an non-specific substance-related side effect.

3. Controls

Appropriate controls are an integral part of every antisense experiment and a prerequisite for the publication of antisense work in scientific journals (10). Controls are necessary to evaluate which of the observed biochemical or biological effects are caused by a sequence-specific antisense mechanism and which effects are due to sequence-related and substance-related side effects. There are two types of control experiments: negative and positive.

Negative controls serve to rule out the possibility that the effects of a (chemically modified) antisense ODN are caused by non-sequence-specific mechanisms. Negative control ODNs are normally designed in such a way that they are unable to hybridize specifically to the desired genetic target in the cell. Thus all biological effects observed in such control experiments have to be attributed to non-specific side effects like cross-hybridization, protein binding or toxicity. Common design criteria for negative control ODNs are:

- length and hybridization characteristics equal to those of the corresponding antisense ODN
- identical chemical modifications in antisense and control ODNs
- reduced or no ability to hybridize to the antisense target
- no (complementary) homology to other cellular mRNAs
- critical motifs, such as a G-quartet, must be equally present or absent in both antisense and control molecules

Positive controls are ODNs that provide additional evidence that a true antisense effect is the reason for the observed biological effects. Many different types of controls have been proposed and used in the past, each with its own advantages and disadvantages. As there is no single ideal control, a combination of two or more different controls is recommended. The following paragraphs describe the most widely used and accepted types of controls.

3.1 Sense controls

These are ODNs that have a sequence complementary to that of the antisense ODN (*Figure 2*). Sense controls have a sequence identical to the mRNA target which is also 'sense'. Therefore these ODNs are unable to hybridize to the target. This type of control is still the most widely used. Sense ODNs are readily designed and usually have hybridization characteristics very similar to those of their antisense counterparts due to the equal content of G–C and A–T bases. For these reasons, they have long been regarded as the ideal and logical type of control. In many cases, however, we and other researchers have found that sense controls produce biological effects of their own at a frequency that cannot be attributed to substance-related side effects alone. One possible explanation was that sense ODNs may interact with the antisense strand of the DNA. But given the highly complex structure of nuclear DNA, it seems very unlikely that a short ODN can separate the double helix and bind to one strand tightly enough to stop the transcription of a gene. We have therefore analyzed the sense counterparts of many of our antisense sequences which had been shown to be specific with other types of controls. We found that many sense sequences had an unexpectedly high (complementary) homology to completely unrelated genes. This is due to the non-random nature of sense sequences and may explain the biological activity of many sense controls. Even more importantly, as described in Section 2.2, certain sequence motifs—such as a G-quartet—can cause pronounced sequence-related biological effects. A CCCC motif in an antisense sequence would thus generate a GGGG motif in the sense control and produce effects that are not seen with the antisense ODN. Conversely, if an antisense ODNs contains a GGGG motif, it will show biological effects that are not sequence-specific. The sense control—which would have a CCCC instead—would lack these non-specific effects, and thus lead to the misinterpretation that the effect of the antisense ODN is a true antisense effect.

(a)

5′ GAATCACTGGAGCTACCT 3′

5′ AGGTAGCTCCAGTGATTC 3′

(b)

5′ TCAGGAACCCCTTGCAGA 3′

5′ TCTGCAAGGGGTTCCTGA 3′

Figure 2. Example of sense controls. (a) Example of an antisense sequence (top) the sense counterpart of which (bottom) contains no problematic motifs. (b) Antisense sequence complementary to human PKC-γ (top) and its respective sense control (bottom). Note that the base composition changes and a GGGG motif appears in the control sequence.

Before using a sense control, a homology search in a sequence database like EMBL or GenBank should be conducted in order to assess the likelihood of unintended cross-hybridization with other mRNA species. If no such cross-homologies are found and the sequence does not contain problematic motifs, sense ODNs can provide a valid and recommended type of control.

Sense controls

Advantages

- readily designed
- hybridization properties nearly identical to those of the antisense counterpart
- widely accepted

Disadvantages

- high incidence of non-specific cross-hybridization
- may contain problematic motifs which are not present in antisense
- questionable interaction with DNA antisense strand

Design method

1. Revert the sequence of the antisense ODN into its complementary sense counterpart.
2. Check both sense and antisense sequences carefully for problematic motifs, such as GGGG, 2 × GGG or CpG. Use as the control only if such motifs are absent.
3. Check sense control for unexpected sequence homologies in a sequence database like GenBank or EMBL.

3.2 Random controls

Randomized controls, which are also termed 'nonsense' or 'scrambled', can be obtained by mixing up the bases of an antisense ODN in a randomized fashion. The rationale behind this approach is that a random sequence would lack any specific information and that the biological effects of such an ODN would reflect the non-sequence-specific or substance-related side effects of an ODN. In this respect it is important to realize that even a random sequence may have unexpected homologies, and that there is probably no such thing as a completely 'nonsense' sequence (*Figure 3*).

The hybridization properties of random sequences may differ from those of the antisense ODN. A balanced distribution of A/T and G/C bases along the length of of an antisense ODN may become very lopsided in a random sequence. For statistical reasons this is particularly likely to happen in short ODNs.

Some authors have proposed a completely random mixture of ODNs of length n as a control, where n is the length of the corresponding antisense ODN. These ODNs are synthesized with all four bases (A, C, G and T) present in each coupling step. This yields a mixture of all possible sequences antisense sequence:

5′ TCAGGAACCCCTTGCAGA 3′

Step 1: generate 10-20 random sequences with same base composition as antisense sequence (5xA, 6xC, 4xG, 3xT)

1 TATCCGAGCCAAGTCGAC
2 GGTTCCACTACCCGAAAG
3 CCTCAGGCATACCTAGAG
4 AGACTCAGGCCTAGCTAC
5 AGTGCCACTATGCCACAG
. .
. .
. .
10 CATAGGCTCCAGGCATAC

Steps 2 & 3: check each random sequence for cross homologies in a sequence database like GenBank or EMBL.
Sequence 2 has a 15 base homology to c-myc mRNA and is discarded

~~GGTTCCACTACCCGAAAG~~

Step 4: check remaining sequences for problematic sequence motifs. Sequence 1 contains 2 CpG motifs which may cause unspecific stimulation of immune cells.

~~TATCCGAGCCAAGTCGAC~~

Step 5: select the control sequence which most closely resembles the antisense with respect to the distribution of A-T vs. G-C bases (sequence 4 in this example).

AGACTCAGGCCTAGCTAC

Figure 3. Example of selection of a randomized control sequence.

of length n, i.e. 4^n different ODNs. In theory, ODNs with problematic sequences would comprise only a minute fraction and the gross biological effect of the mixture would reflect just the substance-related side effects. We have tested such mixtures of 14- and 18-mer phosphorothioate ODNs in a number of different mammalian cell lines at concentrations between 1 and 4 μM. This treatment led to massive signs of toxicity in all cells (unpublished observations). Our hypothesis to explain this effect is that a completely random mix contains ODNs that hybridize to virtually every mRNA present in the cell. Even if only a fraction of each mRNA is blocked, this is obviously sufficient to cause massive toxicity. There have been studies in which no toxicity has been reported with random mixtures of unmodified ODNs. This may have been due to insufficient stability of these ODNs, which were probably degraded before they could have detrimental effects on the cells.

In our own work we generally use selected random controls. These controls are obtained by mixing the bases of the antisense sequence in a random fashion and thus produce 10–20 different candidate control sequences. For each of these sequences a homology search against all eukaryotic sequences in the EMBL database is run. The random sequences with the lowest degree of cross-homology to sequences in the database are then compared with the antisense ODN and the sequence that most closely resembles the antisense ODN with respect to the distribution of A/T and G/C bases, sequence motifs, etc., is chosen.

Random controls

Advantages	*Disadvantages*
• good indicators of substance-related side effects • may be used for multiple antisense sequences	• laborious design

Design method (see Figure 3)

1. Generate 10–20 random sequences using the bases of the antisense ODN.
2. Check each candidate control sequence for unexpected cross-homologies in a sequence database like GenBank or EMBL.
3. Discard candidates with cross-homologies to other genes.
4. Discard all sequences that contain problematic sequence motifs that are not present in the antisense molecule.
5. Of the remaining candidates, select the control sequence that most closely resembles the antisense with respect to the distribution of A/T and G/C bases.

3.3 Reverse controls

Reverse controls are obtained by reversing the antisense sequence with respect to its 5′–3′ orientation (*Figure 4*). This sequence is unable to hybridize to the antisense mRNA target. Reverse ODNs have several advantages over sense controls:

- the base composition remains exactly the same
- the hybridization characteristics and free energy parameters remain the same
- most sequence motifs, which may cause non-specific effects (such as G-quartet or palindromes), are conserved. Thus, reverse controls can be used to determine whether these motifs do, indeed, produce non-specific effects in the biological system under study.
- reverse sequences seem to have a lower tendency towards 'accidental' cross-homologies than do sense controls. This became apparent when we analyzed over 200 of our antisense sequences which targeted mammalian mRNAs. The sense and reverse counterparts of these antisense sequences were checked for cross-homologies with related and unrelated sequences and, surprisingly, the incidence of cross-homologies was significantly lower with the reverse sequences (unpublished results). The absence of unwanted cross-homologies, however, must be checked for each individual 'reverse control' by a database search as described for random controls.

```
5′  TCAGGAACCCCTTGCAGA  3′

5′  AGACGTTCCCCAAGGACT  3′
```

Figure 4. Antisense sequence (top) and reverse control (bottom), which is obtained by reversing the 5′–3′ orientation of the antisense.

Reverse controls

Advantages

- readily designed
- same hybridization characteristics as antisense
- problematic motifs are often retained

Disadvantages

- must be individually prepared for each antisense sequence
- cannot be used if cross-homologies occur

Design method

1. Generate the reverse sequence of the antisense ODN.
2. Check reverse control for unexpected sequence homologies in a sequence database such as GenBank or EMBL.

The fact that reverse controls usually have exactly the same binding and hybridization characteristics as the respective antisense sequence makes them an excellent and highly valid type of control which in our laboratory is often used as the next in line after initial experiments with a random control.

3.4 Mismatch controls

Mismatch controls are generated by introducing one or more deliberate mismatches into an antisense sequence (*Figure 5*). Theoretically, the more mismatches an antisense sequence has with respect to the target mRNA, the less stably it should bind and hence inhibit the expression of the target gene. Generally this assumption holds true, but it is of importance where the mismatches are located, what type of bases are mismatched and in what sequence context the mismatch occurs. In the following we will discuss each of these factors separately, but it should be kept in mind that each mismatch will cause a combination of these effects and the results cannot be predicted in detail.

1. *Location of the mismatch*: mismatches around the centre of ODNs have more effect than peripheral mismatches. A mismatch at the 5′ or 3′ end will only shorten the effective ODN length by one base, causing little effect especially in ODNs of ≥18 bases. A mismatch in the centre of a 15-mer, on the other hand, can completely abolish the efficacy of an antisense ODN. If more than one mismatch is introduced, spacing these out along the ODN will have more effect than a cluster of mismatches.
2. *Type of base*: it is important which base is changed, and for what base it is exchanged. As a rule of thumb, the magnitude of the effect of base changes is as follows: G to A/T > C to A > G/C to C/G > A/T to G > A to C > A/T to T/A.

Mismatch controls can also be used to estimate the specificity of an antisense ODN. If one mismatch in an antisense sequence completely abolishes the biological activity, partial hybridization of the antisense ODN to unrelated mRNAs is unlikely to cause any side effects. If, however, pronounced effects are still observed with an antisense sequence, bearing three or more mismatches, the specificity of this antisense is questionable.

```
5′  TCAGGAACCCCTTGCAGA  3′
5′  TCCGGAACCACTTCCAGA  3′
```

Figure 5. Antisense sequence (top) and mismatch control (bottom). The highlighted bases are different from those in the antisense sequence.

Mismatch controls

Advantages	*Disadvantages*
• readily designed • can be used to estimate specificity of corresponding antisense	• must be individually designed for each antisense sequence

Design method

1. As rule of thumb, use two mismatches in 14- to 16-mers and three mismatches in 17- to 20-mers.
2. Space mismatches evenly along the length of the ODN.
3. Position mismatches at least two bases away from each end.
4. Keep the overall G–C *vs* A–T content of the ODN unchanged.
5. Do not introduce problematic motifs into the sequence through a mismatch.

3.5 Non-expressing control cells

Sequence-related or non-specific effects of an antisense ODN can be evaluated by treating cells that are known not to express the mRNA against which the ODN is targeted. In such cells the antisense ODN should have no biological effect. The test system to be used should be carefully chosen in order to obtain meaningful results. Ideally the control cells should be identical to the original cells except that they do not express the target gene. As this will hardly ever occur in natural systems, less closely related cell types usually have to serve as control system. One alternative is to use cells from a different tissue which do not express the target gene; the other is to use the same cell type from a different species. The latter alternative, however, is only suitable if the target mRNAs in both species are sufficiently divergent, to exclude the possibility of an effective cross-reaction of the antisense ODN. It is also important to check whether the rate and amount of ODN uptake into control cells is comparable to that in the original target cells. Non-expressing control cells are useful for estimating the non-specific side effects that an antisense compound may have and are thus especially suited for the early phases of antisense drug development.

Non-expressing control cells

Advantages	*Disadvantages*
• the antisense sequence serves as its own control • no separate ODN necessary • very valid control	• suitable control cells may be difficult to find • control cells may have different biological properties

Non-expressing control cells *Continued*

Selection criteria for control cells

- control cells should not express the target gene
- ODNs should be taken up by control cells at a rate similar to that in target cells
- control cells should be cultivated under similar conditions (plus or minus serum, etc.)
- control cells should divide at a similar rate to target cells

3.6 Second antisense

A second ODN, directed against a different part of the target mRNA, can serve as a positive control. Especially in those cases where there is no suitable antibody available to show reduction of the respective protein product, and if there is no reduction in target mRNA levels, a second ODN can provide good circumstantial evidence for a true antisense mechanism. In order to draw such conclusions, however, a number of factors should be carefully considered:

1. Both antisense ODNs should be effective in inhibiting target mRNA expression. If a biological effect cannot be reproduced with a second ODN, this may be because the original ODN did not act via a true antisense mechanism or because the second ODN was poorly designed, and therefore ineffective. Thus a number of secondary ODNs may need to be tested.
2. The two ODNs should target different parts of the mRNA and share neither sequence homology nor sequence motifs that are known to cause non-sequence-specific effects.
3. Often two ODNs are not equally effective. In this case the magnitude of the biological response may be different, but the type of response, such as reduced proliferation or cell differentiation, should be identical.
4. Each ODN should be individually tested against an appropriate negative control.

Second antisense

Advantages

- good alternative if gene product cannot be assayed directly

Disadvantages

- often need to design several ODNs to find a pair of active ones
- each ODN must be tested against a negative control

Design method

Similar to that for first antisense.

4. Assay systems

The antisense-mediated gene-inhibitory effect of every ODN should be confirmed by appropriate biochemical and biological assays. As it is not possible to directly visualize the sequence-specific hybridization of an antisense ODN to its target, circumstantial evidence from one or more indirect assays has to serve as 'proof' that an antisense mechanism is the reason for the observed biological effects. One or more of the following procedures can be employed to produce such circumstantial evidence. The assays are discussed with respect to their usefulness in evaluating antisense effects. Detailed protocols for these techniques would be beyond the scope of this chapter—for all of these standard manuals and protocols are available in volumes of the 'Practical Approach' series and other literature.

4.1 Measurement of target mRNA levels: Northern blots and RT-PCR

Unmodified DNA-ODNs and some types of chemically modified ODNs such as phosphorothioates and phosphoramidates are potential substrates for RNase H, an enzyme that cleaves the RNA strand of a DNA–RNA hybrid (11). In biological systems, where RNase H plays a role, for example *Xenopus* oocytes (12), and when using compatible substrate ODNs, the selective decrease of the targeted mRNA species is a strong indicator for a sequence-specific antisense effect. The antisense-mediated cleavage of a target mRNA should result in two mRNA fragments which can be specifically detected by Northern blot analysis or reverse transcription–polymerase chain reaction (RT-PCR).

In Northern blots, one or two additional shorter bands should appear, which represent the mRNA fragments. The ratio between full-length mRNA and fragments can be an indicator of antisense efficiency. However, this ratio may not reflect the rate of target mRNA cleavage correctly, since the cleaved mRNA fragments are often substantially less stable than full-length mRNA and thus are quickly degraded.

RT-PCR can be used as an alternative to Northern blots. With PCR, even minute amounts of fragmented target mRNA should be detectable. An RT-PCR control system consists of three different primers (*Figure 6*), one reverse and two nested forward primers. The reverse primer should be located approximately 300–500 bases downstream of the antisense target site. One of the forward primers (Primer 1) is also located downstream of the antisense site, the other one (Primer 2) is located upstream. For the RT-PCR reaction, the reverse transcription is done with the common reverse primer. Both cleaved and non-cleaved target mRNA are transcribed. After the reverse transcription step, the reaction is split into two aliquots which are amplified separately, each using one of the forward primers. The reaction containing forward Primer 1 amplifies the cleaved and the non-cleaved mRNA, while Primer 2 will only amplify the non-cleaved fraction. The difference between the signals produced by the Primer 1 reaction compared with the Primer 2 reaction allow an estimate of the amount of target mRNA cleavage by the antisense ODN.

The specific inhibition of target mRNA levels is strong evidence for a true sequence-specific antisense effect. Conversely, however, unchanged target mRNA levels do not necessarily mean that an antisense ODN did not work (13). In the latter case, other assays must be used to confirm an antisense effect.

Measurement of target mRNA levels

Advantages

- highly valid
- standard method
- hybridization probes (ODNs) and primers readily available

Disadvantages

- only applicable for RNase H-mediated antisense effects

Method for RT-PCR

1. Design a reverse PCR primer, located 300–500 bases downstream of the antisense target site.
2. Design two forward primers, Primer 1 located just downstream of the antisense target site and Primer2 located upstream of the target site.
3. Treat target cells with antisense ODN for the desired time.
4. Extract total RNA from treated cells.
5. With an aliquot of the RNA, perform a reverse transcription reaction (see a general PCR manual for details) with double the reagents and volume.
6. After the reverse transcription step, split the reaction into two separate PCR tubes and add forward Primer 1 to one tube and forward Primer 2 to the other.
7. Perform the PCR amplification reaction.
8. Run aliquots of each reaction on an agarose gel and compare the intensities of bands produced by the two reactions.

4.2 Measurement of protein levels

It is the aim of any antisense approach, irrespective of the type of antisense molecule used, specifically to inhibit the expression of a protein. Thus, measuring the level of this protein at different time points following antisense treatment provides the most straightforward evidence for the efficacy of an antisense compound. Direct proof that the protein product of the targeted gene is down-regulated or completely suppressed should be given wherever possible. Suitable assays for changes in specific protein levels are Western blots, ELISAs and immunoprecipitation.

Western blots are the preferred method, since they provide information on the approximate molecular weight of the detected protein and allow differentiation between signals produced by antibody binding to the specific protein and signals caused by cross-reactivity of the antibody with other proteins. The drawbacks of Western blots are that a relatively large number of cells is needed for each assay and that the method is laborious and time consuming, making repeated measurements at different time points or experimental conditions difficult.

If an established ELISA is available for the protein under investigation, this is a good alternative for testing many different samples. Only small amounts of protein are needed for each assay, the method is rapid and, in many cases, even quantitative. A disadvantage is that specific signals cannot be differentiated from signals that are caused by cross-reactivity of the primary antibody.

If many time points or experimental conditions are to be tested, a combination of both methods is recommended: first run a Western blot and an ELISA for two or three experimental points in parallel to demonstrate the specificity of the antisense ODN and to show that there is a good correlation between the results obtained by either method. Further experiments can be done using ELISA assays alone.

A very important factor for protein assays in antisense experiments is the time that lies between the beginning of the antisense treatment and the lysis of cells for protein extraction. From our own experience, it takes most cells about 6–8 h to incorporate sufficient amounts of (phosphorothioate) ODNs for an effective inhibition. After that period, antisense inhibition affects only *de novo* protein synthesis. Thus it is very helpful to know the approximate half-life and/or turnover rate of the protein that is to be inhibited. A continuous inhibition for one or two half-life periods is often the minimum required to get a clearly detectable decrease in protein levels. Waiting too long, on the other hand, can mean that the antisense ODN is no longer active and that temporarily decreased protein levels have returned to normal. Immunoprecipitation is a good alternative if the half-life and turnover of the target protein are very uncertain. Here, only proteins that are newly synthesized after the addition of labeled methionine are detected. Thus any time point after adding the labeled methionine will reflect the degree of specific protein inhibition at that time. The fact that cells have to be grown in the presence of radiolabeled methionine limits the use of immunoprecipitation to cell culture facilities that are suitably equipped to handle such materials safely.

Western blotting

Advantages

- gives direct evidence of protein inhibition
- very specific
- shows approximate molecular weight of detected protein
- semi-quantitative

Disadvantages

- a suitable antibody must be available
- a large number of cells is needed for each assay
- laborious and time consuming

ELISA assay

Advantages

- direct evidence of protein inhibition
- a small number of cells is needed for each assay
- many samples can be processed simultaneously
- quantitative

Disadvantages

- a suitable antibody and protein standard must be available
- no information on size of detected protein
- specificity depends on quality of ELISA kit used

Immunoprecipitation

Advantages

- direct evidence of protein inhibition
- detects only newly synthesized proteins
- small number of cells needed for each assay
- semi-quantitative

Disadvantages

- a suitable antibody must be available
- use of potentially hazardous materials ($[^{35}S]$methionine) in cell cultures

4.3 Biochemical assays

The level of many proteins with a catalytic function can be assayed by monitoring their biochemical activity with suitable substrates. Examples of such proteins are enzymes or receptors that have a protein kinase domain (13). Biochemical assays are usually very sensitive, so cells grown in a single microtiter well or a small specimen from a defined area of the CNS are often sufficient for one measurement, and even small deviations in activity can be detected. Furthermore, most assays can be easily performed in larger numbers. These factors make biochemical assays a good choice in cases where many different conditions are to be tested, for example to establish dose–response curves for an antisense drug. Biochemical assays bear, however, the risk of misinterpretation. They should be evaluated with caution and a clear understanding of the enzyme/substrate system used is necessary. Many substrates can be processed by different (iso-)enzymes or catalytic protein domains. Thus, many biochemical assays are not absolutely target-specific. Furthermore, the activity of enzymes and other catalytic proteins is often up-

or down-regulated transiently via reactions like phosphorylation and dephosphorylation. In that case, changes in biochemical activity do not reflect changes in protein level.

The validity of every biochemical assay should be demonstrated in conjunction with at least one direct method such as Northern or Western blots or by a positive antisense control. In cases where there is good correlation between the results obtained by each method under some exemplary experimental conditions, biochemical assays can be regarded as valid for the measurement of antisense effects.

Biochemical assays

Advantages

- sensitive
- many samples can be processed easily
- small number of cells needed for each assay
- semi-quantitative

Disadvantages

- only suitable for proteins with a catalytic or enzymatic domain
- changes in activity can be misinterpreted as changes in protein level
- limited specificity (iso-enzymes)

4.4 Binding assays

Receptor binding assays can be viewed as a special form of biochemical assay. Binding assays monitor the degree of binding of a ligand to a (receptor) protein binding site (14). The specificity of the method depends largely on the specificity of the ligand for its receptor. The affinity between receptor and ligand can vary significantly under different conditions (15), thus care must be taken to ascertain that a change in the number of binding sites actually reflects a change in receptor protein levels. Often radiolabeled ligands are used that can be either detected quantitatively by scintillation counting or visualized *in situ* by autoradiography. The latter has the added advantage of excellent spatial resolution, which is especially useful for analysing antisense effects in various regions of the brain.

Binding assays

Advantages

- specific (depending on ligand)
- rapid
- allows quantification and visualization

Disadvantages

- only useful for receptor proteins
- (radiolabeled) ligand needed
- changes in affinity can mimic a decrease in receptor density

4.5 Cell proliferation

In neurobiology, the manipulation (induction or inhibition) of cell proliferation by antisense ODNs has not been attempted often. Proliferation assays are easily performed, however, either by manual counting on small samples or by automation using a cell counter. Proliferation assays are not limited by the need for special reagents like specific antibodies or receptor ligands. Changes in cell proliferation rates are, however, a very general phenomenon which can be induced by a wide variety of events, ranging from specific antisense-mediated gene inhibition over sequence-related and unrelated side effects to the simple fact that an ODN preparation may be toxic due to inadequate purification. ODNs or their breakdown products may interfere with some indirect proliferation assay such as [^{3}H]thymidine and BrdU incorporation (16). The most reliable assay seems to be the direct counting of cell numbers.

Cell proliferation

Advantages	*Disadvantage*
• easy to perform • can be automated • no need for specific antibodies or receptor ligands	• not very specific

4.6 Morphological analysis

In some instances morphological changes of cultured cells, especially of neurons, can be used to monitor an antisense effect. This applies mainly to the inhibition of structural proteins (17) or factors that induce gross morphological changes like cell differentiation (18). In cell cultures, morphological changes can be monitored over an extended period without disturbing the culture itself, thus allowing repeated measurements in the same culture. If the specificity of an antisense ODN for the inhibition of its target mRNA has been demonstrated by other, more direct methods, morphological analysis can be an excellent way to monitor antisense effects over extended periods of time under many different conditions.

Morphological analysis

Advantages	*Disadvantage*
• easy to perform • repeated measurements in same cell culture possible	• not very specific • sequence-related and toxic effects can also cause morphological changes

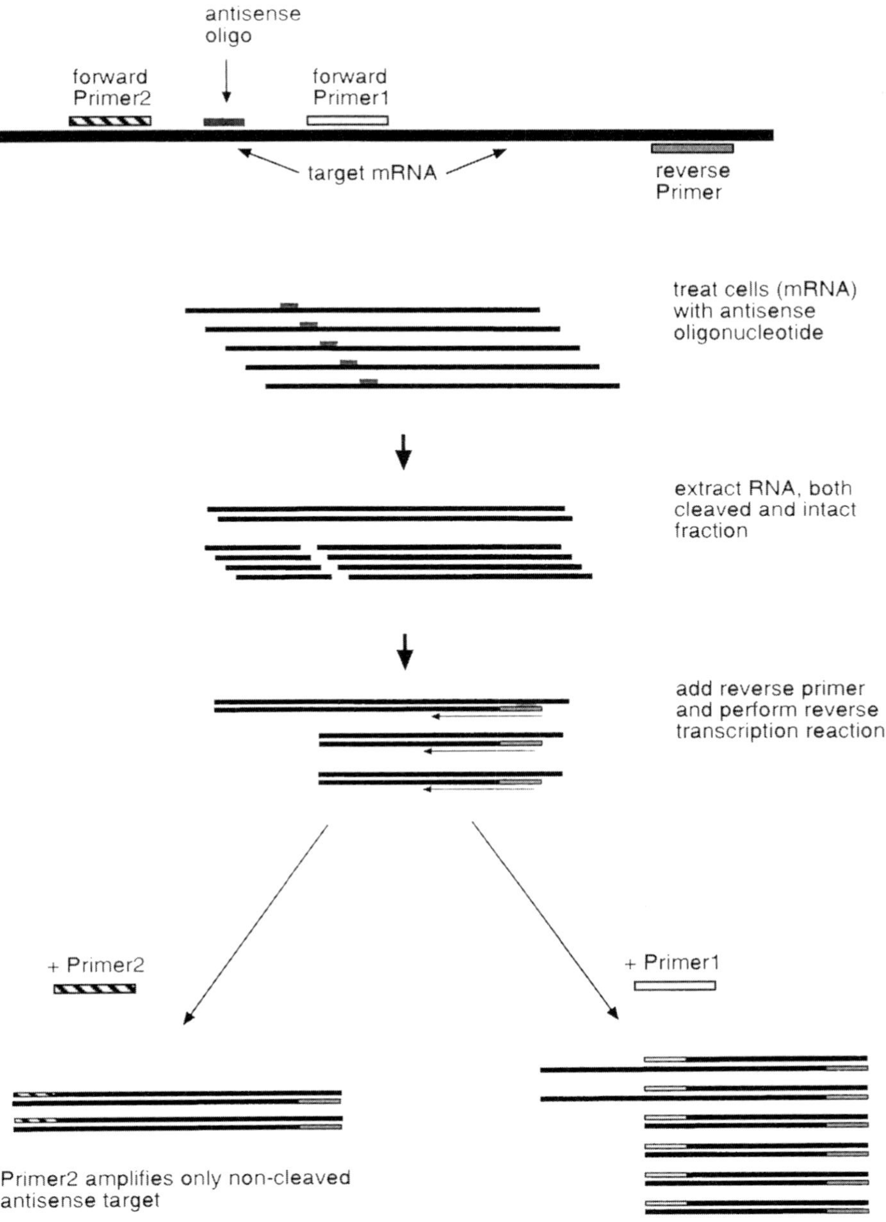

Figure 6. Evaluating the rate of target mRNA degradation by a specific antisense ODN using RT-PCR.

4.7 Functional assays

The inhibition of many proteins can be monitored by functional assays. Especially in neurobiology, where the shape, magnitude and duration of many electrophysiological signals is characteristic for certain ion channels or receptors, the changes of such signals may be closely correlated with changes in respective protein levels (19,20).

Antisense inhibition of a receptor can be functionally monitored by comparing cells that have been treated with a specific antisense, a control ODN and no ODN. If these cells are then exposed to the respective receptor agonist (e.g. a growth factor, cytokine, neurotransmitter or hormone), a strongly diminished or absent cellular response to this stimulus, if present only in the antisense-treated cells, is highly indicative of a specific inhibition of the respective receptor protein (21). Functional assays are a key procedure in the development of antisense drugs, since it is at this point that an ODN must prove to be superior to other drugs either in efficacy or specificity.

Functional assays

Advantages

- specific
- many key proteins in neurobiology can be analyzed
- highly relevant parameter in drug development

Disadvantage

- gene function must be known beforehand

References

1. Woolf, T. M., Melton, D. A. and Jennings, C. G. (1992). *Proc. Natl Acad. Sci. USA*, **89**, 7305.
2. Yaswen, P., Stampfer, M. R., Ghosh, K. and Cohen, J. S. (1993). *Antisense Res. Dev.*, **3**, 67.
3. Kadonga, J. T. (1991). *Methods Enzymol.*, **208**, 10.
4. Krieg, A. M., Yi, A. K. , Matson, S., Waldschmidt, T., Bishop, G. A., Teasdale, R., Koretzky, G. A. and Klinman, D. M. (1995). *Nature*, **374**, 546.
5. Branda, R. F., Moore, A. L., Lafayette, A. R., Mathews, L., Hong, R., Zon, G., Brown, T. and McCormack, J. J. (1996). *J. Lab. Clin. Med.*, **128**, 329.
6. Wang, K. Y., McCurdy, S., Shea, R. G., Swaminathan, S. and Bolton, P. H. (1993). *Biochemistry*, **32**, 1899.
7. Venczel, E. A. and Sen, D. (1993). *Biochemistry*, **32**, 6220.
8. Wyatt, J. R., Vickers, T. A., Robertson, J. L., Buckheit, R. W., Klimkait, T., DeBeates, E., Davis, P. W., Rayner, B., Imbach, J. L. and Ecker, D. J. (1994). *Proc. Natl Acad. Sci. USA*, **91**, 1356.
9. Tanaka, H., Vickart, P., Bertrand, J. R., Rayner, B., Morvan, F., Imbach, J. L. and Paulin, D. (1994). *Nucleic Acids Res.*, **22**, 3069.

10. Stein, C. A. and Krieg, A. M. (1994). *Antisense Res. Dev.*, **4**, 67.
11. Crouch, R. J. and Dirksen, M. L. (1982). In: Roberts, R. J. (Ed.), *Nucleases*, p. 56. Cold Spring Harbor Laboratory Press, Cold Spring Harbor, NY.
12. Dagle, J. M., Weeks, D. L. and Walder, J. A. (1991). *Antisense Res. Dev.*, **1**, 11.
13. Brysch, W., Magal, E., Louis, J. C., Kunst, M., Klinger, I., Schlingensiepen, R. and Schlingensiepen, K. H. (1994). *Cancer Gene Ther.*, **1**, 99.
14. Zang, Z., Florijn, W. and Creese, I. (1994). *Biochem. Pharmacol.*, **48**, 225.
15. Bylund, D. B. and Toews, M. L. (1993). *Am. J. Physiol.*, **265**, L421.
16. Matson, S. and Krieg, A. M. (1992). *Antisense Res. Dev.*, **2**, 325.
17. Osen-Sand, A., Catsicas, M., Staple, J. K., Jones, K. A., Ayala, G., Knowles, J. and Grenningloh, G. (1993). *Nature*, **364**, 445.
18. Schlingensiepen, K. H., Schlingensiepen, R., Kunst, M., Klinger, I., Gerdes, W., Seifert, W. and Brysch, W. (1993). *Dev. Genet.*, **14**, 305.
19. Campbell, V., Berrow, N. and Dolphin, A. C. (1993). *J. Physiol.* (London), **470**, 1.
20. Brussaard, A. B. and Baker, R. E. (1995). *Neurosci. Lett.*, **191**, 111.
21. Tseng, L. F., Collins, K. A. and Kampine, J. P. (1994). *Eur. J. Pharmacol.*, **258**, R1.

4

Modulation of gene expression in the CNS as a tool in behavioral pharmacology

WOLFGANG SOMMER and MARKUS HEILIG

1. Introduction

Antisense oligodeoxynucleotides (ODNs) are widely used in the nervous system as a tool to understand basic mechanisms of neural functioning. They often serve as an essential substitute when conventional pharmacological tools are lacking (e.g. for transcription factors) or when their specificity is inadequate to discriminate between individual components of a particular system (e.g. receptor subtypes of a specific class). Based on the specificity inherent in the genetic code, antisense technology may allow for a better functional analysis. Antisense studies can thereby facilitate costly and often capricious drug development efforts, and delineate targets where such efforts may later be justified. An additional exciting prospect of this research is that DNA analogs may be developed that are themselves efficient as therapeutic agents.

In this chapter we will first give a brief overview of some recent discoveries on the function of G-protein-coupled receptors (dopamine receptors and neuropeptide Y (NPY) receptors) and on the function of the inducible transcription factor c-Fos that have become possible through the use of antisense technology. After each review section we give practical experimental protocols for the use of antisense technology which have emerged as particularly useful in our laboratory. We also focus on the issue of how to analyze the pharmacokinetics of antisense oligonucleotides in the CNS.

2. Functional analysis of G-protein-coupled receptors

2.1 The Y1 subtype of NPY receptors

In a line of studies based on agonist administration, we obtained evidence that central neuropeptide Y (NPY) acts as an endogenous anti-anxiety signal by activating a Y1 subtype of NPY receptor in the amygdala (1–4). Useful receptor antagonists were not available, preventing attempts to establish whether the anti-anxiety actions of exogenous NPY and its analogs reflect a physiological role of the endogenous peptide. When the Y1 receptor was cloned (5–7), the sequence information necessary for antisense ODN design became available. Using a combined *in vitro*/*in vivo* approach, we then demonstrated (8,9) that:

1. In cortical neurons from rat embryos cultured in the presence of antisense ODNs, the density of Y1 receptors was decreased by approximately 60%.
2. The decrease in Y1 receptor density was accompanied by a comparable decrease in the second messenger response to NPY (i.e. inhibition of forskolin-induced cAMP accumulation.
3. Repeated intracerebroventricular (i.c.v.) administration of 50 μg of the antisense ODN every 12 h for 2 days produced a selective loss of cortical Y1-binding density by approximately 60%.
4. The loss of Y1 receptors *in vivo* was followed by a marked increase in experimental anxiety as tested in the elevated plus-maze, a model where central NPY administration acts in the opposite way. In a follow-up study (10), this approach was used to resolve whether food intake stimulation, another prominent effect of central NPY (11), was mediated by Y1 receptors. Y1 antisense ODN treatment not only did not suppress food intake, but increased it, so it seemed likely that another NPY receptor subtype was responsible for the latter action of the peptide. Consistent with this prediction, a Y5 NPY receptor subtype, which appears to mediate feeding effects of NPY, was subsequently cloned (12). Thus, the utilization of antisense ODNs helped clarify a heterogeneity which might be beneficial for future drug design efforts.

2.2 The dopamine D_2 receptor family: different roles of D_2 and D_3 subtypes

Receptor knockdown by antisense methodology has been validated in systems where an extensive conventional pharmacological characterization is available. Convincing evidence of this type has been obtained by several laboratories for dopamine D_2 receptors. Five distinct subtypes of dopamine receptor have been cloned in recent years. Subtypes D_1 and D_5 belong to the D1 family, while subtypes D_2, D_3 and D_4 are members of the D2 family. Zhang and Creese (13; see also Chapter 6) found that i.c.v. infusion of a phosphorothioate antisense ODN, corresponding to the rat D_2 receptor mRNA, reduced rat striatal D_2 receptors by approximately 50%, while D_1, muscarinic and serotonin 5-HT_2 receptors were unaffected. D_2 receptor autoradiography indicated a D_2 receptor down-regulation of about 50%

throughout the striatum and over 70% in the nucleus accumbens; reversibility after 5 days was also demonstrated. A random control ODN was inactive. The antisense treatment inhibited locomotion induced by the D_2 receptor agonist quinpirole, without altering behavior induced by a D_1 receptor agonist. Antisense treatment also elicited catalepsy and reduced spontaneous locomotor activity. Thus the profile of D_2 antisense action was virtually identical to that observed with classical competitive D_2 antagonists. Similar data have been obtained in mice by Weiss and collaborators, although the reductions in receptor density were lower in these studies (14–16). A 20-mer phosphorothioate D_2 antisense ODN, administered by this group i.c.v. or directly into the striatum to mice with unilateral 6-hydroxydopamine lesions of the corpus striatum, inhibited rotations induced by D_2 dopamine receptor agonists but did not block rotations induced by D_1 or muscarinic cholinergic receptor stimulation. This behavioral effect was dose- and time-related and was reversed upon cessation of antisense treatment. Repeated administration of D_2 antisense ODN specifically reduced the levels of D_2 dopamine receptors and D_2 dopamine receptor mRNA; D_1 receptors were unaffected.

The dopamine D_3 receptor subtype (17) has attracted particular interest due to its largely limbic distribution, and its possible involvement in mediating the abuse potential of central stimulants (18). The lack of selective, high-affinity D_3 antagonists has, however, prevented the latter hypothesis from being examined. Recently, we developed a phosphorothioate 15-mer targeted at the D_3 transcript which inhibits D_3 receptor expression both *in vitro* in stable transfected CHO cells (19; also see below) and *in vivo* in the rat striatum (20). Although the lack of selective D_3 ligands prevents precise quantification of receptor loss, conservative indirect estimation suggests significant B_{max} reduction of the binding of the combined $[D_2 + D_3]$ ligand spiperone in the limbic forebrain, where D_3 receptors are relatively abundant, but not in the neostriatum, where D_2 receptors dominate and D_3 receptors are sparse. The reduction in D_3 receptors was accompanied by a marked increase of dopamine synthesis in the nucleus accumbens, suggesting that D_3 receptors may influence dopamine synthesis by acting as presynaptic inhibitory autoreceptors. Functional observations were consistent with this conclusion, as D_3 receptor knockdown was accompanied by marked suppression of exploratory locomotor activity (19).

These findings are in agreement with the more detailed elucidation of dopamine D_2 and D_3 function presented by the Creese laboratory, which elegantly demonstrated that both D_2 and D_3 receptors act as autoreceptors in nigrostriatal dopamine neurons. D_2 or D_3 receptor binding in the substantia nigra was specifically suppressed by intranigral administration of antisense ODNs to D_2 or D_3 receptor mRNA, respectively. Either treatment attenuated the ability of the direct dopamine agonist apomorphine to inhibit nigrostriatal dopamine neurons, and simultaneous D_2 and D_3 treatment potentiated this effect (21; see Chapter 6).

2.3 Practical considerations in the antisense suppression of G-protein-coupled receptors

Receptor proteins generally have a much slower turnover than, for example, inducible transcription factors. Also, the magnitude of their inducibility on the transcriptional level is generally lower. Because of this, receptor knockdown requires prolonged antisense ODN application times. While earlier works used repeated intermittent ODN injections, in recent protocols continuous infusion has been employed. In this way, superior brain tissue distribution and concentrations are achieved. The most practical method for this purpose is the delivery of the ODN by osmotic minipumps (*Protocol 1*).

Protocol 1. Continuous ODN infusion into the rat brain

Equipment and reagents

- Oligodeoxynucleotide
- Sterile Ringer's solution
- Saline
- Stereotaxic frame
- Brain infusion kit (Alza Corp., Palo Alto, CA, USA)
- Osmotic minipump, model 2001 (Alza Corp.)

Method

1. Dissolve ODN in sterile Ringer's solution. Doses between 30 and 40 nmol/day i.c.v. have been found to be effective. The pumping rate is 1 μl/h, which translates into concentrations of 1.25–1.7 nmol/μl.
2. Cut tubing of the brain infusion kit to the appropriate length to avoid bending when pump assembly is put in place. Load the pump and the brain infusion kit separately, then connect the two to avoid formation of air bubbles. Put the pump in saline overnight in order to prime it.
3. The following day, place the cannula of the brain infusion kit into the desired position using standard procedures for stereotaxic operation. With a hemostat, bluntly dissect a subcutaneous cavity from the caudal limit of the incision and down between the scapulae. Place the pump in the cavity, taking care not to bend the tubing. Close the incision with sutures or Wachenfelt clips, taking care not to puncture the tubing.
4. Postoperatively, give antibiotics systemically (e.g. 200 000 U benzylpenicillin).
5. Perform functional analysis on days 3–6 after beginning the infusion.

As stated elsewhere in this volume, if antisense technology is used for functional studies it is imperative that the efficiency is demonstrated at the protein level. For receptors, this is most appropriately done by assaying binding density. However, since the antisense approach has mostly been chosen because there are no specific pharmacological tools, the efficiency of the treatment will be difficult to demonstrate in a binding assay where selective ligands will also be likely to be lacking. Tissue culture may be necessary to circumvent this problem. Our recent work on the dopamine D_3 receptor subtype illustrates this approach. Established ligands, such as spiperone, label both D_2 and D_3 receptor sites. Using stably transfected cell lines expressing either D_2 or D_3 receptors, it was demonstrated that the antisense D_3 ODN suppressed the expression of its target while leaving the closely related D_2 subtype unaffected (*Protocol 2*).

Protocol 2. Antisense blockade of D_2 and D_3 receptors in stably transfected cell lines

Equipment and reagents

- Chinese hamster ovary (CHO) cells, stably expressing D_3 or D_2 receptors
- Alpha-MEM (Biochrom, Berlin, Germany) supplemented with 10% fetal calf serum, 100 U/ml penicillin G, 100 μg/ml streptomycin and 2 mM L-glutamine
- 50 mM Tris–HCl
- Glacial acetic acid
- 6-well plates
- 100 mm Petri dishes
- binding buffer (50 mM Tris, 4 mM $MgCl_2$, 1.5 mM $CaCl_2$, 5 mM KCl, 1 mM EDTA, 129 mM NaCl, 0.05 mg/ml BSA, 0.1 mg/ml ascorbic acid)
- [^{3}H]Spiperone (95 Ci/mmol, Amersham; labels both D_3 and D_2 receptors)
- Trypsin/EDTA solution (Gibco BRL)
- Liquid scintillation cocktail (e.g. Ready Safe, Beckman)
- Liquid scintillation counter

Method

1. Plate out 2×10^3 stably transfected CHO cells in 10 ml of medium in a 100 mm Petri dish.
2. After 2 days, replace the medium with an equal volume of fresh medium containing oligonucleotides at a concentration of 4 μM; replace oligonucleotide-containing medium every day.
3. Dissociate the cells after 2 days' incubation with the oligonucleotides, using trypsin/EDTA solution and replate into 6-well plates at a density of 1.5×10^3 cells/well. Continue changing the oligonucleotide-containing medium every day.
4. After a further 3 days' incubation with the oligonucleotide, wash the cells with PBS (2×2.0 ml), then add the ligand, in 1 ml of binding buffer, in nine different concentrations (0.078 + 5.2 nM final, triplicates). For each concentration, non-specific binding is determined in separate wells in the presence of unlabeled reagents.
5. Incubate for 60 min at room temperature; stop the incubation by washing in 50 mM Tris–HCl (5×5 ml).
6. Add 500 μl of glacial acetic acid to each well; aliquot in triplicate 100 μl samples from each well, add to a scintillation vial containing 5 ml liquid scintillation cocktail and count bound radioactivity.
7. To control for effects on cell viability and/or proliferation, use separate wells for each treatment to determine cell numbers and Trypan Blue exclusion.

3. Functional role of c-*fos* in the adult CNS

Inducible transcription factors are encoded by immediate–early genes (IEGs) and, upon stimulation of a neuron, link transient changes in second messenger systems with long-term changes in the cell, i.e. induce or suppress transcriptional processes in the nucleus (22–25). The *fos* and *jun* families of IEGs have been extensively studied. Fos and its relatives bind to members of the Jun family through a leucine zipper motif to form heterodimers called activator protein-1 (AP-1) complexes which bind specific DNA sequences in gene promoter regions. Once there, they can induce or inhibit transcription, depending on the genetic loci of the binding site and the composition of the AP-1 protein.

The expression of c-*fos* is induced in the CNS by a vast array of physiological and pathological stimuli. Its induction has been widely used as a marker of neuronal activation. However, since there are no pharmacological tools that allow a specific blockade or stimulation of c-*fos*, its role in complex brain functions remained a matter of speculation. In the next section we will review recent progress in characterizing the role of c-*fos* in the CNS which has become possible by the use of antisense oligonucleotide technology. The feasibility of time- and dose-dependently blocking c-*fos* expression in the brain by a single injection of a phosphorothioate antisense ODN directly into the target area was first demonstrated by Robertson and colleagues (26).

3.1 Antisense blockade of c-*fos* expression in selected regions of the brain

3.1.1 c-*fos* and emotional responses

The amygdala is a limbic structure which has been associated with emotional integration of fear and anxiety. As numerous stressors have been shown to increase the expression of IEGs, including c-*fos*, in this region, it is thought that these genes play a role in mediating limbic responses (27). We investigated the role of c-*fos* in anxiety disorders using a modified version of a punished drinking conflict test, a pharmacologically validated animal model of anxiety. It was shown that administration of c-*fos* antisense ODNs into the amygdala attenuated c-*fos* expression and produced a marked release of punished responding, an effect normally obtained with anxiety-reducing compounds (28).

3.1.2 c-*fos* in the control of motor behavior

Besides the amygdala, we have also studied the function of the c-*fos* transcript in the basal ganglia. These ganglia participate in sensorimotor integration and motor-associated learning. Expression of c-*fos* in striatal GABA-ergic neurons is induced by systemic administration of amphetamine or cocaine via dopamine D1 receptors, and is associated with increased locomotor activity and stereotypic behavior, e.g. focused sniffing, or rearing (29–31). We, and others, have demonstrated that infusions of c-*fos* antisense ODNs into the striatum can suppress *d*-amphetamine- and cocaine-induced expression of this gene (2,26,32).

There are several biochemical and behavioral consequences of antisense blockade of c-*fos* expression in the striatum:

1. Following unilateral infusion of anti-c-*fos* and also anti-*ngfi*-a ODNs into the neostriatum or the globus pallidus, animals treated with *d*-amphetamine show rotational behavior towards the side of suppression (32–35). Bilateral injections of c-*fos* antisense ODNs into either the nucleus accumbens or the neostriatum block the motor activation induced by cocaine and amphetamine (2,36). Moreover, rats injected with c-*fos* antisense into the medial prefrontal cortex display decreased locomotor activity when exposed to novel environments (37). Thus, within cortical and basal ganglia structures involved in the control of motor functions, namely the medial prefrontal cortex, the core region of the nucleus accumbens, the neostriatum and the globus pallidus, the blockade of c-*fos* expression leads to inhibition of motor programs and, therefore, the c-Fos protein might facilitate a common pathway in these neurons.
2. The unexpectedly rapid onset of behavioral c-*fos* antisense actions in relation to an inducing stimulus suggests that low-level, basal expression of c-*fos* may be involved in ongoing regulation of a number of downstream genes. Thus, it is the interference with this basal expression that is responsible for observed c-*fos* antisense effects. In fact, we found increased levels of c-*fos*, *jun*B and *ngfi*-a mRNA in the striatum shortly (90 min) after intrastriatal infusions of c-*fos* antisense ODNs (38). These findings suggest an inhibitory role of basal Fos protein levels on the expression of certain genes in the striatum and a cross-talk mechanism between IEG transcription factors.
3. Suppression of basal c-*fos* expression by antisense ODNs in striatal neurons significantly reduces the release of the neurotransmitter γ-aminobutyric acid (GABA) in the substantia nigra, the major projection area of the D1 receptor-containing striatal neurons (*Figure 1*). These results provide evidence for a facilitatory role of a c-*fos*-regulated mechanism in the control of GABA transmission (38,39).
4. In theory, any of a vast number of genes containing AP-1-binding sites in their promoter regions could be influenced by changes in the expression of c-*fos*. These potential targets include genes that encode enzymes (e.g. tyrosine hydroxylase or glutamic acid decarboxylase) that are involved in the synthesis of neurotransmitters (e.g. norepinephrine, dopamine or GABA), peptides (e.g. cholecystokinin, enkephalin, dynorphin or neurotensin), growth factors (e.g. nerve growth factor), transcription factors (e.g. those encoded by *jun*B or *ngfi*-a) and others (23). We found that c-*fos*

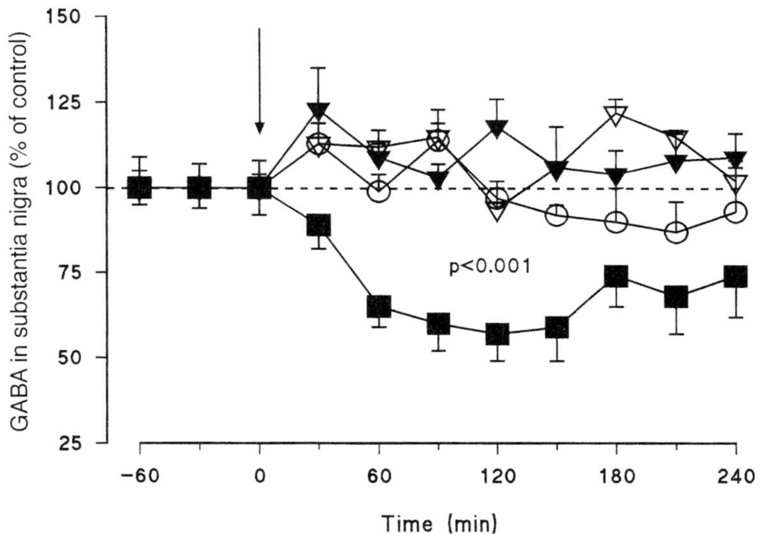

Figure 1. Rapid antisense effects on neuronal activity. Release of the neurotransmitter γ-aminobutyric acid (GABA) in the substantia nigra of awake, freely moving rats, intrastriatally injected with c-*fos* antisense, sense and random oligonucleotides (ODNs) (2 nmol, partially phosphorothioate modified). The sham group was infused with Ringer's solution alone. The rats were implanted with microdialysis probes 2 days before the experiment. The vertical arrow indicates the onset of the intrastriatal injection of the ODNs. The results are expressed as a percentage of three basal values of 30 min perfusate fractions measured prior to the ODN infusion. The c-*fos* antisense ODN decreased GABA release in the ipsilateral substantia nigra significantly within 1 h. The maximal effect was observed 2 h after the onset of the ODN infusion. In the same animal the GABA release in the ipsilateral globus pallidus was unaffected (not shown). These results provide evidence for a facilitatory role of c-*fos* in the control of striatal GABA transmission (38).

antisense blocks the caffeine-induced increase in mRNA levels of the peptide precursors for neurotensin and substance P while leaving preproenkephalin and preprodynorphin mRNA levels unaffected (40). Inhibition of neurotensin expression by c-*fos* antisense has also been found by others (41,42). Although it is unknown whether these changes in peptide expression account for the behavioral effects produced by intrastriatal infusions of c-*fos* antisense ODNs, they provide evidence for biochemical disturbances produced by these agents.

3.1.3 Epileptogenesis

Kindling is an animal model of epileptogenesis where repeated subconvulsive electrical stimulation of 'seizure-responsive' regions of the brain (i.e. amygdala and hippocampus) eventually produce full generalized seizures (43,44). A single kindling stimulus produces focal seizure activity or an after-discharge that is essential for kindling to occur. A single after-discharge in the amygdala results in IEG induction in the amygdala, claustrum, piriform cortex and the perirhinal cortex (45,46). Experiments have shown that repeated infusion of antisense ODNs to c-*fos* into the amygdala can suppress the expression of this gene and significantly accelerate the rate of kindling in rats (47). Considering our findings on a reduced GABA release after c-*fos* antisense treatment (see above), the increased kindling rate may result from reduction in inhibitory GABA-ergic neurotransmission in this region, which in turn would facilitate excitatory transmission of seizure-producing neurons.

3.1.4 Behavioral studies in c-*fos* knockout mice

Knockout experiments of IEG transcription factors can be classified into two groups. Null mutations within the *jun* family are lethal during embryogenesis and demonstrate the absolute requirement of these genes for development. In contrast, c-*fos* and *fosB* knockout mice do not show phenotypic alterations in their nervous system. However, both c-*fos* and *fosB* knockout mice do present with a variety of more subtle behavioral abnormalities. For example, c-*fos* knockout mice are much less responsive to external stimuli or stress than wild-type animals and are unable to learn complex tasks (48–50), whereas *fosB* knockout mice show alterations in nursing behavior and in their behavioral responses to cocaine (51,52). Moreover, c-*fos* knockout mice seem to have an alteration in their molecular clock, as light-induced phase shifts of the circadian rhythm are attenuated in these animals (53). Antisense treatment (a cocktail of antisense ODNs to c-*fos* and *junB* was given i.c.v.) produced a similar effect on the cyclicity of the circadian rhythm (54). Further, it has been shown that null mutants for c-*fos* exhibit an attenuation of kindling development (55), while *fosB* knockout mice are particularly susceptible to seizure activity (56). The reason for the discrepancy between kindling in c-*fos* knockout animals and those receiving intramygdalar infusion of c-*fos* antisense ODNs is unclear. However, the global absence of c-*fos* during development and in adulthood in knockout animals probably produces different alterations in cerebral physiology than does the localized suppression of this gene by antisense ODNs. Thus, one must be cautious when interpreting the differences between the two models, as they do not represent equivalent paradigms in which to investigate the role of a particular gene. In any case, these studies suggest that the Fos proteins may play a role in determining the threshold for seizure development.

In summary, the behavioral and biochemical alterations observed after both antisense treatment and permanent gene knockouts suggest that members of the Fos family may not be essential for neural function, but appear to increase the potential for differentiated responses to specific stimuli. The antisense studies of c-*fos* function illustrate the most striking advantages of this approach over gene knockouts, namely that it allows spatial and temporal control of genetic manipulation and that species other than mouse become accessible for the analysis of gene function.

3.1.5 Practical considerations in the antisense blockade of c-*fos* in distinct regions of the brain

A single injection is sufficient to block the expression of proteins that have a high turnover or are rapidly induced by certain stimuli such as IEGs. Over time, the original treatment protocols have been improved in order to enhance reliability (*Protocol 3*). In this protocol, the use of implanted guide cannulas minimizes the stress caused by operation and anesthesia on the day of the experiment. Animals are consistently handled, since inconsistent handling can lead to inter-individual differences in stress response, IEG transcription factor levels and behavioral response. Animals can move freely during the injection, avoiding restraint stress. In this way the infusion rate can be decreased to 0.25 μl/min in order to reduce reagent loss and tissue damage produced by forced injections. When possible, i.e. in short treatment protocols such as the analysis of turning behavior, the degree of sulfur modification in each molecule should probably be reduced by using partially modified ODNs (see below). Freely moving animals also allow better assessment of toxicity or seizure development eventually caused by the oligonucleotides. Such effects may be masked if animals are anesthetized during the administration of the ODNs.

Protocol 3. Injection of antisense oligonucleotides into freely moving rats

Equipment

- Stereotaxic frame
- Stainless steel microinjection guide cannula (e.g. from Plastics One, Roanoke, VA, USA)
- CMA/100 microinjection pump (CMA)
- Microsyringe (Hamilton), Model 801, 10 μl

Method

1. Using standard procedures for stereotaxic operation, place the guide cannula into the desired position. Seal the guide with a dummy cannula.
2. Allow at least 1 week recovery before injection of ODN. Handle animals consistently, since inconsistent handling can cause inter-individual differences in stress responses, IEG transcription factor levels and behavioral responses. Habituate animals to the short restraint period during the placement of the injector cannula. **Important**: make sure that cannula caps screw on smoothly. IEGs are easily induced by a variety of manipulations, including even mild stressors such as restraint. Habituation may eliminate this IEG induction, but it is necessary to include sham treatments as an extra control.

Protocol 3. *Continued*

3. Use at least 1 m of flexible tubing. Connect the infusion cannula, tubing and microsyringe, and rinse with sterile water, taking care not to leave any air bubbles in the tubing. Withdraw an appropriate volume of dissolved oligonucleotides, thereby leaving a *ca.* 1–2 mm air bubble between the injection solution and the water. Place the microsyringe into the pump. Adjust syringes when using two or more simultaneously.
4. Insert the injection cannula into the guide while gently holding the animal, and fix in position (we use custom-made dust caps). We normally infuse a 1–2 mM solution (water, saline or Ringer's) at 0.25 μl/min for injections into the parenchyma and at 5 μl/30 s for i.c.v. injections. Leave the injection cannula in place for another 1–2 min. Seal with a dummy cannula. During the infusion observe the animals for signs of pathology and keep the connection tubing clear.
5. Analyze 1–12 h after oligonucleotide injection for antisense effects.

Suppression of c-*fos* expression in the striatum also induces marked increases in c-Fos and Ngfi-a protein and in mRNA levels in the ipsilateral globus pallidus and in certain thalamic areas (15; Sommer, unpublished observations). In a recent study, Hebb and Robertson (57) found that in the superior colliculus, a brain region involved in postural control, there was a marked increase in c-Fos protein levels after intrastriatal c-*fos* antisense treatment that was significantly correlated to the intensity of rotation. These studies demonstrate that suppression of c-*fos* expression in a certain brain area produces subsequent changes of neuronal activity in distal regions that are innervated by the neurons of the treated area. These phenomena may serve as excellent markers to study the neuronal circuitry underlying the behavioral response.

4. Pharmacokinetics of oligonucleotides in the brain

Knowledge about the fate of the oligonucleotides after their administration into the brain is crucial for effective antisense application, since it may lead to information necessary for the design of the study or for the interpretation of the results. Thus, it is necessary to demonstrate clearly whether ODNs reach the targeted region in the brain, penetrate targeted cells and remain inside the cell for a certain period of time without degradation. For example, the primary difference between the effects of partially modified ODNs and those of fully modified ODNs is that the former have a shorter latency of onset and duration of action. As a result of this, the time course of the behavioral effects of intrastriatally injected antisense ODNs to c-*fos* can vary between 1 and 10 h

(32,35,38,58). As for the use of any new kind of drug, there is no substitute for systematically testing parameters of regional pharmacokinetics.

An extensive discussion of these issues has been published (59,60). The purpose of this section is to focus on the technical aspects of how to study the pharmacokinetics of ODNs in the brain. Their spread, uptake and elimination *in vivo* during the experiment/treatment can be monitored using markers that allow microscopic detection in brain sections or detection in brain homogenates using electrophoresis. Despite the concern that marker molecules may modify the physicochemical properties of the oligonucleotides and thus may affect the mechanism of distribution or cellular uptake, in a number of studies labeling with fluorescence, biotin, digoxygenin, 5-bromdeoxyuridine or radioactive markers shows a very similar distribution in the brain when compared with each other (59,61–66).

Oligonucleotides are exposed outside and within the cellular environment to metabolic activity. The majority of *in vivo* studies using antisense ODNs have used phosphorothioate derivatives of phosphodiester ODNs, since this modification makes the molecules resistant to nuclease attack, the primary source of ODN degradation, and increases the toxic potential and the binding affinity for proteins (67). To minimize these disadvantages, recent studies have employed ODNs containing the thioate modification only at a few of the internucleoside linkages, i.e. partially phosphorothioate-modified ODNs. These modifications are commonly placed at the termini of the molecules. It has been reported that repeated infusions of phosphorothioate ODNs into the amygdala produced marked cellular damage, whereas the same treatment with partially modified ODNs did not (47). Compared with unmodified ODNs, phosphorothioate ODNs have a reduced tissue penetration when infused into the ventricles (65,66). Oligonucleotide uptake was markedly decreased in regions remote from the ependymal surface. Consequently, either continuous infusion or frequent i.c.v injections may be necessary to maximize antisense effects and especially to block the synthesis of constitutively expressed gene products.

Other potential sources of artefacts in light microscopic analysis occur in the preparation of the tissue and in the method of visualization of the label. The possibility of diffusion processes in liquid phases crossing cellular compartments or tissue borders should always be kept in mind. Post-mortem changes in the distribution of the oligonucleotide have to be accounted for in the experimental protocol. The use of radioactive markers allows very short tissue-processing times since sections taken on a cryostat can be exposed directly to autoradiographic film. For the study of intracellular localization, however, fluorescent labeling is much more suitable. In our hands, stable fixation for histology, including immunolabeling, can be achieved by adding glutaraldehyde to the 4% paraformaldehyde fixative and by performing all necessary incubations or washing steps at 40 °C.

In our analysis of the role of the IEG c-*fos* in the striatum, it was essential to know how far the antisense ODNs spread after a single injection into the neostriatum and what kind of cells were taking up the ODNs (38). We found that completely phosphorothioate-modified ODNs (c-*fos* antisense), end-labeled with either radioactive or fluorescent markers, could be recovered intact from tissue extracts up to 24 h after injection into the striatal region of the brain (*Figure 2*, *Protocol 4*). However, 20 min after the injection, the majority of the injected substance had already disappeared. Together with other studies, this was interpreted as evidence for rapid clearance of the ODNs into the circulation or into the ventricular system (59,68). As a consequence of these findings, we changed our injection protocol to use much slower infusion rates (0.25 μl/min). The spread of radiolabeled ODNs in the brain was monitored by autoradiography (*Figure 3*). Our results demonstrated that the ODNs, injected in a volume of 1 μl, spread throughout this relatively large region within 20 min, and diffusion appeared to be restricted by the corpus callosum and the ventral borders of the striatum. While there was no generalized distribution throughout the brain, even after 24 h, a sub-

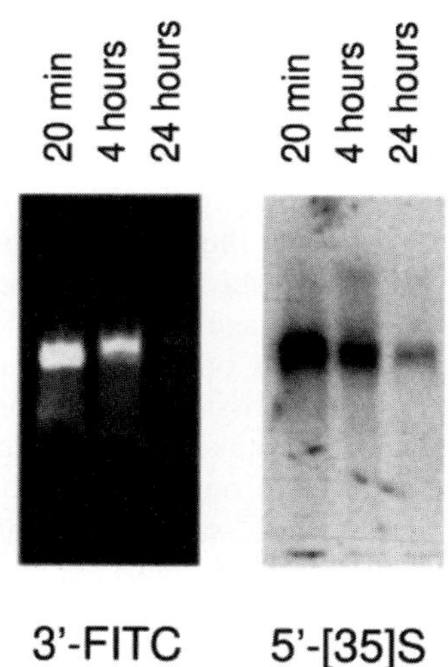

Figure 2. Stability of oligonucleotides after injection into the rat brain. Phosphorothioate-modified ODNs (24-mer) were simultaneously labeled at both ends with a radioactive marker ([^{35}S]ATP-γS) placed at the 5′ end and a fluorescent marker (FITC) at the 3′ end of the molecule. Animals were injected into the striatum with 5×10^5 c.p.m. radioactively 5′-end-labeled phosphorothioate-modified ODNs diluted in 1 nmol of cold compound. Striatal tissue was obtained 20 min, 4 h and 24 h after the injection and analyzed for the presence of the injected material. The radioactive and the fluorescent signals both gave rise to a single band of exactly the same size and decreasing signal intensity in the electrophoretic analysis (12% polyacrylamide gel), demonstrating that intact ODNs could be recovered up to 24 h after microinjection into the striatum. Most of the injected radioactivity disappeared 20 min after the injection, which may reflect a rapid clearance of the phosphorothioate-modified ODNs into the circulation or the ventricles. The absence of breakdown products in both detection methods points towards exonuclease activity as the major source of ODN degradation in brain tissue.

stantial amount of the ODNs appeared in the major projection regions of the striatal neurons within hours. For example, the ODNs were detected in the globus pallidus within 30 min following infusion into the striatum. Within 4 h they were detectable in the substantia nigra, approximately 5–6 mm distal from the injection site. Thus, ODNs that are infused locally into the brain may exert effects in regions relatively distant from the initial site of administration.

Protocol 4. Spread of oligonucleotides after their injection into the brain

Equipment and reagents

- Radiolabeling buffer
- T4 polynucleotide kinase
- Minigel (12% polyacrylamide)
- Tracking dye (bromophenol blue)
- Vertical slab gel unit (e.g. Pharmacia Biotech)
- $[^{35}S]ATP$-γS (10 mCi/ml, 600 Ci/mmol; Amersham)
- Hyperfilm (Amersham)
- Speedvac (Savant)
- Injection solution (e.g. artificial CSF, 0.9% saline, Ringer acetate)
- Extraction buffer (50 mM Tris pH 8.8, 1 mM EDTA, 0.5% Tween 20%, 0.5 mg/ml Proteinase K)
- Phenol/chloroform/isoamylalcohol (25:24:1 by volume; pH 8.0)

A. *Radiolabeling of oligonucleotides at the 5′ end*

1. Mix 0.5 nmol of oligonucleotide and 5 μl of $[^{35}S]ATP$-γS in 30 μl reaction volume together with buffer and T4 polynucleotide kinase according to the supplier's protocol (e.g. either Promega or Gibco).
2. Incubate at 37 °C for 1–3 h.
3. Load the whole reaction on to a 12% polyacrylamide minigel and run until the oligonucleotide has migrated approximately 3 cm into the gel. The position of the oligonucleotide may be estimated from the position of the tracking dye. In a 12% polyacrylamide minigel, bromophenol blue co-migrates with oligonucleotides of about 15 bases in length.
4. Expose the gel for several hours to X-ray film. Cut out the band and elute the oligonucleotides in 400 μl sterile water at 60 °C for several hours to overnight.
5. Transfer solution to a fresh tube; use 1 μl to measure the amount of incorporated radioactivity by scintillation counting. Store at –20 °C until use.

Note: when using phosphorothioate modified oligonucleotides we have found that extended incubation times (up to 3 h at 37 °C) resulted in substantial increases of labeled end-products of the reaction. Usually, we elute approximately 12×10^6 cpm from labeling reactions using phophorothioate-modified oligonucleotides.

B. *Injection into the brain*

1. Calculate 5×10^5 cpm per injection and dry the appropriate amount of the radiolabelled oligonucleotide under vacuum in a Speedvac (Savant).

Protocol 4. *Continued*

Dissolve the radioactivity in injection solution containing the same amount of cold oligonucleotides as used in the functional studies.

2. Inject the oligonucleotides into the desired brain region according to the protocol used for the functional experiments. Keep some of the radiolabeled oligonucleotides for gel analysis.
3. After the given amount of time, kill the animals by decapitation.
4. Freeze the brains in isopentane at –40 °C for sectioning on a cryostat.
5. Expose slides to X-ray film.
6. As an alternative to section 4, dissect out brain regions, cut them into small pieces and store the tissue at –70 °C for further analysis.

C. *Recovery of injected oligonucleotides from brain tissue*

1. Homogenize the tissue in 10 volumes (w/v) of extraction buffer by gentle agitation at 50 °C for 3 h. Initially disrupt the tissue by triturating the suspension several times through a 1 ml pipette tip.
2. Extract the lysate three times with one volume of phenol/chloroform/isoamylalcohol (25:24:1 by volume; pH 8.0).
3. Centrifuge.
4. Add to the supernatant a solution containing 0.3 M NaCl and 10 mM $MgCl_2$ plus 10 μg yeast tRNA per ml.
5. Precipitate with 3 volumes of ethanol at –70 °C overnight.
6. Centrifuge at maximum speed and resuspend the resulting pellet in 50 μl water.
7. Load aliquots on to a 12% non-denaturing polyacrylamide gel.
8. Expose gel to X-ray film.

Equally important to the question of regional spread is to determine which brain cell types take up antisense ODNs. Simultaneous immunolocalization of neuron-specific antigens and fluorescently tagged ODNs confirmed that these molecules were being incorporated into neurons after intrastriatal infusions, while glial uptake was much more sparse and slower (59; *Figure 4*, *Protocol 5*). Similar findings on differences in neuronal and glial uptake of ODNs have been reported by others (69). Nevertheless, there are several reports describing antisense activities on genes, such as angiotensinogen or the glutamate transporter subtypes GLAST and GLT-1, which are mainly or exclusively expressed in glial cells (70,71).

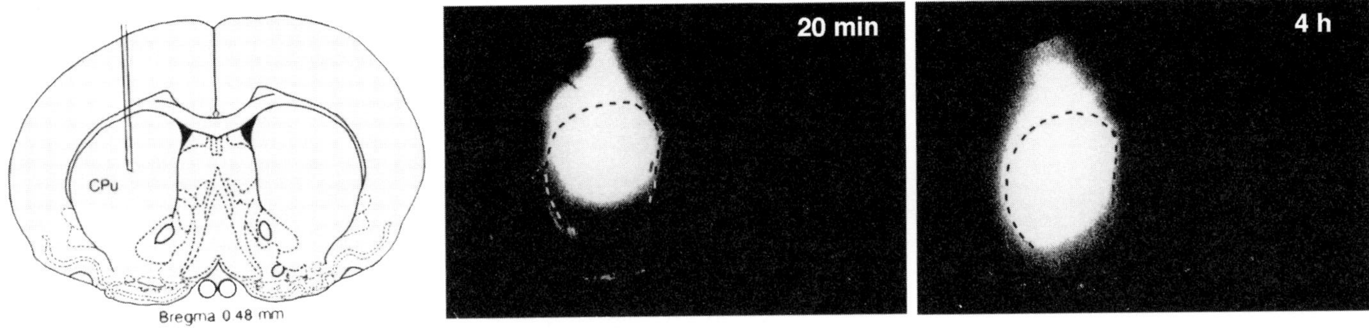

Figure 3. Spread of oligonucleotides after direct injection into the striatum. Autoradiograph showing the distribution of [^{35}S]ATP-γS-labeled c-*fos* antisense phosphorothioate ODNs 20 min and 4 h after a single injection (1 μl) into the striatum. The ODNs spread throughout the dorsal part of the striatum within 20 min after the injection and the entire dorsal striatum is labeled within 4 h. In the rostro-caudal dimension the signal is visible within the entire caudate putamen, extending into the medial forebrain bundle. In addition, dorsal cortical areas, initially the part around the cannula tract and the corpus callosum, become labeled with increasing intensity over the time course of the experiment. The labeling was restricted to the injected side even after 24 h (not shown). The border of the striatum is outlined on the autoradiograms (hatched line). The placement of the injection cannula is shown in the scheme on the left (38).

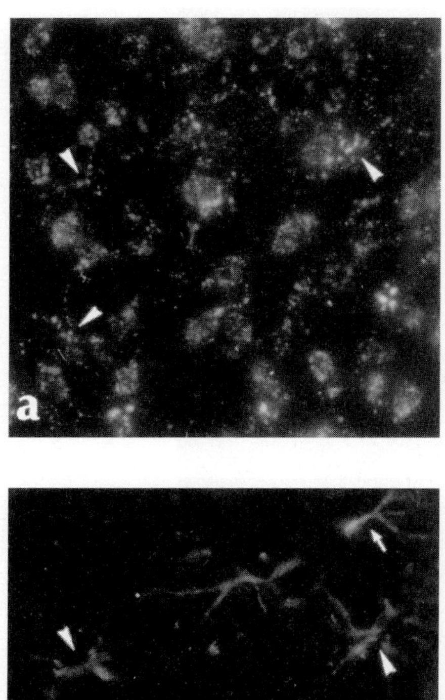

Figure 4. Uptake of FITC-conjugated oligonucleotides after injection into the brain. Photomicrographs of FITC 3′-conjugated c-*fos* antisense phosphorothioate ODN-labeled neurons and glial cells 24 h after the injection (1 nmol/1 μl) into the striatum (a). At this time point the appearance of the intracellular FITC signals was punctate. In addition to the predominant neuronal uptake early after the injection, there was now also staining of glial cells by the ODNs. Astrocytes were identified by staining with a rabbit antiserum to glial fibrillary acidic protein (GFAP) followed by detection with a rhodamine-labeled anti-rabbit antibody (b). Arrowheads point to double-labeled cells. Magnification ×200.

Protocol 5. Cellular uptake of oligonucleotides after their injection into the brain

Equipment and reagents

- Injection solution (e.g. artificial CSF, 0.9% saline or Ringer acetate)
- 0.9% NaCl
- Fixative containing 4% paraformaldehyde and 0.25% (v/v) glutaraldehyde in 0.1 M phosphate-buffered saline (PBS)
- 10% Phosphate-buffered sucrose
- PBS containing 0.25% Triton-X
- Glycerol/PBS solution (3:1, v/v)
- Antiserum to a cell-type specific marker, e.g. glial fibrillary acidic protein (GFAP) (1:500, DAFO)
- Fluorescently conjugated antibody, e.g. rhodamine-conjugated anti-rabbit antibody (1:40, Amersham).
- Cryostat
- Epifluorescence microscope with filters that allow switching between 365 nm and 550–580 nm illumination

A. *Injection and tissue preparation*

1. Dissolve FITC-labeled oligonucleotides in the appropriate injection solution at 1 nmol/μl.
2. Inject the oligonucleotides into the desired brain region according to the protocol used for the functional experiments.
3. At the chosen time point, kill the rats by overdose of pentobarbital anesthesia and perfuse, through the left cardiac ventricle, 200 ml 0.9% NaCl followed by 300 ml fixative containing 4% paraformaldehyde and 0.25% (v/v) glutaraldehyde in 0.1 M PBS.
4. Keep the brains for 2 h in fixative and then transfer to 10% phosphate-buffered sucrose for 1–2 days.
5. Freeze the brains and take sections (14 μm thick) on a cryostat.
6. Coverslip with glycerol/PBS solution (3:1, v/v) and evaluate under an epifluorescence microscope.

B. *Simultaneous immunolocalization of cell type-specific antigens and fluorescently tagged ODNs*

1. Incubate sections with antiserum to a cell-type specific marker, e.g. glial fibrillary acidic protein (GFAP) (1:500, DAFO), in PBS containing 0.25% Triton-X at 4°C.
2. Wash several times with cold PBS.
3. Incubate for indirect immunofluorescence with the appropriate fluorescently conjugated antibody (e.g. rhodamine-conjugated anti-rabbit antibody, 1:40, Amersham).
4. Wash several times with cold PBS.
5. Coverslip and evaluate under an epifluorescence microscope.
6. Examine oligonucleotide uptake and cell type by switching between 365 nm and 550–580 nm illumination.

5. Summary and perspectives

Specific antisense blockade of expression is now an established neuropharmacological tool for targeting neurotransmitter receptors and inducible transcription factors. In its short history, however, antisense methodology has also acquired a reputation for being somewhat capricious. Antisense experiments have to be carefully designed and appropriate controls need to be used (for detailed discussion of these problems see earlier chapters of this volume). In this sense, knowledge about the pharmacokinetics of ODNs after their administration into the brain may be of great value in planning efficient antisense experiments as well as for the proper interpretation of the results.

The CNS has not yet become a primary target for ODN-based therapeutic strategies, mainly because, under normal conditions, ODNs do not cross the blood–brain barrier and virtually no ODNs can be detected in the brain after systemic administration (72). The increased appreciation of antisense ODNs as a tool in neuropharmacology may inspire further exploration in ODN chemistry and thus overcome some of the pharmacokinetic and pharmacodynamic obstacles of this technology. It may, therefore, not be long before these agents are developed into a whole new class of neuropharmaceuticals.

References

1. Heilig, M., Koob, G. F., Ekman, R. and Britton, K. T. (1994) *Trends Neurosci.*, **17**, 80.
2. Heilig, M., McLeod, S., Brot, M., Heinrichs, S. C., Menzaghi, F., Koob, G. F. and Britton, K. T. (1993) *Neuropsychopharmacology*, **8**, 357.
3. Heilig, M., McLeod, S., Koob, G. K. and Britton, K. T. (1992) *Regul. Peptides*, **41**, 61.
4. Heilig, M., Soderpalm, B., Engel, J. A. and Widerlov, E. (1989) *Psychopharmacology*, **98**, 524.
5. Eva, C., Keinanen, K., Monyer, H., Seeburg, P. and Sprengel, R. (1990) *FEBS Lett.*, **271**, 81.
6. Herzog, H., Hort, Y. J., Ball, H. J., Hayes, G., Shine, J. and Selbie, L. A. (1992) *Proc. Natl Acad. Sci. USA*, **89**, 5794.
7. Larhammar, D., Blomqvist, A. G., Yee, F., Jazin, E., Yoo, H. and Wahlested, C. (1992) *J. Biol. Chem.*, **267**, 10935.
8. Heilig, M., Pich, E. M., Koob, G. F., Yee, F. and Wahlested, C. (1992) *Soc. Neurosci. Abs.*, **642**, 18.
9. Wahlestedt, C., Pich, E. M., Koob, G. F., Yee, F. and Heilig, M. (1993) *Science*, **259**, 528.
10. Heilig, M. (1995) *Regul. Peptides*, **59**, 201.
11. Stanley, B. G. (1993) In: Wahlestedt, C. and Colmers, W. F. (Eds), *The Biology of Neuropeptide Y and Related Peptides*, pp. 457–509. Humana Press, Totowa, NJ.
12. Gerald, C., Walker, M. W., Criscion, L., Gustafson, E. L., Batzlhartmann, C., Smith, K. E., Vayesse, P., Durkin, M. M., Laz, T. M., Linemeyer, D. L.,

Schaffhauser, A. O., Whitebread, S., Hofbauer, K. G., Taber, R. I., Branchek, T. A. and Weinshank, R. L. (1996) *Nature*, **382**, 168.

13. Zhang, M. and Creese, I. (1993) *Neurosci. Lett.*, **161**, 223.
14. Weiss, B., Zhou, L. W., Zhang, S. P. and Qin, Z. H. (1993) *Neuroscience*, **55**, 607.
15. Zhou, L. W., Zhang, S. P., Qin, Z. H. and Weiss, B. (1994) *J. Pharmacol. Exp. Ther.*, **268**, 1015.
16. Zhou, L. W., Zhang, S. P. and Weiss, B. (1996) *Neurochem. Int.*, **29**, 583.
17. Sokoloff, P., Giros, B., Martres, M. P., Bouthenet, M. L. and Schwartz, J. C. (1990) *Nature*, **347**, 146.
18. Caine, S. B. and Koob, G. F. (1993) *Science*, **260**, 1814.
19. Ekman, A., Nissbrandt, H., Heilig, M., Dijkstra, D. and Eriksson, E. (1998) *Naunyn-Schmiedelberg's Arch. Pharmacol.*, in press.
20. Nissbrandt, H., Ekman, A., Eriksson, E. and Heilig, M. (1995) *Neuroreport*, **6**, 573.
21. Tepper, J. M., Sun, B. C., Martin, L. P. and Creese, I. (1997) *J. Neurosci.*, **17**, 2519.
22. Curran, T. and Morgan, J. I. (1995) *J. Neurobiol.*, **26**, 403.
23. Hughes, P. and Dragunow, M. (1995) *Pharmacol. Rev.*, **47**, 133.
24. Morgan, J. I. and Curran, T. (1991) *Trends Pharmacol. Sci.*, **12**, 343.
25. Robertson, H. A. (1992) *Biochem. Cell. Biol.*, **70**, 729.
26. Chiasson, B. J., Hooper, M. L., Murphy, P. R. and Robertson, H. A. (1992) *Eur. J. Pharmacol.*, **227**, 451.
27. Honkaniemi, J., Kainu, T., Ceccatelli, S., Rechardt, L., Hokfelt, T. and Pelto-Huikko, M. (1992) *Neuroreport*, **3**, 849.
28. Moller, C., Bing, O. and Heilig, M. (1994) *Cell. Mol. Neurobiol.*, **14**, 415.
29. Cole, A. J., Bhat, R. V., Patt, C., Worley, P. F. and Baraban, J. M. (1992) *J. Neurochem.*, **58**, 1420.
30. Graybiel, A. M., Moratalla, R. and Robertson, H. A. (1990) *Proc. Natl Acad. Sci. USA*, **87**, 6912.
31. Paul, M. L., Graybiel, A. M., David, J. C. and Robertson, H. A. (1992) *J. Neurosci.*, **12**, 3729.
32. Sommer, W., Bjelke, B., Ganten, D. and Fuxe, K. (1993) *Neuroreport*, **5**, 277.
33. Dragunow, M., Lawlor, P., Chiasson, B. and Robertson, H. (1993) *Neuroreport*, **5**, 305.
34. Hebb, M. O. and Robertson, H. A. (1997) *Mol. Brain Res.*, **48**, 97.
35. Hebb, M. O. and Robertson, H. A. (1997) *Mol. Brain Res.*, **47**, 223.
36. Umekage, T., Namima, M., Fukushima, K., Sugita, S. and Watanabe, Y. (1997) *Neuroreport*, **8**, 407.
37. Persico, A. M., Schindler, C. W., Davis, S. C., Ambrosio, E. and Uhl, G. R. (1998) *Neuroscience*, **82**, 1115.
38. Sommer, W., Rimondini, R., O'Connor, W., Hansson, A. C., Ungerstedt, U. and Fuxe, K. (1996) *Proc. Natl Acad. Sci. USA*, **93**, 14134.
39. Sommer, W. and Fuxe, K. (1997) *Neurochem. Int.*, **31**, 425.
40. Svenningsson, P., Georgieva, J., Kontny, E., Heilig, M., Fredholm, B. B., Sasa, H., Umekage, T., Namima, M., Arimura, S., Nakata, H., Watanabe, Y. and Kobayashi, M. (1997) *Eur. J. Neurosci.*, **9**, 2135.
41. Merchant, K. M. (1994) *Mol. Cell Neurosci.*, **5**, 336.
42. Robertson, G. S., Tetzlaff, W., Bedard, A., St-Jean, M. and Wigle, N. (1995) *Neuroscience*, **67**, 325.
43. Goddard, G. V., McIntyre, D. C. and Leech, C. K. (1969) *Exp. Neurol.*, **25**, 295.

44. Racine, R., Okujava, V. and Chipashvili, S. (1972) *Electroencephal. Clin. Neurophysiol.*, **32**, 295.
45. Chiasson, B. J., Dennison, Z. and Robertson, H. A. (1994) *Mol. Brain Res.*, **29**, 191.
46. Dragunow, M. and Robertson, H. A. (1987) *Nature*, **329**, 441.
47. Chiasson, B. J., Hong, M. G. and Robertson, H. A. (1997) *Neurochem. Int.*, **31**, 459.
48. Johnson, R. S., Spiegelman, B. M. and Papaioannou, V. (1992) *Cell*, **71**, 577.
49. Paylor, R., Johnson, R. S., Papaioannou, V., Spiegelman, B. M. and Wehner, J. M. (1994) *Brain Res.*, **651**, 275.
50. Wang, Z. Q., Ovitt, C., Grigoriadis, A. E., Mohle-Steinlein, U., Ruther, U. and Wagner, E. F. (1992) *Nature*, **360**, 741.
51. Brown, J. R., Ye, H., Bronson, R. T., Dikkes, P. and Greenberg, M. E. (1996) *Cell*, **86**, 297.
52. Hiroi, N., Brown, J. R., Haile, C. N., Ye, H., Greenberg, M. E. and Nestler, E. J. (1997) *Proc. Natl Acad. Sci. USA*, **94**, 10397.
53. Honrado, G. I., Johnson, R. S., Golombek, D. A., Spiegelman, B. M., Papaioannou, V. E. and Ralph, M. R. (1996) *J. Comp. Physiol. Sens. Neural. Behav. Physiol.*, **178**, 563.
54. Wollnik, F., Brysch, W., Uhlmann, E., Gillardon, F., Bravo, R., Zimmermann, M., Schlingensiepen, K. H. and Herdegen, T. (1995) *Eur. J. Neurosci.*, **7**, 388.
55. Watanabe, Y., Johnson, R. S., Butler, L. S., Binder, D. K., Spiegelman, B. M., Papaioannou, V. E. and McNamara, J. O. (1996) *J. Neurosci.*, **16**, 3827.
56. Mandelzys, A., Gruda, M. A., Bravo, R. and Morgan, J. I. (1997) *J. Neurosci.*, **17**, 5407.
57. Hebb, M. O. and Robertson, H. A. (1997) *Soc. Neurosci. Abstr.*, **23**, 467.
58. Hooper, M. L., Chiasson, B. J. and Robertson, H. A. (1994) *Neuroscience*, **63**, 917.
59. Sommer, W., Cui, X., Erdmann, B., Wiklund, L., Bricca, G., Heilig, M. and Fuxe, K. (1998) *Antisense Nucleic Acid Res. Dev.*, **8**, 75.
60. Sommer, W., Pfaff, D. W. and Ogawa, S. (1998) In: McCarthy, M. M. (Ed.), *Modulating Gene Expression by Antisense Oligonucleotides to Understand Neural Functioning,* Kluwer Academic Publishers, Norwell, pp. 9–26.
61. Ogawa, S., Olazabal, U. E., Parhar, I. S. and Pfaff, D. W. (1994) *J. Neurosci.*, **14**, 74.
62. Sakai, R. R., Ma, L. Y., Zhang, D. M., McEwen, B. S. and Fluharty, S. J. (1996) *Neuroendocrinology*, **64**, 425.
63. Schlingensiepen, K. H. and Heilig, M. (1997) In: Schlingensiepen, R., Brysch, W. and Schlingensiepen, K. H. (Eds), *Antisense—from Technology to Therapy*, pp. 186–223. Blackwell Science, Berlin.
64. Tischmeyer, W., Grimm, R., Schicknick, H., Brysch, W. and Schlingensiepen, K. H. (1994) *Neuroreport*, **5**, 1501.
65. Whitesell, L., Geselowitz, D., Chavany, C., Fahmy, B., Walbridge, S., Alger, J. R. and Neckers, L. M. (1993) *Proc. Natl Acad. Sci. USA*, **90**, 4665.
66. Yee, F., Ericson, H., Reis, D. J. and Wahlestedt, C. (1994) *Cell. Mol. Neurobiol.*, **14**, 475.
67. Stein, C. A. and Cheng, Y. C. (1993) *Science*, **261**, 1004.
68. Szklarczyk, A. and Kaczmarek, L. (1997) *Neurochem. Int.*, **31**, 413.

69. McCarthy, M. M., Schlenker, E. H. and Pfaff, D. W. (1993) *Endocrinology*, **133**, 433.
70. Rothstein, J. D., Dykes-Hoberg, M., Pardo, C. A., Bristol, L. A., Jin, L., Kuncl, R. W., Kanai, Y., Hediger, M. A., Wang, Y., Schielke, J. P. and Welty, D. F. (1996) *Neuron*, **16**, 675.
71. Wielbo, D., Sernia, C., Gyurko, R. and Phillips, M. I. (1995) *Hypertension*, **25**, 314.
72. Pardridge, W. M. (1994) *Trends Biotechnol.*, **12**, 239.

5

Behavioral and neuroendocrine effects of antisense targeting in the rat

R. LANDGRAF

1. Introduction

Research focused on interactions between behavioral and neuroendocrine parameters is multidisciplinary. One strategic aim is to observe and quantify behavior in animals and to relate this behavior to specific processes in the brain. In this context, an approach often used is to induce deficits in either the animals' behavior or in an intracerebral neuroendocrine pathway. However, even if the latter is well characterized, it is difficult to define its causal behavioral consequences. This is particularly true when attempting to study substrates of cognitive processes, as learning and memory cannot be measured directly but only inferred from their consequences. These, however, measured as behavioral alterations, are regulated by multiple pathways and a deficit in one of them may be counter-regulated by others or may trigger a plethora of secondary changes and is, therefore, not necessarily directly attributable to an altered behavioral performance.

No matter how complex the mechanisms underlying behavioral regulation may be from a theoretical point of view and, thus, how blurred their interactions necessarily are, the ultimate proof of their utility to the organism requires the demonstration of a robust relationship between the neurobiological process and behavior. A number of techniques are currently available to identify whether specific neuroendocrine changes are causal to, or are merely correlated with, behavioral changes. Among them, antisense targeting provides a much needed alternative to current approaches including receptor antagonist treatment or germline null mutation (knockout) strategies in analysing the role of defined gene products (e.g. neuropeptides, receptors) in specific behaviors. In this context it is important to note that the use of antisense oligodeoxynucleotides (ODNs) in adult animals circumvents the problems of genetic linkage and background genotypes (7), irreversible developmental defects (8) and compensations (13) that *a priori* confound the interpretation of behavioral studies using knockout mice. A particularly important feature for application to behavioral and neuroendocrine studies is that antisense techniques can be applied to rats as well as mice. Furthermore, despite the limitations mentioned above, the use of antisense ODNs may enable the spatial and temporal specificity critical for behavioral studies. Antisense targeting, however, has its own pitfalls and drawbacks that have to be considered to bring its advantages into play. Focusing on behavioral and neuroendocrine effects of antisense targeting in the rat, this chapter will discuss some of these methodological and conceptional issues and will review some successful and unsuccessful efforts, including our own.

2. Methodological considerations

2.1 Controls

Several possible molecular mechanisms have been proposed to explain the consequent down-regulation of protein synthesis (16,18,26,29,48). These include translational arrest through steric blockade, inhibition of RNA processing and RNase cleavage of the DNA–mRNA duplex. In theory, any peptide or protein, if a portion of its transcript sequence is known, can be specifically targeted for down-regulation, even if other very similar sequences are expressed. The complementary base binding of antisense targeting offers a unique degree of specificity that cannot be achieved with conventional pharmacological strategies. Sequence specificity, however, is not easy to achieve and corresponding efforts are often limited by the time, resources and money available. In testing for antisense-specific effects the minimum requirement is to have vehicle and scrambled-sequence ODNs as controls. Although sense instead of scrambled sequence ODNs have frequently been and are still being used as negative controls (11,15,23,46,49,50), their use is not recommended because a sense ODN may form a triplex with DNA or bind to proteins needed for the expression of the target genes. For example, in our studies with the vasopressin receptor antisense ODN (17), the sense ODN used showed a similar, though weaker, effect to that of the antisense ODN. Furthermore, Georgieva *et al.* (6) presented evidence from a recent study that sense and antisense ODNs may even be equipotent.

Furthermore, whenever possible, specificity controls should include both chemical and biological controls. More than just one chemical modification of the antisense ODN may be a useful chemical control. Molecular, cellular or behavioral responses similar to those with the phosphorothioated version would confirm an antisense mechanism of action rather than other (toxic) effects related to the chemical modification. This was the case in two recent papers. In the first, we succeeded in showing that effects of an end-capped phosphorothioate vasopressin V1 receptor antisense ODN on social short-term memory could be confirmed by using an inverted 3′–3′-internucleotide linkage modification (17). Partial modification with sulphur substitution solely at 5′- and 3′-terminal phosphate groups would provide these end-capped molecules with sufficient nuclease resistance while minimizing their toxicity in the brain. In the second paper, Guzowski and McGaugh (9) used end-capped ODNs in addition to fully phosphorothioate-substituted ODNs with both chemical modifications inducing similar effects.

A more biological control would be an antisense ODN directed towards another mRNA which, although related to the mRNA of interest, should not be involved in the regulation of the respective neuroendocrine or behavioral parameter of interest. This approach to confirm the specificity of an antisense ODN in *in vivo* studies is, in other words, to determine the specificity of the behavioral and neuroendocrine effects. Neumann *et al.* (28), for example, measured a significant reduction in the number of milk ejection reflexes as well as in the weight gain of the litter in response to oxytocin, but not vasopressin, antisense ODN treatment. Similarly, Liebsch *et al.* (20) compared corticotropin-releasing hormone (CRH)-1 and CRH-2 antisense ODNs. Whereas the former reduced anxiety-related behavior but not the coping strategy during forced swimming, the latter facilitated active coping without affecting the emotionality of the animals. Furthermore, biological controls could also include the measurement of neuropeptides or receptor proteins related to those of interest but not targeted by the antisense ODN or of the targeted gene product in another brain area. Karle *et al.* (14), for instance, have down-regulated a $GABA_A$ receptor subunit by infusing the respective antisense ODN continuously into the right hippocampus of rats. They used the left hippocampus as internal control and estimated the binding to the acetylcholine receptor which had not been targeted by the antisense treatment. Similarly, Reul *et al.* (34) detected a marked decline in hippocampal mineralocorticoid receptor after antisense treatment; simultaneously measured glucocorticoid receptor levels remained unaffected by this treatment. In another study (17) a significant down-regulation of the vasopressin receptor in the septum was not accompanied by similar changes in closely related brain areas such as the bed nucleus of the stria terminalis and the amygdala, indicating a high degree of site specificity. With regard to the pitfalls and limitations of antisense targeting, however, exclusive reliance on antisense results to reveal the physiological significance of certain gene products may be misleading. Convincing verification would come from the confirmation of antisense results by another, more traditional approach such as antagonist administration. By doing so, we could confirm effects of a vasopressin receptor antisense ODN on anxiety-related behavior (17) by administration of a V1 receptor antagonist (21).

2.2 Homology

One should not ignore the homology with other mRNAs that, although being ‘weak’ or ‘not showing significant matches in the database’ in most cases, cannot necessarily guarantee full specificity. The problem is that ODNs, even those with minimal homology, may also block an additional (i.e. non-targeted) mRNA that is directly or indirectly involved in the neuroendocrine or behavioral effects measured. A higher degree of homology, on the other hand, may be functionally inert as the additionally targeted mRNA does not play a critical role in the functional alterations observed after antisense treatment. Hence, the degree of homology alone is not crucial to distinguish sequence-specific from gene-specific effects. Most studies have been carried out with ODNs between 15 and 20 nucleotides in length. Longer ODNs, although less likely to hybridize to unintended target sequences, would have a poorer penetration into the neurons. In general, the factors that make an ODN biologically active still remain largely theoretical and various parameters that have been examined are unable to predict fully which of the ODNs will function specifically. On the basis of their secondary and tertiary structure and complex inter- and intracellular compartments, only a few binding sites are accessible on a given (and ideally unique) transcript and these have to be identified by screening, i.e. by trial and error. This can be a time-consuming and expensive procedure.

2.3 Specificity

The actions of an antisense ODN are not generally specific or non-specific. Rather, specificity is a feature strictly related to the experimental conditions used, including animal model, brain area, survival time, etc. Therefore it has to be established afresh each time, even if the same ODN has been used repeatedly before. As mentioned above, in a recent study Neumann *et al.* (28) described specific effects of an oxytocin antisense ODN on suckling-related parameters in the rat. Infusion of an oxytocin antisense ODN directly into the supraoptic nucleus of conscious, lactating rats resulted in reduced oxytocin levels in the blood during the suckling stimulus, indicating a specific inhibition of peptide secretion. Similarly, electrical stimulation of the pituitary stalk had to be approximately three times higher in both phosphorothioated and 3′–3′ end-inverted oxytocin antisense ODN-treated rats than in controls in order to raise the intramammary pressure. The blunted secretory and electrophysiological response in oxytocin antisense-treated animals in response to stimulation occurred at a time when intraneuronal neuropeptide stores were not reduced or even depleted. These findings, sufficiently validated by proper chemical and biological controls, suggest short-term effects not primarily related to, for instance, translational arrest and depletion of the gene product. For reasons not yet fully understood, these non-antisense mechanisms of action may be extraordinarily sequence-specific and, therefore, have to be carefully distinguished from non-specific effects.

Using the same neuropeptide antisense ODN, however, no sequence-specific antisense effects could be observed in another series of experiments.The central and peripheral release of both vasopressin and oxytocin was measured by simultaneous microdialysis in the hypothalamus and the blood in rats treated with antisense, scrambled sequence or vehicle. Whereas the rise in blood vasopressin in response to osmotic stimulation could be selectively prevented from occurring only in antisense-treated animals, the intrahypothalamic rise was inhibited equally in both antisense- and scrambled sequence-treated rats. These findings indicate that end-capped phosphorothioated ODNs *per se* non-specifically affected intrahypothalamic, but not peripheral, peptide release, even after the administration of one fifth of the original dose, i.e. 0.4 μg/0.5 μl per hypothalamic supraoptic nucleus. In another attempt to down-regulate intrahypothalamic neuropeptide release patterns, we confirmed Neumann's result by obtaining similar effects in both antisense- and scrambled sequence-treated rats. Furthermore, the same vasopressin antisense ODN that consistently increased water consumption and urine osmolality after intracerebroventricular infusion (43) failed to induce these effects if administered bilaterally into the supraoptic nucleus. We do not know the reasons for these negative findings, but would like to issue a word of caution regarding extrapolating and generalizing antisense or non-antisense effects. As demonstrated in the example mentioned above, even effects in the same neuroendocrine system may be contradictory. Thus, the more parameters measured and the more controls involved, the higher the likelihood of revealing multiple effects after antisense treatment. Unequivocal results, in other words, often just reflect our inability to reveal the plethora of subtle antisense-induced changes at multiple levels of the organism rather than the simplicity and unambiguity of such an effect *per se*.

Some recent studies have reported non-specific effects including sequence-independent effects of ODNs in cultured primary cells (32) and toxic hematological and histopathological effects of phosphorothioated ODNs in mice (38). In the latter study, ODN-treated mice were described as consuming less food and as weak and cachectic. We ourselves have sometimes observed motor irritations after intracerebroventricular administration of ODNs, but only if they were phosphorothioated throughout and given in a high dose (i.e. 50 μg). To elucidate non-specific effects further, we administered various ODNs intracerebroventricularly, including complete phosphorothioated antisense (vasopressin, oxytocin) and sense sequences as well as complete phosphorothioated scrambled sequences and scrambled sequences with 3′–3′-inverted internucleotide linkages (Schöbitz, Engelmann, Landgraf, Montkowski, Reul, Skutella, Wotjak, Holsboer and Spanagel, unpublished observations). Interestingly, regardless of their sequence and chemical modification, the ODNs transiently elevated body temperature, suppressed food and fluid intake, inhibited locomotor activity and induced expression of interleukin-6 after a single infusion into the lateral ventricle of the rat brain, this last effect indicating that the ODNs were endowed with pro-inflammatory properties. Additional purification of the commercially purchased ODNs by ion exchange chromatography did not reduce these side effects, which strongly suggests that either nucleic acids or their metabolites, but not the by-products of the chemical synthesis, caused the autonomic and behavioral effects measured. That behavioral depression as a possible result of sequence-independent effects of ODNs might mask sequence-specific effects has, therefore, to be taken into account. To clarify this issue further and to examine whether the outcome of behavioral tests is really affected by non-specific effects of the ODNs, we conducted the following series of experiments. Again, various completely phosphorothioated ODNs were administered intracerebroventricularly to rats which were then tested in different behavioral paradigms known to be sensitive to sickness. Although signs of sickness and lethargy were detectable in the animals, the social investigation of a conspecific juvenile was not altered, indicating unchanged olfactory-mediated short-term memory. This is an unexpected observation as:

(1) ODN-treated rats showed discrete signs of sickness including ruffling of the fur and a curled posture.

(2) The increase in body temperature was found to be at a maximum during the period of behavioral testing.

(3) As first introduced by Dantzer *et al.* (4), the social investigatory behavior is a well-established test of sickness behavior in rodents.

Similarly, the behavioral performance of the rats in the elevated plus-maze, an index of anxiety-related behavior, remained virtually unaffected by ODN treatment. Neither the time spent in the closed arms and the number of entries in the closed arms, which reflects the level of anxiety, nor the numbers of total arm entries, used as a parameter of general activity, were found to be altered. Furthermore, this test is sensitive to sickness induced by the pro-inflammatory and pyrogenic interleukin-1β as high doses of this cytokine alter the number of closed-arm entries. Thus, although ODNs infused intracerebroventricularly may produce a number of non-specific effects that warrant caution, they do not necessarily influence robust (for instance spontaneously ongoing) or stimulated behaviors.

In the same study, another test was used that is sensitive to sickness, namely food-reinforced behavior. This test, which is widely used to study reinforcement, yielded ambiguous results. Despite a non-specific reduction in the number of food-motivated lever presses in scrambled sequence-treated rats, we were able to demonstrate specific suppression of reinforced behavior by a tyrosine hydroxylase antisense ODN, which was caused by the inhibition of the central catecholaminergic system. This specificity could further be increased by local infusion into the ventral tegmental area, where dopaminergic fibers of the mesolimbic system are known to originate.

Taking all these data into account, it can be stated that ODNs do not necessarily influence the outcome of behavioral paradigms in a non-specific manner if:

(1) proper chemical and biological controls are used, the former including at least scrambled sequence and vehicle;

(2) non-specific effects of ODNs on body temperature and general locomotion are taken into account;

(3) as low a dose as possible is administered, and

(4) ODNs are preferentially locally infused, i.e. directly into the brain area of interest.

2.4 Administration

Periventricular brain structures appear to be readily influenced by the intracerebroventricular antisense approach. However, as deeper structures may not be as susceptible to the antisense treatment, a local infusion directly into

Table 1. Selected examples of neuroendocrine and behavioural effects after acute (single or repeated) antisense administration

Target mRNA (Reference)	Brain Area	Modification Controls	Effects
c-fos (Hebb and Robertson, 1997)	striatum	endcapped phosphorothioate; scrambled sequence	reduced c-fos expression, ipsiversive rotation following D-amphetamine
Oxytocin (Neumann *et al.*, 1994, 1995)	supraoptic nucleus	scrambled sequence; vasopressin antisense, vehicle	less plasma oxytocin, reduced number of milk ejection reflexes and weight gain of the litter, unaltered peptide content in neurohypophysis
cAMP response element binding protein (CREB) (Guzowski and McGaugh, 1997)	dorsal hippocampus	endcapped phosphorothioate; scrambled sequence, vehicle	impaired memory consolidation
Corticotropin-releasing hormone (CRH), vasopressin and oxytocin (Landgraf *et al.*, 1997)	paraventricular nucleus	endcapped phosphorothioate; scrambled sequence, vehicle	reduced plasma ACTH in response to stressor
Angiotensin II-1-receptor (Meng *et al.*, 1994)	icv	phosphorothioate; scrambled sequence	decreased AngII-1 receptor binding, reduced drinking response to Ang II
Mineralocorticoid receptor (Sakai *et al.*, 1996)	amygdala	phosphorothioate; scrambled sequence, vehicle	decreased mineralo- but not glucocorticoid receptors in amygdala

the area of interest is to be preferred. This is supported by numerous findings indicating that antisense ODNs have the potential of reversibly down-regulating or even disrupting the expression of proteins in a fully differentiated brain without disturbing its genetically specified neuronal or synaptic architecture. In any case, the (empirically determined) minimum dose of antisense ODN and the minimum number of injections required for a discernible effect should be used. There are only a few reports comparing single acute, repeated acute and continuous infusions of ODNs. The results of some studies using either acute or continuous infusions are shown in *Tables 1* and *2*. In general, the length of antisense treatment depends on the turnover of the targeted peptide or protein. Along with other workers, we prefer to use continuous administration if proteins with a relatively long turnover time have to be targeted. Antisense effects have been reported, for instance, after 2 days for neuropeptide Y receptors in the cortex (47), after 3–5 days for opioid receptors in the spinal cord (45) and after 4 days for the vasopressin V1 receptor in the septum (17). This, however, merely means that effects were measurable at

Table 2. Selected examples of neuroendocrine and behavioural effects after continuous antisense administration via osmotic minipumps

Target mRNA (Reference)	**Brain Area**	**Modification Controls**	**Effects**
Prodynorphin (Georgieva *et al.*, 1995)	dorsal striatum	phosphorothioate; scrambled sequence, sense	reduced dynorphin levels
Tyrosine hydroxylase (Skutella *et al.*, 1997)	substantia nigra	unmodified; scrambled sequence, vehicle	reduced tyrosine hydroxylase protein content, ipsilateral turning behaviour
Dopamine transporter (Silvia *et al.*, 1997)	substantia nigra	phosphorothioate; scrambled sequence, sense	reduced transporter protein, dopamine overflow
CRH1 receptor (Liebsch *et al.*, 1995)	central nucleus of the amygdala	endcapped phosphorothioated; scrambled sequence, vehicle	Reduced anxiety-related behaviour, unchanged short-term memory
V1 vasopressin receptor (Landgraf *et al.*, 1995)	septum	endcapped phosphorothioated; scrambled sequence, sense, vehicle	Reduced septal V1 receptor, reduced short-term memory and anxiety-related behaviour
Growth hormone receptor (Pellegrini *et al.*, 1996)	icv	not mentioned; prolactin antisense, vehicle	increase in growth hormone peak amplitude and number of peaks
Mineralocorticoid receptor (Reul *et al.*, 1997)	icv	endcapped phosphorothioated; scrambled sequence, vehicle	decline in hippocampal mineralo- but not glucocorticoid receptor density

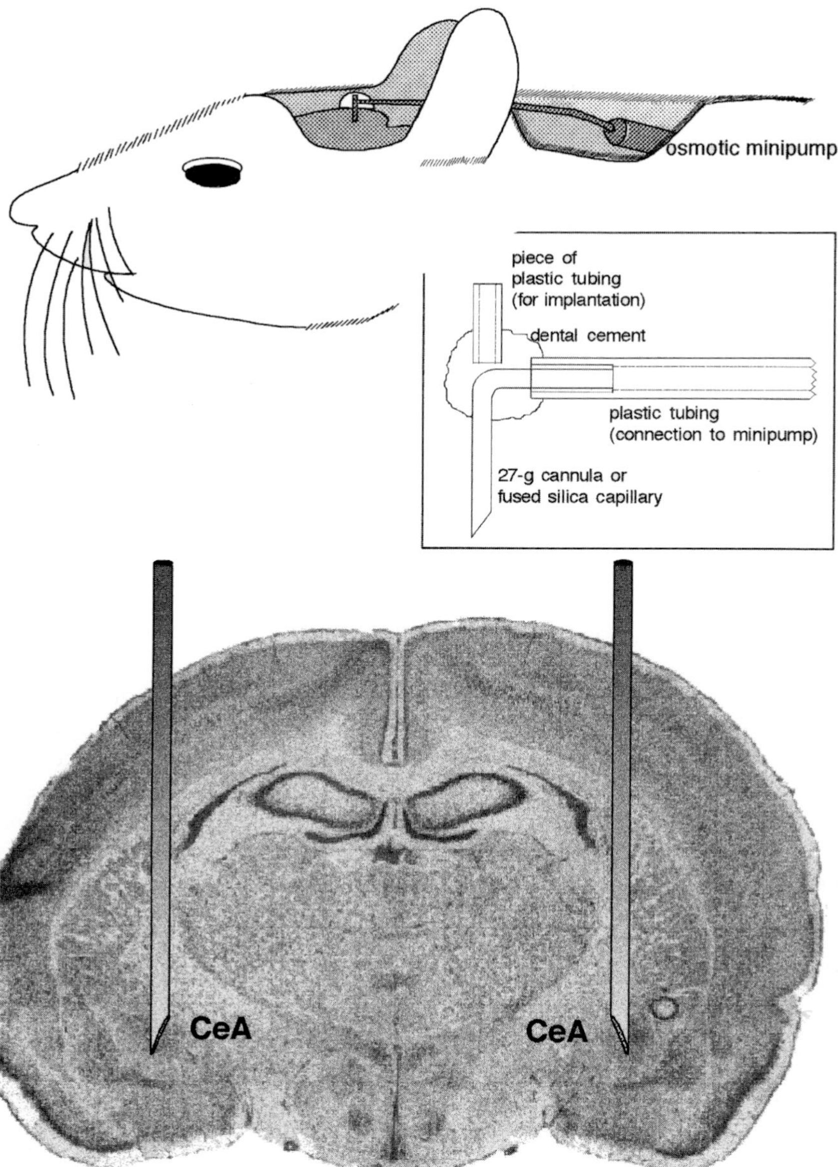

Figure 1. Bilateral oligonucleotide infusion into the central nucleus of the amygdala via osmotic minimpumps. The entire device, i.e. the infusion cannula (fused silica capillary for very small brain loci or 27-g cannula if the solution has to be delivered into a larger brain area) already connected to the plastic tubing and the pump, is implanted. The plastic tubing (and if necessary the pump itself) is filled with either the antisense or a control solution. We usually use a relatively long plastic tubing and insert a very small air bubble near the pump to control for the rate of delivery *post mortem*.

this time point and does not reflect the underlying dynamics. In addition to the targeted gene product, the mode of administration is determined by the behavioral test after antisense treatment. If, for instance, unstressed animals have to be tested, infusion via osmotic minipumps is likely to be better than (often stressful) acute infusions. Using both plasma corticotropin (ACTH) and oxytocin as stress indices, we measured basal peptide levels in rats implanted with osmotic minipumps delivering the solutions into either the amygdala (*Figure 1*) or the septum or intracerebroventricularly and established that this administration procedure *per se* is not stressful to the animals. For acute infusions, animals should be equipped with guide cannulae at least 4 days prior to infusion and must be carefully handled so that they become familiar with the infusion procedure. We usually use 27g guide cannulae and fused silica capillaries with an outer diameter of 140 μm for infusion. Well-handled (and preferentially sleepy) rats even tolerate bilateral infusions of, for example, 0.5 μl without becoming restless or showing other signs of arousal and stress.

3. Antisense effects on behavioral and neuroendocrine regulation

Whenever possible, to reveal ODN effects on neuroendocrine parameters, peptides or receptor proteins should be measured in a physiologically relevant context. A peptide ligand, for example, becomes biologically active only after its release into the extracellular fluid, where the dynamics of its concentration have to be determined. Better than the measurement of neuropeptide content in homogenized brain tissue, therefore, is the detection of the biologically active signal after its release into the extracellular space (be it the systemic circulation or the extracellular fluid of a distinct brain area) and the assessment of the functional consequences. In this way, an antisense-induced deficit in vasopressin secretion may become evident as increased water consumption (43), a deficit in oxytocin secretion as reduced milk ejection (28) and a deficit in CRH, vasopressin and oxytocin as diminished secretion of ACTH from the adenohypophysis (18).

The above-mentioned and other findings leave no doubt that the peptides are causally and critically involved in the respective physiological and endocrine consequences. As already mentioned in the introduction, the involvement of endogenous substances and pathways in the regulation of behavior is generally less unequivocal as there is certainly hardly any intracerebral ligand or receptor that is not directly or indirectly involved in its control. Despite this rather blurred relationship between an antisense-induced deficit and behavioral performance, there are several arguments supporting the measurement of behavioral parameters following antisense treatment. Independent of the targeted transcript, it is of particular interest to measure behavior as the 'endpoint' of all regulative patterns. The more robust the antisense-induced

Table 3. Selected behavioural effects of antisense treatment

Effects on	**Target mRNA Administration Brain area**	**Controls**	**Reference**
Learning and memory	cAMP response element binding protein (CREB), acute into dorsal hippocampus	scrambled sequence, vehicle	Guzowski and McGaugh, 1997
	shaker-like Kv 1.1 potassium channel, repeated icv	fully degenerated oligo, vehicle	Meiri *et al.*, 1997
	insulin-like growth factor (IGF-1), acute into inferior olive	sense, vehicle	Castro-Alamancos and Torres-Aleman, 1994
Emotionality	vasopressin V1 receptor, via osmotic minipumps into septum	scrambled sequence, vehicle	Landgraf *et al.*, 1995
	corticotropin-releasing hormone (CRH), acute icv	sense, vehicle	Skutella *et al.*, 1994a
	CRH1 receptor, via osmotic minipumps into central nucleus of amygdala	scrambled sequence, vehicle	Liebsch *et al.*, 1995
Antinociception	MOR-1 receptor, acute icv	scrambled sequence, vehicle	Rossi *et al.*, 1997
	mu-opioid receptor, repeated icv	scrambled sequence, sense, vehicle	Chen *et al.*, 1995
	cannabinoid receptor, repeated icv	scrambled sequence	Edsall *et al.*, 1996
Feeding and Drinking	neuropeptide Y, repeated injections into arcuate nucleus	sense, vehicle	Akabayashi *et al.*, 1994
	vasopressin, acute icv	scrambled sequence, sense, vehicle	Skutella *et al.*, 1994b
	corticotropin-releasing hormone (CRH), repeated icv	scrambled sequence	Hulsey *et al.*, 1995
Reproductive behaviour	progesterone receptor, acute injection into ventromedial hypothalamus	scrambled sequence	Ogawa *et al.*, 1994
	oxytocin, acute injection into supraoptic nucleus	scrambled sequence, vasopressin antisense, vehicle	Neumann *et al.*, 1994
	glutamic acid decarboxylase, crystalline oligos into medial hypothalamus	scrambled sequence	McCarthy *et al.*, 1994

effect, the more likely are behavioral correlates. Furthermore, many behavioral paradigms can easily be done without additionally treating and stressing the animal. Again, the problems necessarily associated with the blurred relationship between an antisense-induced deficit and behavioral performance can best be handled if the former is as specific as possible, reversible, restricted to a distinct brain area, and sufficiently validated by proper chemical and biological controls.

The use of antisense ODNs designed to hybridize with and thus to neutralize specific sequences of mRNA has helped to elucidate the role of many gene products in behavioral and neuroendocrine regulation by down-regulating or even blocking their production at source. A large number of antisense ODNs targeting behaviorally and neuroendocrinologically important peptides and proteins have already been studied; some specific examples of these and of our own experiments are provided below.

Selected examples of antisense effects on either behavioral or neuroendocrine parameters are given in *Tables 3* and *4*. Even though behavioral and neuroendocrine effects of antisense ODNs are not measured together very often, they are generally closely interrelated. An example of antisense

Table 4. Selected neuroendocrine effects of antisense treatment

Effects	Target mRNA Administration Brain Area	Controls	Reference
Reduced plasma ACTH in response to stressor	corticotropin-releasing hormone (CRH), vasopressin and oxytocin; repeated injections into paraventricular nucleus	scrambled sequence, vehicle	Landgraf *et al.*, 1997
Dose-related reduction of dynorphin A levels in the striatum	prodynorphin, over 3 days via osmotic minipump into dorsal striatum	scrambled sequence, sense, vehicle	Georgieva *et al.*, 1995
Increase in growth hormone peak amplitude and number of peaks, reduction in binding sites	growth hormone receptor, over 7 days via osmotic minipumps icv	prolactin antisense, vehicle	Pellegrini *et al.*, 1996
Changed circadian rhythm of corticosterone secretion	vasoactive intestinal peptide (VIP), acute infusion into supra-chiasmatic nucleus	scrambled sequence	Scarbrough *et al.*, 1996
Decline in hippocampal mineralo- but not glucocorticoid receptor concentrations, higher plasma ACTH in response to stress	mineralocorticoid receptor, over 7 days via osmotic minipumps icv	scrambled sequence, vehicle	Reul *et al.*, 1997

effects on both behavioral and neuroendocrine parameters is given by Guzowski and McGaugh (9). These authors concentrated on the cAMP response element binding (CREB) protein, a constitutively expressed regulatory transcription factor. Recent experimental evidence suggests that CREB and other cAMP response element binding transcription factors are involved in synaptic activity-dependent, long-term neuronal plasticity as well as long-term memory formation in animals. Intrahippocampal infusion of CREB antisense ODNs to inhibit CREB protein turnover in the dorsal hippocampus produced both a specific, local and transient disruption of CREB protein levels and an impaired 48 h retention in a water maze task without affecting acquisition or memory for up to 4 h. These findings suggest that hippocampal CREB influences long-term memory by regulating learning-induced gene expression required for memory consolidation. In this well-designed study, antisense ODNs were compared with scrambled ODNs and vehicle. Furthermore, two different chemical modifications were used, fully phosphorothioated ODNs displaying a specificity and an efficacy similar to those of end-capped ODNs.

Another study of combined behavioral and neuroendocrine antisense effects focused on angiotensin (41). To determine whether angiotensin of brain origin influences neuronal circuits subserving fluid intake, antisense ODNs were intracerebroventricularly administered and the drinking response to a number of well-characterized dipsogenic stimuli was monitored. Compared with multiple controls, an antisense ODN encompassing the translation start site of angiotensin mRNA induced a pronounced inhibitory effect on water drinking triggered by either intracerebroventricular renin or peripheral isoproterenol. The effect of the former is consistent with the notion that the antisense ODN targets angiotensin mRNA and decreases peptide synthesis, thereby reducing the amount of substrate available for renin to act on. However, in contrast to the antisense-induced decrease in water intake, but consistent with the findings of Neumann *et al.* (28) after oxytocin antisense treatment, the authors were not able to detect a concurrent decrease in angiotensin content. Interestingly, peripheral antisense administration failed to inhibit the drinking response, and other antisense ODNs targeting other nucleotide sequences of angiotensin mRNA showed no discernible effect on water intake.

To specifically deplete postsynaptic striatal D_2 dopamine receptors, an antisense ODN was infused bilaterally into the striatum of adult rats (33). The diminished binding of a receptor ligand was accompanied by a suppression of apomorphine-induced stereotypic sniffing. Silvia *et al.* (40) reported that intranigral administration of dopamine transporter antisense via osmotic minipumps produces reductions in transporter mRNA and protein levels as well as an altered rotational activity. Another approach to the nigrastriatal dopamine system has been described by Skutella *et al.* (44). Minipump administration of tyrosine hydroxylase antisense ODN into the substantia nigra resulted in a reduced enzyme protein content and dopamine levels;

furthermore, antisense-treated rats showed ipsilateral turning behavior, these behavioral asymmetries not being observed in control animals.

Our own efforts to induce both behavioral and neuroendocrine antisense effects were successful after minipump infusion of antisense ODNs to vasopressin V1 receptor mRNA into the rat septum (17). The significantly reduced receptor density in the septum, but not in related brain areas, resulted in a diminished ability of the rats to store juvenile-related olfactory information in the social recognition test. Furthermore, antisense-treated rats, unlike the control animals, showed signs of a reduced anxiety-related behavior, an effect that was subsequently confirmed by intraseptal administration of a V1 receptor antagonist (21). In a similar study we focused on the mineralocorticoid receptor (34). Intracerebroventricular administration of an antisense ODN via minipumps resulted in a decrease in hippocampal mineralocorticoid, but not glucocorticoid, receptor concentrations. As in our vasopressin receptor study, mineralocorticoid mRNA levels were found to be increased in antisense-treated animals indicating translational arrest and ongoing transcription. Although no changes in anxiety-related behavior were observed, antisense animals had markedly higher plasma levels of ACTH than rats treated with scrambled sequence or with vehicle, suggesting an enhanced responsiveness of the hypothalamo-pituitary-adrenal axis to stressful situations.

Finally, we tried to down-regulate the CRH-1 and CRH-2 receptor subtypes in the rat. Following the example of others (28,31,37), we used the comparison of two different antisense ODNs as an additional control. Beginning on day 3, various behavioral tests were conducted during intracerebroventricular adminstration via osmotic minipumps. Whereas CRH-1, but not CRH-2, receptor antisense treatment diminished the anxiety-related behavior on the elevated plus-maze (*Figure 2*), the CRH-2, but not CRH-1, receptor

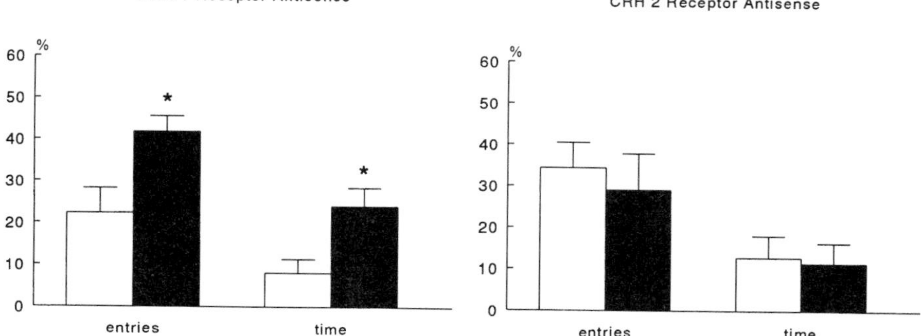

Figure 2. Percent entries the rats made into the open arms and percent time the rats spent in the open arms of the elevated plus-maze. The animals were chronically (intracerebroventricularly via osmotic minipumps) infused with scrambled sequence (white columns, $n = 8$ each) or antisense oligonucleotides targeting either CRH 1 receptor mRNA or CRH 2 receptor mRNA (black columns, $n = 8$ each). $*p < 0.05$. Adapted from Liebsch *et al.* (1998).

antisense ODN reduced the mobility of animals in the forced swim test, indicating a shift towards passive stress coping (20). No antisense effects were observed in the social discrimination test (olfactory short-term memory) or in the open field (locomotor activity). Unfortunately, as already described in a previous paper (19), the density of both receptor subtypes in almost all brain areas was too low to detect a further reduction in response to antisense treatment.

As mentioned in the introduction, the necessarily blurred relationship between a neuroendocrine alteration and behavioral regulation limits corresponding experimental approaches *a priori*. Nevertheless, even from this very brief review, one can justifiably conclude that, if properly used, antisense ODNs targeted to transcripts encoding neuropeptides or receptor proteins in the brain hold great promise for selectively altering their function and, thus, for studying their physiological involvement in behavioral and neuroendocrine regulation.

References

1. Akabayashi, A., Wahlestedt, C., Alexander, J. T. and Leibowitz, S. F. (1994) *Mol. Brain Res.*, **21**, 55.
2. Castro-Alamancos, M. A. and Torres-Aleman, I. (1994) *Proc. Natl Acad. Sci. USA*, **91**, 10203.
3. Chen, X. H., Adams, J. U., Geller, E. B., Deriel, J. K., Adler, M. W. and Liu-Chen, L. Y. (1995) *Eur. J. Pharmacol.*, **275**, 106.
4. Dantzer, R., Bluthé, R. M. and Kelley, K. W. (1991) *Brain Res.*, **557**, 115.
5. Edsall, S. A., Knapp, R. J., Vanderah, T. W., Roeske, W. R., Consroe, P. and Yamamura, H. I. (1996) *Neuroreport*, **7**, 593.
6. Georgieva, J., Heilig, M., Nylander, I., Herrera-Marschitz, M. and Terenius, L. (1995) *Neurosci. Lett.*, **192**, 69.
7. Gerlai, R. (1996) *Trends Neurosci.*, **19**, 177.
8. Grant, S. G. N., O'Dell, T. J., Karl, K. A., Stein, P. L., Soriano, P. and Kandel, E. R. (1992) *Science*, **258**, 1903.
9. Guzowski, J. F. and McGaugh, J. L. (1997) *Proc. Natl Acad. Sci. USA*, **94**, 2693.
10. Hebb, M. O. and Robertson, H. A. (1997) *Brain Res.*, **48**, 97.
11. Hou, W., Shyu, B.-C., Chen, T.-M., Lee, J.-W., Shieh, J.-Y. and Sun, W.-Z. (1997) *Eur. J. Pharmacol.*, **329**, 17.
12. Hulsey, M. G., Morris Pless, C. and Martin, R. J. (1995) *Regul. Peptides*, **59**, 241.
13. Hummler, E., Cole, T. J., Blendy, J. A., Ganss, R., Aguzzi, A., Schmid, W., Beermann, F. and Schutz, G. (1994) *Proc. Natl Acad. Sci. USA*, **91**, 5647.
14. Karle, J., Witt, M. R. and Nielsen, M. (1997) *Brain Res.*, **765**, 21.
15. Lamprecht, R. and Dudai, Y. (1996) *Learning and Memory*, **3**, 31.
16. Landgraf, R. (1996) *J. Endocrinol.*, **151**, 333.
17. Landgraf, R., Gerstberger, R., Montkowski, A., Probst, J. C., Wotjak, C. T., Holsboer, F. and Engelmann, M. (1995) *J. Neurosci.*, **15**, 4250.
18. Landgraf, R., Naruo, T., Vecsernyes, M. and Neumann, I. (1997) *Eur. J. Endocrinol.*, **137**, 326.

19. Liebsch, G., Landgraf, R., Gerstberger, R., Probst, J. C., Wotjak, C. T., Engelmann, M., Holsboer, F. and Montkowski, A. (1995) *Regul. Peptides*, **59**, 229.
20. Liebsch, G., Landgraf, R. and Holsboer, F. (1999) *J. Psych. Res.*, **33**, 153
21. Liebsch, G., Wotjak, C. T., Landgraf, R. and Engelmann, M. (1996) *Neurosci. Lett.*, **217**, 101.
22. McCarthy, M. M., Masters, D. B., Rimvall, K., Schwartz-Giblin, S. and Pfaff, D. W. (1994) *Brain Res.*, **636**, 209.
23. Meeker, R., LeGrand, G., Ramirez, J., Smith, T. and Shih, Y.-H. (1995) *J. Neuroendocrinol.*, **7**, 419.
24. Meiri, N., Ghelardini, C., Tesco, G., Galeotti, N., Dahl, D., Tomsic, D., Cavallaro, S., Quattrone, A., Capaccioli, S., Bartolini, A. and Alkon, D. L. (1997) *Proc. Natl Acad. Sci. USA*, **94**, 4430.
25. Meng, H., Wielbo, D., Gyurko, R. and Phillips, M. I. (1994) *Regul. Peptides*, **54**, 543.
26. Neumann, I. (1997) *Neurochem. Intl*, **31**, 363.
27. Neumann, I., Kremarik, P. and Pittman, Q. J. (1995) *Neuroscience*, **69**, 997.
28. Neumann, I., Porter, D. W. F., Landgraf, R. and Pittman, Q. J. (1994) *Amer. J. Physiol.*, **267**, R852.
29. Nicot, A. and Pfaff, D. W. (1997) *J. Neurosci. Methods*, **71**, 45.
30. Ogawa, S., Olazábal, U. E., Parhar, I. S. and Pfaff, D. W. (1994) *J. Neurosci.*, **14**, 1766.
31. Pellegrini, E., Bluet-Pajot, M. T., Mounier, F., Bennett, P., Kordon, C. and Epelbaum, J. (1996) *J. Neurosci.*, **16**, 8140.
32. Perez, J. R., Li, Y., Stein, C. A., Majumder, S., van Oorschot, A. and Narayanan, R. (1994) *Proc. Natl Acad. Sci. USA*, **91**, 5957.
33. Rajakumar, N., Laurier, L., Niznik, H. B. and Stoessl, A. J. (1997) *Synapse*, **26**, 199.
34. Reul, J. M. H. M., Probst, J. C., Skutella, T., Hirschmann, M., Stec, I. S. M., Montkowski, A., Landgraf, R. and Holsboer, F. (1997) *Neuroendocrinology*, **65**, 189.
35. Rossi, G. C., Leventhal, L., Pan, Y.-X., Cole, J., Su, W., Bodnar, R. J. and Pasternak, G. W. (1997) *J. Pharmacol. Exp. Ther.*, **281**, 109.
36. Sakai, R. R., He, P. F., Yang, X. D., Ma, L. Y., Guo, Y. F., Reilly, J. J., Moga, C. N. and Fluharty, S. J. (1994) *J. Neurochem.*, **62**, 2053.
37. Sakai, R. R., Ma, L. Y., Zhang, D. M., McEwen, B. S. and Fluharty, S. J. (1996) *Neuroendocrinology*, **64**, 425.
38. Sarmiento, U. M., Perez, J. R., Becker, J. M. and Narayanan, R. (1994) *Antisense Res. Dev.*, **4**, 99.
39. Scarbrough, K., Harney, J. P., Rosewell, K. L. and Wise, P. M. (1996) *Amer. J. Physiol.*, **270**, R283.
40. Silvia, C. P., Jaber, M., King, G. R., Ellinwood, E. H. and Caron, M. G. (1997) *Neuroscience*, **76**, 737.
41. Sinnayah, P., McKinley, M. J. and Coghlan, J. P. (1997) *Clin. Exp. Hypertension*, **19**, 993.
42. Skutella, T., Montkowski, A., Stöhr, T., Probst, J. C., Landgraf, R., Holsboer, F. and Jirikowski, G. J. (1994) *Cell. Mol. Neurobiol.*, **14**, 579.
43. Skutella, T., Probst, J. C., Engelmann, M., Wotjak, C. T., Landgraf, R. and Jirikowski, G. F. (1994) *J. Neuroendocrinol.*, **6**, 121.

44. Skutella, T., Schwarting, R. C. W., Huston, J. P., Sillaber, I., Probst, J. C., Holsboer, F. and Spanagel, R. (1997) *Eur. J. Neurosci.*, **9**, 210.
45. Standifer, K. M., Chien, C. C., Wahlestedt, C., Brown, G. P. and Pasternak, G. W. (1994) *Neuron*, **12**, 805.
46. Umekage, T., Namima, M., Fukushima, K., Sugita, S. and Watanabe, Y. (1997) *Neuroreport*, **8**, 407.
47. Wahlestedt, C., Merlo Pich, E., Koob, G. F., Yee, F. and Heilig, M. (1993) *Science*, **259**, 528.
48. Weiss, B., Davidkova, G. and Zhang, S.-P. (1997) *Neurochem. Intl*, **31**, 321.
49. Wu, H. C., Chen, K. Y., Lee, W. Y. and Lee, E. H. Y. (1997) *Neuroscience*, **78**, 147.
50. Zapata, A., Capdevila, J. L., Tarrason, G., Adan, J., Martinez, J. M., Piulats, J. and Trullas, R. (1997) *Brain Res.*, **745**, 114.

6

Electrophysiological and behavioral effects of dopamine receptor knockdown in the brain

SIMRANJIT KAUR, IAN CREESE and JAMES M. TEPPER

1. Introduction

The functions of dopamine, both physiological and pathological, have been extensively studied in the central nervous system (CNS). Dopamine has been found to be involved in the regulation of motor behaviors, in emotion, in learning and memory and also in the pathophysiologies of conditions such as Parkinson's disease (1–3), Huntington's chorea (4), schizophrenia (5,6) and drug abuse and addiction (7,8).

Dopamine is the neurotransmitter in a number of CNS pathways, including the nigrostriatal pathway, which originates in the substantia nigra pars compacta (A9) and innervates the dorsal striatum (9–11), and the mesocorticolimbic pathway, which originates in the ventral tegmental area (VTA; A10) and projects to limbic areas, such as the ventral striatum, nucleus accumbens, the olfactory tubercle and the medial prefrontal, cingulate and entorhinal cortices (12).

Dopamine was previously thought to act at just two receptors, the dopamine D_1 and D_2 receptors. This classification was based on biochemistry, anatomical localization and pharmacological affinities (13). However, recent molecular cloning studies have demonstrated the existence of at least five distinct dopamine receptors, the D_1 (14), D_2 (15), D_3 (16), D_4 (17) and D_5 (18) receptors. These receptors have been subdivided into two families based on amino acid sequences, pharmacological affinities and G-protein associations; the dopamine D1-like receptor family, which comprises the D_1 and D_5 receptors, and the dopamine D2-like receptor family, comprising the D_2, D_3 and D_4 receptors (19,20).

D1-like receptors stimulate adenylyl cyclase via interactions with the G protein, G_s (19,21) while D_2 receptors inhibit adenylyl cyclase via the G protein, G_i (19,22) among actions at other effector mechanisms. The D_3 and D_4 receptors are also known to be coupled to G proteins (23,24).

Due to the lack of selective pharmacological agents acting solely at the individual dopamine receptors, antisense technology is an ideal method with which to investigate the functions of these receptors. Administering antisense oligodeoxynucleotides (ODNs) into a given brain region would result in a specific knockdown of receptors to which the antisense is targeted in that region only, without causing changes in other receptors or an up-regulation in receptor number, a problematic consequence of pharmacological interventions (25).

In this chapter we will discuss electrophysiological data, especially with regard to D_2 and D_3 autoreceptors, and behavioral data obtained in dopamine receptor antisense knockdown studies as well as present new data on the spread of the antisense ODNs and effects on tyrosine hydroxylase after D_2 antisense treatment.

2. Antisense technology applied to dopamine receptor research

Antisense ODNs are sequences of single-stranded DNA that are taken up into the cell by receptor-mediated endocytosis or non-selective pinocytosis, and are designed to hybridize by Watson–Crick base pairing to complementary sequences within the targeted mRNA. This then prevents translation of the mRNA to the functional protein. The precise mechanism by which this occurs is unclear, but the antisense ODNs may act by interfering with ribosome binding and processing of mRNA, interfering with mRNA conformation or mRNA splicing and ribonuclease H (RNase H) activation of mRNA digestion.

The majority of the research done with antisense technology has been *in vitro*, but recent studies have investigated the effects of antisense treatment *in vivo*, including applications in the CNS. Antisense administration *in vivo* has been used to inhibit the expression of neurotransmitter receptors, including several subtypes of dopamine receptors (26–30), NMDA (31,32), neuropeptide Y (33) and vasopressin receptors (34); proteins such as SNAP-25 (35) and neuropeptide Y (36); enzymes such as tyrosine hydroxylase (37) and immediate–early gene products such as c-Fos (38,39).

The premise behind the use of antisense technology is that it is a relatively simple and highly specific method with which to investigate the functions of individual proteins. The functions, physiological or pathological, of the individual dopamine receptors have not been ascertained conclusively due to the absence of selective agonists or antagonists that can discriminate among the different receptor subtypes within the D_1-like or D_2-like receptor families under physiological conditions. The pharmacological agents in use currently can discriminate only between the dopamine receptor families but not the receptor subtypes within those families. For example, sulpiride, which is used as a 'selective' D_2 receptor antagonist, does not discriminate between D_2 and

D_3 receptors, while SCH 23390, used as a 'selective' D_1 receptor antagonist, does not differentiate between D_1 and D_5 receptors.

However, the advent of antisense technology has provided a useful method with which to study dopamine receptors. Antisense administration has produced successful specific and functional knockdowns of dopamine receptor subtypes. One of the major advantages of using antisense knockdown over transgenic knockout animals is that in transgenic animals, developmental changes may occur to compensate for the reduction in receptor number and these changes may have a far-reaching effect on steps downstream of the receptor activation and possibly also on associated neurotransmitter systems while antisense ODNs can be applied directly into the mature CNS. Also, the reduction in receptor number induced by antisense administration can be both local and reversible, allowing the animals to serve as their own controls.

The length of sequence, dose, route and duration of administration of the ODNs as well as the choice of control must all be taken into consideration to ensure optimal effectiveness. The ODNs are usually 15–30 base pairs in length. ODNs of this length should only hybridize to the sequence they are directed at. Shorter sequences, <14 base pairs long, tend to lack specificity while long sequences, >50 bases, may bind to short alternative sequences to which they are partially complementary. The melting temperature of the ODNs should be high, so that they are stable at body temperature. The likelihood of the formation of secondary structures, such as a hairpin within the molecule itself, should be low. Such formations would reduce the ability of the ODN molecule to hybridize with the target sequence. Appropriate controls must also be chosen to ensure that the knockdown observed is specific. The controls commonly used include mismatched ODNs, random ODNs or the 'sense' ODNs. The amino acid sequences of the controls should be checked in GenBank to ensure that these sequences do not inadvertently act as antisense to other known sequences. Until the complete genome is sequenced, though, hydridization may still occur to unknown sequences.

The antisense ODNs used in our laboratory are the 'S'-modified phosphorothioate ODNs which have enhanced nuclease-resistance. They are 19 base pairs in length. We use random ODNs as our controls. These are not truly random: they contain the same nucleotides as the antisense, but in a randomized order. As the antisense ODNs are inefficient in crossing the blood–brain barrier, acute administration or chronic injections or infusions into the brain structures of interest or into the lateral cerebral ventricles results in sufficient uptake into neurons. In this laboratory we chronically infuse the ODNs, either via micro-osmotic ALZET pumps or motorized syringe pumps, over a period of a few days. In studies using irreversible antagonists, the half-life of dopamine D_2 receptors was found to range from 8 to 160 h depending on the conditions of the study, which is ideal for our purposes (40–42).

Although there are many benefits of using antisense technology, there are also some disadvantages. Due to the presence of spare receptors, it is difficult to correlate the amount of receptor knockdown with functional consequences. However, studies using irreversible dopamine antagonists suggest that 70–90% of dopamine receptors need to be occupied to produce a behavioral effect (43–46). Also, Qin *et al.* (47) reported that a small reduction in dopamine D_2 receptor number after D_2 antisense administration in the mouse striatum did produce behavioral alterations.

As antisense ODNs cross the blood–brain barrier poorly and have potential toxic effects, it is unlikely that antisense technology as it stands currently will be used clinically for CNS disorders (48). At present, direct administration of the antisense into the CNS is required. In studies carried out in our laboratory, chronic infusions of D_2 antisense into the substantia nigra produced marked reductions in D_2 receptor number without any accompanying toxicity (26).

2.1 Spread of D_2 receptor antisense oligodeoxynucleotides in the brain

Tepper *et al.* (26) showed that there was no retrograde transport into the striatum of the D_2 antisense after administration into the substantia nigra and only the number of receptors in the substantia nigra was reduced with no change seen in D_2 receptor number in the striatum. Thus, local infusion of antisense ODNs can be used to selectively target pre-synaptic or post-synaptic receptors depending on the site of administration. Such restricted receptor manipulation cannot currently be achieved with pharmacological agents or in transgenic knockout animals.

Tepper *et al.* (26) also noticed that the receptor knockdown produced by the D_2 antisense was heterogeneous in the substantia nigra. The areas close to the site of administration exhibited a larger reduction in D_2 receptor number than did sites further away. This heterogeneity was not noticed by Zhang and Creese (29), who reported that the decrease in D_2 receptor number produced by intracerebroventricularly administered D_2 antisense was homogeneous throughout the striatum.

The intracranial spread of the antisense ODNs is relatively restricted in a functional sense, since dopaminergic neurons recorded contralateral to a unilateral substantia nigra administration of D_2 or D_3 receptor antisense for 3 days display normal electrophysiological and pharmacological properties (26). The effective extent of the antisense knockdown in the brain can be estimated by examining the spread of fluorescently labeled ODNs, which also appears to be relatively restricted, as illustrated in *Figure 1*. When infused through a 32g cannula at 100 nl/h for 24 h, 10 μg/μl fluorescently labeled D_2 antisense ODN diffuses in a roughly spherical pattern out to a diameter of 600–1000 μm as illustrated for two representative infusions in *Figure 1*. Even several hundred micrometers from the center of the injection, cell bodies can be seen to contain relatively high and homogeneous levels of fluorescent signal (*Figure 1C*). However, a few hundred micrometers away from this

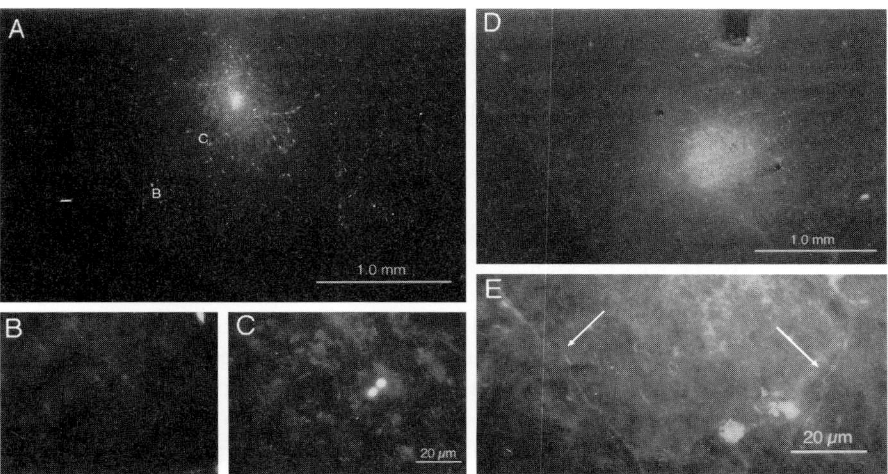

Figure 1. (A) Low-magnification photomicrograph of a 60 μm coronal section through the ventral midbrain of a rat illustrating the spread of a rhodamine-labeled D_2 dopamine receptor antisense ODN after local infusion (10 μg/μl at 100 nl/h for 24 h). The volume over which the ODN spreads exhibits a relatively sharp border. (B) The neuropil only 500 μm ventrolateral to the periphery of the injection site (area indicated by B in panel A) is completely devoid of any labeling. (C) Neurons at the periphery of the injection site (area indicated by C in panel A) are lightly but unmistakably labeled with the fluorescent ODN (arrows). (D) Low-magnification photomicrograph of a 60 μm coronal section through the ventral midbrain of a rat illustrating the spread of an FITC-labeled D_2 dopamine receptor antisense ODN after local infusion (10 μg/μl at 100 nl/h for 24 h). The bulk of the ODN is constrained to a sphere $<$1.0 mm in diameter. (E) High magnification photomicrograph of an area on the periphery of the injection sites showing two dendrites (arrows) labeled with the fluorescent ODN indicating that the ODN fills not only cell somata but also dendrites. This suggests that antisense ODNs may be able to inhibit dendritic as well as somatic protein synthesis.

point, no labeling at all is visible (*Figure 1B*), suggesting that the intracellular concentration of the ODN falls off fairly rapidly with distance. High magnification images reveal fluorescent signal in the dendrites as well as the cell bodies (*Figure 1E*), suggesting that even if some dopamine receptors are translated in the dendrites, as other proteins have been shown to be (49), antisense administration could block their synthesis as well.

3. Electrophysiological consequences of antisense knockdown

3.1 Antisense knockdown of presynaptic D_2 receptors

The effects of antisense knockdown of nigral dopamine D_2 autoreceptors were investigated using electrophysiological techniques. This laboratory reported that infusing D_2 antisense ODNs unilaterally into the substantia nigra for 3–6 days resulted in a functional knockdown of D_2 autoreceptors in the ipsilateral substantia nigra without affecting post-synaptic striatal D_2 dopamine receptors or nigral D_1 or D_3 receptors (26,50). D_2 antisense markedly attenuated the inhibitory effect of apomorphine on dopaminergic neurons *in vivo*. The inhibition of nigrostriatal neurons seen after the administration of low-dose apomorphine has been attributed to action at the somatodendritic autoreceptors (51,52).

However, there was no change in the rate or pattern of the spontaneous activity of the antisense-treated neurons when compared with the controls. The somatodendritic and terminal excitability, as assessed electrophysiologically, was found to be greater in the antisense-treated neurones than in the controls. These data show that D_2 receptors are present on somatodendritic and axon terminal regions of nigrostriatal neurons but suggest that endogenous dopamine acting at somatodendritic autoreceptors has little or no effect on the rate or pattern of spontaneous neuronal activity in anesthetized rats.

Some of the findings obtained by Tepper *et al.* (26) are consistent with the data obtained by Silvia *et al.* (53). Silvia *et al.* (53) found that administering D_2 antisense unilaterally into the substantia nigra induced contralateral rotations in response to cocaine. The ability of sulpiride, a D_2 receptor antagonist, to increase electrically-stimulated dopamine release was attenuated in striatal slices from the antisense-treated side which was consistent with a decrease in the number of striatal D_2 autoreceptors. The administration of D_2 antisense in this study produced a 40% reduction in the number of nigral D_2 receptors on the treated side compared with the untreated side, similar to the reduction reported by Tepper *et al.* (26). However, Silvia *et al.* (53) reported there were no spontaneous rotations in the antisense-treated whereas Tepper *et al.* (26) observed very modest contralateral rotations which were attributed to a reduction in terminal autoinhibition of dopamine release. As these rotations were not very pronounced (<1 rotation/min), it is possible that Silvia *et al.* (53) did not notice them.

3.2 Antisense knockdown of D_3 autoreceptors

There is considerable evidence showing that D_2 autoreceptors are located in the substantia nigra (54–59) but some studies have suggested on pharmacological grounds that a proportion of the autoreceptors may actually be D_3 receptors. Dopamine has been shown to bind to D_3 receptors with 20-fold higher affinity than D_2 receptors and high-affinity agonist binding is a characteristic of autoreceptors (16). Also, it has been reported that the ability of agonists to inhibit dopaminergic neurons correlates with their affinities for the D_3 receptor (60–65). Nissbrandt *et al.* (64) reported that D_3 antisense administration increased dopamine synthesis in the substantia nigra and the nucleus accumbens, also suggesting that a subpopulation of D_3 receptors act as autoreceptors and have a tonic inhibitory action on dopamine synthesis.

When D_3 receptor antisense was infused into the substantia nigra, it produced similar effects to D_2 antisense, i.e. an attenuation of the inhibitory effect of apomorphine on nigral dopaminergic neurons as well as an increase in somatodendritic and terminal excitability (26). Interestingly, an additive effect was seen after the simultaneous administration of both D_2 and D_3 antisense. These data suggest that D_3 receptors are also expressed on the somatodendritic as well as axon terminal regions of the nigral dopaminergic neurons and are important in the modulation of the excitability of dendritic regions and the modulation of terminal excitability and inhibition of dopamine release respectively.

However, a recent study in D_3 transgenic knockout mice reported contrasting results. In the D_3 transgenic mice, while there were increases in dopamine release, there was no apparent effect on the function of dopamine autoreceptors measured electrophysiologically. There was also no difference in the basal firing rates of midbrain dopaminergic neurons between the transgenic knockout animals and the wild-type mice, as reported by Tepper *et al.* (26) after D_3 (or D_2) antisense knockdown. However, the putative selective D_3 receptor agonist, PD 128907 inhibited the activity of nigral and VTA dopaminergic neurons and the release of dopamine as shown by *in vivo* microdialysis, to the same extent in both the wild-type and transgenic animals. The authors suggest that this is due to PD 128907 acting at D_2 and not D_3 receptors (66). Koeltzow *et al.* (66) concluded that, even though D_3 receptors play a role in dopamine release, they are not involved in dopamine autoreceptor function but instead they may be involved in the post-synaptically activated short-loop feedback modulation of dopamine release.

One reason for the discrepancies within these two studies may be the different models used. The study carried out by Tepper *et al.* (26) was done in the substantia nigra of anesthesized rats in which receptor knockdown was achieved by antisense treatment, while Koeltzow *et al.* (66) used D_3 receptor-deficient mice. Due to developmental changes which may occur in the D_3 knockout transgenic mice in order to compensate for the loss of receptors, it may not be possible to directly compare data from these two models.

Koeltzow *et al.* (66) assert that, due to the low density of D_3 receptors in the substantia nigra, these receptors do not play a role in regulating dopaminergic neuronal activity. The authors cite studies showing that high densities of D_3 receptors are only found in limbic areas such as the nucleus accumbens shell, olfactory tubercle, the ventral pallidum, the amygdala and islands of Calleja (16,67,68). A number of studies, however, have detected moderate amounts of D_3 receptor mRNA in the rat substantia nigra (16,67,69,70). Bancroft *et al.* (71) also observed moderate levels of [^{3}H]PD 128907 and [^{3}H](+)-7-OHDPAT binding, representing D_3 receptor sites, in the substantia nigra.

Studies using 6-hydroxydopamine-induced lesions have also shown that D_3 receptors are present on the dopaminergic neurons themselves and that these receptors may play the role of autoreceptors (16). It is, however, possible that due to the relative abundance of D_2 receptor mRNA in the substantia nigra (72), it may be difficult to detect D_3 mRNA signal.

There have also been a number of pharmacological studies, using agonists and antagonists with affinities at the dopamine D_3 receptors, suggesting that these receptors do function as autoreceptors and regulate dopaminergic cell firing. Lejeune and Millan (62) reported that the firing rate of VTA neurons was dose-dependently inhibited by 7-OHDPAT, a D_3 receptor-preferring agonist, and that (+) S 14297, a D_3 receptor antagonist, attenuated the inhibitory effect of 7-OHDPAT. The authors concluded that inhibitory dendritic D_3 autoreceptors regulate the activity of VTA dopaminergic neurons. Pramipexole, a D_3 receptor agonist, was found by Piercey *et al.* (73) to depress dopamine neuron firing when administered in gradually accumulating doses, while Kreiss *et al.* (61) reported that when the potencies for *in vivo* inhibition of substantia nigra pars compacta dopaminergic single cell firing were determined for a number of D_2 and D_3-preferring agonists, significant correlation was found between the potencies of these compounds and the *in vitro* binding affinities at D_3 receptors.

Koeltzow *et al.* (66) indicate in their study that PD 128907 acts not at the D_3 receptor but at D_2 receptors due to the similar responses seen after the administration of PD 128907 in wild-type and D_3 knockout transgenic mice. A number of studies report that PD 128907 acts selectively at the dopamine D_3 receptor (74–77) with K_i values of 1.43 nM and 413 nM for the high- and low-affinity D_3 receptors respectively (75). However, a few studies have reported that PD 128907, as suggested by Koeltzow *et al.* (66), may actually be acting at dopamine D_2 receptors. A drug-discrimination study investigating the apomorphine-like discriminative stimulus effects of PD 128907 showed that they were antagonized more potently by the D_2 receptor antagonist, haloperidol, than by the putative D_3 antagonists (78). Bowery *et al.* (79) found that PD 128907 inhibited cell firing in the VTA as well as in the substantia nigra pars compacta and that these effects were antagonized by L-741,626, a selective D_2 receptor antagonist. These studies indicate that PD 128907 acts at dopamine D_2 and not D_3 receptors. Thus, it is conceivable that the conclusions arrived at using PD 128907 may pertain to dopamine D_2 and not D_3 receptors. Thus, as mentioned previously, it is difficult to draw definite conclusions from pharmacological studies, due to the non-specificity of most currently available pharmacological agents and this is where antisense technology comes in useful. Antisense administration only produces reductions of the receptors at which it is targeted, resulting in specific knockdowns, thereby avoiding effects produced by actions at other receptors.

4. Behavioral consequences of antisense knockdown of dopamine receptors

4.1 Antisense knockdown of dopamine D_1 receptors

Pharmacological studies have shown that D_1-like receptors are involved in grooming behaviors and need to be co-stimulated with D_2-like receptors to induce stereotypy. Zhang *et al.* (30) administered D_1 antisense intracerebroventricularly and observed diminished grooming behavior induced by the D_1-like receptor agonist, SKF 38393, but the stereotyped activity induced by the D_2-like agonist, quinpirole, was unaffected. The reduction in grooming behavior was directly related to the length of time for which the D_1 antisense was administered. The D_1 antisense treatment also reduced the number of rotations occurring after SKF 38393 treatment in mice lesioned striatally with 6-hydroxydopamine (6-OHDA) but the rotations seen after treatment with quinpirole or oxotremorine, a muscarinic agonist, were unaffected. When the antisense treatment was stopped, the rotations returned to their normal levels.

The data obtained in these studies correspond to data obtained previously in pharmacological studies (80,81). The administration of D_1-like agonists induces grooming behavior while the administration of D_1-like antagonists has the opposite effect (82,83). Waddington *et al.* (83) also showed that in D_1 receptor knockout transgenic mice, spontaneous grooming behavior was attenuated.

4.2 Antisense knockdown of dopamine D_2 receptors

A study done in this laboratory infused D_2 antisense into the lateral cerebral ventricle for 3 days and saw reductions of approximately 50% and 70% in the number of striatal and nucleus accumbens D_2 receptors respectively (29). These reductions in D_2 receptor number translated into an attenuated locomotor response to quinpirole but the grooming behavior induced by the D_1-like agonist, SKF 38393, was unchanged. D_2 antisense treatment also induced catalepsy as well as reduced spontaneous locomotion. A more recent study done in this laboratory (84) corroborated the previous findings and also showed that D_2 antisense did not affect the locomotor response to low-dose amphetamine or the stereotyped response to high-dose amphetamine. These findings indicate that the locomotor response to amphetamine was less sensitive to D_2 antisense treatment than spontaneous locomotor activity. Earlier pharmacological studies and more recent studies done with D_1 receptor-deficient transgenic animals have also shown differential effects within spontaneous locomotion and drug-induced locomotion (85–89).

Studies done by other groups have also shown specific knockdown of dopamine D_2 receptors with D_2 antisense and behavioral consequences arising from these knockouts. Weiss *et al.* (28) and Zhou *et al.* (90) reported specific knockdown of dopamine D_2 receptors after the administration of D_2 antisense to mice with unilateral 6-OHDA lesions of the corpus striatum and also observed an inhibition in rotational behavior induced by quinpirole but not that induced by SKF 38393 or by the muscarinic receptor agonist, oxotremorine. Qin *et al.* (47) found that although there was only a small reduction in the number of dopamine D_2 receptors in the mouse striatum produced by the administration of intracerebroventricular D_2 antisense, the restoration of the behavioral alterations induced by the irreversible D_2-like antagonist, fluphenazine-*N*-mustard (FNM), such as catalepsy and an attenuation of quinpirole-induced stereotyped activity, was delayed. The authors concluded that the administration of D_2 antisense decreased the rate of recovery of D_2 receptors and inhibited the recovery of D_2 receptor-mediated behaviors after irreversible receptor inactivation.

These studies corroborate findings of previous pharmacological studies using antagonists acting primarily at the D_2 receptor (81,91) as well as data obtained in D_2 receptor knockout transgenic mice (92). Baik *et al.* (92) reported that the absence of the D_2 receptor caused the animals to be akinetic and bradykinetic and these mice showed significantly reduced spontaneous movements.

4.3 Antisense knockdown of dopamine D_3 receptors

D_3 antisense infused intracerebroventricularly produced a specific knockdown of striatal D_3 receptors and also induced behavioral alterations such as increased spontaneous locomotion and but did not induce catalepsy (84). D_3 receptor knockdown also attenuated the stereotyped activity induced by amphetamine but had no effect on amphetamine-induced locomotion, which indicates that D_3 receptors are involved in stereotyped behavior. Another study which corroborates this observation showed that unilateral intrastriatal administration of D_3 antisense did not induce ipsilateral rotations after apomorphine or quinpirole administration (50). Nissbrandt *et al.* (64) found that intracerebroventricularly administered D_3 antisense reduced D_3 receptor binding and increased dopamine synthesis in the nucleus accumbens, where D_3 receptors are relatively abundant, suggesting an autoreceptor role for the D_3 receptor on mesoaccumbens dopaminergic neurons. However, there was no effect, either on binding or on dopamine synthesis, in the striatum, where D_3 receptors are sparse. However, this study also found that D_3 antisense did not counteract the effect of apomorphine on dopamine synthesis in the nucleus accumbens. Thus, this study suggests that D_3 receptors are not involved in nigrostriatally driven motor behaviors but are more involved in the behaviors that arise from the stimulation of mesolimbic dopaminergic pathways. The authors suggest that the lack of effect of D_3 antisense on the effect of apomorphine on dopamine turnover in the nucleus accumbens may result from apomorphine also acting at receptors other than the D_3 receptors.

Increased locomotion has also been reported in D_3 receptor knockout transgenic mice (93,94) as well as in pharmacological studies looking at the behavioral effects of antagonists with high affinities for D_3 receptors (76,95,96).

5. The effects of D_2 receptor knockdown on tyrosine hydroxylase expression in substantia nigra

In an earlier study of the electrophysiological effects of antisense knockdown of D_2 receptors in substantia nigra (26), a few sections from D_2 antisense-treated brains were stained for tyrosine hydroxylase (TH) immunocytochemistry to visualize the dopaminergic neurons in order to see if the antisense caused any obvious damage to the neurons. Not only was there no sign of toxicity, but the TH staining appeared darker on the treated side, although no quantification was attempted. This suggested the possibility that, in addition to the well-known regulation of TH activity by dopamine D2-like autoreceptors (59), the actual expression of TH might be regulated by D_2 autoreceptors.

To test this hypothesis, four rats were unilaterally infused supranigrally for 3 days with D_2 antisense and two were infused with D_2 random antisense as previously described (26). At the end of the infusion period, rats were killed and perfused transcardially with saline followed by 4% paraformaldehyde. The brains were removed and 60 μm sections through the midbrain were cut on a Vibratome. The sections were reacted for immunocytochemical visualization of TH using 3,3′-diaminobenzidine as a chromogen as described elsewhere (97). The effects of the ODN infusions on the density of the TH immunostaining were quantified by obtaining images of the stained sections on a Nikon Optiphot microscope using a 1× objective. The images were obtained with a Cohu video camera and digitized by a Data Translation Quick Capture frame grabber. NIH Image 1.6 was used to demarcate equivalent areas of pars compacta on the two sides of the brain for each section (41 sections from D_2 antisense-treated and 57 sections from D_2 random antisense-treated rats) and calculate the optical density of each.

Representative sections from D_2 antisense-treated and D_2 random antisense-treated rats are shown in *Figure 2*. The data were expressed as the ratio of the optical density of the treated side divided by that of the control side. D_2 antisense treatment yielded a ratio of 1.323 ± 0.038 whereas D_2 random antisense treatment yielded a ratio of 1.014 ± 0.003. These were significantly different ($F = 91.7$, df $= 96$, $P < 0.0001$); thus, D_2 antisense treatment increased the density of TH staining by approximately 32%. When examined at high magnification, the increased density of staining did not appear to be due to more cells and/or processes being stained. Rather, the staining intensity of individual cells and their dendrites and axons appeared darker on the treated side, as shown for cells from the D_2-antisense-treated and control sides from one representative rat in *Figure 3*.

The most parsimonious explanation for these data is that, in addition to regulating the synthesis of dopamine by altering the activity of TH (59), D_2 receptor stimulation or blockade is capable of regulating the expression of the

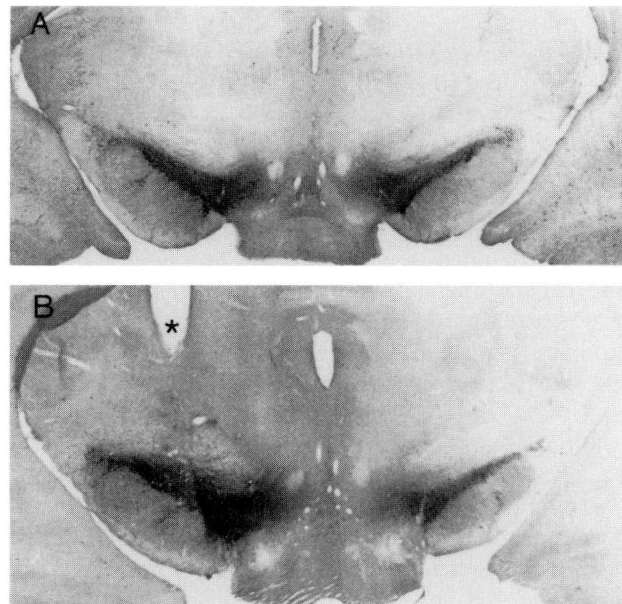

Figure 2. Photomicrographs of two representative sections through substantia nigra stained for tyrosine hydroxylase (TH) immunocytochemistry. (A) The intensity of nigral TH staining in the brain treated for 3 days with D_2 random antisense is equal on both signs of the brain. (B) In contrast, the TH staining in the brain treated for 3 days with D_2 antisense appears much darker on the ipsilateral (left) side.

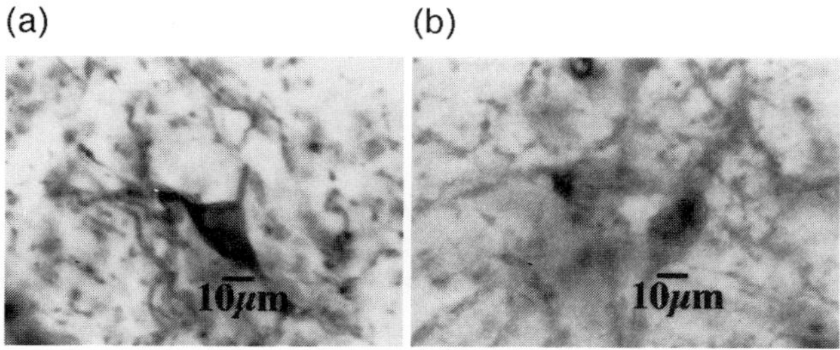

Figure 3. High-magnification photomicrographs of TH-positive neurons ipsilateral (A) and contralateral (B) to a 3 day D_2 antisense infusion. Note how much darker the neuron on the left is compared with either of the neurons on the right.

enzyme itself. This is consistent with the increase in TH mRNA in substantia nigra dopaminergic neurons that was seen after D_2 receptors were irreversibly blocked by FNM (98). The fact that knockdown of D_2 receptors increased TH immunostaining suggests that D_2 autoreceptors are normally stimulated *in vivo* by endogenous dopamine to a sufficient degree to inhibit the expression of TH.

6. Conclusions

Antisense technology has provided a novel and highly specific tool with which to study the functions of the individual dopamine receptors. The knockdowns achieved by local administrations of the antisense ODNs are specific to the receptor at which the antisense is directed, with no effect being seen in adjacent brain regions or in other receptor populations. The antisense ODNs do not diffuse over a large area but remain in a discrete area around the site of administration, thus allowing for discrete receptor populations to be targeted.

In this chapter, we have focused on the electrophysiological consequences of nigral D_2 and D_3 receptor knockdown and provided evidence that both D_2 and D_3 receptors function as autoreceptors in the substantia nigra and are expressed both on somatodendritic nerve terminals as well as on the axon terminal regions. Behaviorally, the antisense studies done to date have corroborated data obtained from pharmacological studies. It also appears that D_2 antisense administration enhances the expression of TH in the substantia nigra, suggesting that dopamine acts at D_2 autoreceptors to inhibit the expression of TH.

Acknowledgements

The fluorescently labeled ODNs were provided by Dr Nicholas Dean, ISIS Pharmaceuticals, CA. We thank Davine Armstrong for quantifying the tyrosine hydroxylase data. This research was supported by the National Institute of Mental Health grants MH 52383 and MH 52450.

References

1. Hornykiewicz, O. (1966) *Pharmacol. Res.*, **18**, 925.
2. Marsden, C. D. (1992) *Sem. Neurosci.*, **4**, 171.
3. Nahmias, C., Garnett, E. S., Firnau, G. and Lang, A. (1985) *J. Neurol. Sci.*, **69**, 223.
4. Klawans, H. L. (1987) *Canadian J. Neurol. Sci.*, **14** (3, *Suppl.*), 536.
5. Carlsson, A. (1988) *Neuropsychopharmacology*, **1**, 179.
6. Davis, K. L., Kahn, R. S., Ko, G. and Davidson, M. (1991) *Amer. J. Psychiatry*, **148**, 1474.
7. Koob, G. F. (1992) *Sem. Neurosci.*, **4**, 139.
8. Koob, G. F. and Bloom, F. E. (1988) *Science*, **242**, 715.
9. Dahlstrom, A. and Fuxe, K. (1964) *Acta Physiol. Scand.*, **232** (*Suppl.*), 1.
10. Ferger, B., Kropf, W. and Kuschinsky, K. (1994) *Psychopharmacology*, **114**, 297.
11. Graybiel, A. M. and Ragadale, C. W. (1983) In: Emson, P. C. (Ed.), *Chemical Neuroanatomy*, pp. 427–504. Raven Press, New York.
12. Bjorklund, A. and Lindvall, O. (1964) In: Bjorklund, A. and Hokfelt, T. (Eds), *Classical Transmitters in the CNS. Handbook of Chemical Neuroanatomy*, pp. 55–122. Elsevier, Amsterdam.

13. Kebabian, J. W. and Calne, D. B. (1979) *Nature*, **277**, 93.
14. Sunahara, R. K., Niznik, H. B., Weiner, D. M., Stormann, T. M., Brann, M. R., Kennedy, J. L., Gelernter, J. E., Rozmahel, R., Yang, Y., Israel, I., Seeman, P. and O'Dowd, B. F. (1990) *Nature*, **347**, 80.
15. Bunzow, J. R., Van Tol, H. H. M., Grandy, D. K., Albert, P., Salon, J., Chisre, M., Machida, C. A., Neve, K. A. and Civelli, O. (1988) *Nature*, **336**, 783.
16. Sokoloff, P., Giros, B., Martres, M.-P., Bouthenet, M.-L. and Schwartz, J..-C. (1990) *Nature*, **347**, 146.
17. Van Tol, H. H. M., Bunzow, J. R., Guan, H.-C., Sunahara, R. K., Seeman, P., Niznik, H. B. and Civelli, O. (1991) *Nature*, **350**, 614.
18. Sunahara, R. K., Guan, H.-C., O'Dowd, B. F., Seeman, P., Laurier, L. G., George, S. R., Torchia, J., Van Tol, H. H. M. and Niznik, H. B. (1991) *Nature*, **350**, 614.
19. Civelli, O. (1995) In: Bloom, F. E. and Kupfer, D. J. (Eds), *Psychopharmacology: The Fourth Generation of Progress*, pp. 155–161. Raven Press, New York.
20. Civelli, O., Bunzow, J. R. and Grandy, D. K. (1993) *Annu. Rev. Pharmacol. Toxicol.*, **32**, 281.
21. Kebabian, J. W. and Greengard, P. (1971) *Science*, **174**, 1346.
22. Onali, P., Olianas, M. C. and Gessa, G. L. (1985) *Mol. Pharmacol.*, **28**, 138.
23. Burris, K. D., Pacheco, M. A., Filtz, T. M., Kung, M.-P., Kung, H. F. and Molinoff, P. B. (1995) *Neuropsychopharmacology*, **12**, 335.
24. Liu, L. X., Monsma, F. J, Jr, Sibley, D. R. and Chiodo, L. A. (1996) *Synapse*, **24**, 156.
25. Weiss, B., Zhang, S.-P. and Zhou, L.-W. (1997) *Life Sci.*, **60**, 433.
26. Tepper, J. M., Sun, B.-C., Martin, L. P. and Creese, I. (1997) *J. Neurosci.*, **17**, 2519.
27. Weiss, B., Zhou, L.-W. and Zhang, S.-P. (1996) In: Raffa, R. B. and Poreca, F. (Eds), *Antisense Strategies for the Study of Receptor Mechanisms*, pp. 71–91. R. G. Landes, Austin, TX.
28. Weiss, B., Zhou, L.-W., Zhang, S.-P and Qin, Z.-H (1993) *Neuroscience*, **55**, 607.
29. Zhang, M. and Creese, I. (1993) *Neurosci. Lett.*, **161**, 223.
30. Zhang, S.-P., Zhou, L.-W. and Weiss, B. (1994) *J. Pharmacol. Exp. Ther.*, **271**, 1462.
31. Standaert, D. G., Testa, C. M., Rudolf, G. D. and Holingsworth, Z. R. (1996) *J. Pharmacol. Exp. Ther.*, **276**, 342.
32. Wahlestedt, C., Golanov, E., Yamamoto, S., Pich, E. M., Koob, G. F., Yee, F. and Heilig, M. (1993) *Nature*, **363**, 260.
33. Wahlestedt, C., Pich, E. M., Koob, G. F., Yee, F. and Heilig, M. (1993) *Science*, **259**, 528.
34. Landgraf, R., Gerstberger, R., Montkowski, A., Probst, J. C., Wotjak, C. T., Holsboer, F. and Engelman, M. (1995) *J. Neurosci.*, **15**, 4250.
35. Catsicas, M., Osen-Sand, A., Staple, J. K., Jones, K. A., Ayala, G., Knowles, J., Grenningloh, G., Pich, E. M. and Catsicas, S. (1996) In: Agrawal, S. (Ed.), *Methods in Molecular Medicine: Antisense Therapeutics,* pp. 57–85. Humana Press, Totowa, NJ.
36. Akabayashi, A., Wahlestedt, C., Alexander, J. T. and Liebowitz, S. F. (1994) *Mol. Brain Res.*, **21**, 55.
37. Skutella, T., Probst, J. C., Jirikowski, G. F., Holsboer, F. and Spanagel, R. (1994) *Neurosci. Lett.*, **167**, 55.
38. Chiasson, B. J., , Hooper, M. L. Murphy, P. R. and Robertson, H. A. (1992) *Eur. J. Pharmacol.*, **227**, 451.

39. Heilig, M., Engel, J. A. and Soderpalm, B. (1993) *Eur. J. Pharmacol.*, **236**, 339.
40. Hall, M. D., Jenner, P. and Marsden, C. D. (1983) *Biochem. Pharmacol.*, **32**, 2973.
41. Leff, S. E., Gariano, R. and Creese, I. (1984) *Proc. Natl Acad. Sci. USA*, **81**, 3910.
42. Norman, A. B., Battaglia, G. and Creese, I. (1987) *J. Neurosci.*, **7**, 1484.
43. Hamblin, M. and Creese, I. (1983) *Life Sci.*, **32**, 2247.
44. Meller, E., Bordi, F. and Bohmaker, K. (1989) *Life Sci.*, **44**, 1019.
45. Saller, C. F., Kreamer, L. D., Adamovage, L. A. and Salama, A. I. (1989) *Life Sci.*, **45**, 917.
46. Seeman, P., Lee, T., Chan-Wong, M., and Wong, K. (1976) *Nature*, **261**, 717.
47. Qin, Z.-H., Zhou, L.-W., Zhang, S.-P, Wang, Y. and Weiss, B. (1995) *Mol. Pharmacol.*, **48**, 730.
48. Gura, T. (1995). *Science*, **270**, 575.
49. Torre E. R. and Steward, O. (1996) *J. Neurosci.*, **16**, 5967.
50. Sun, B.-C., Zhang, M., Ouagazzal, A.-M., Martin, L. P., Tepper, J. M. and Creese, I. (1996) In: Merchant, K. (Ed.), *Pharmacological Regulation of Gene Expression in the CNS*, pp. 51–78. CRC Press, Boca Raton, Florida.
51. Akaoka, H., Charlety, P., Saunier, C.-F., Buda, M. and Chouvet, G. (1992) *Neuroscience*, **49**, 879.
52. Pucak, M. L. and Grace, A. A. (1994) *J. Pharmacol. Exp. Ther.*, **271**, 1181.
53. Silvia, C. P., King, G. R., Lee, T. H., Xue, Z.-Y., Caron, M. G. and Ellinwood, E. H. (1994) *Mol. Pharmacol,*, **46**, 51.
54. Boyar, W. C. and Altar, C. A. (1987) *J. Neurochem.*, **48**, 824.
55. Lacey, M. G., Mercuri, N. B. and North, R. A. (1987) *J. Physiol.*, **392**, 397.
56. Meador-Woodruff, J. H., Mansour, A., Healy, D. J., Kuehn, R., Zhou, Q.-Y., Bunzow, J. R., Akil, H., Civelli, O. and Watson, S. J. (1992) *Neuropsychopharmacology*, **5**, 231.
57. Morelli, M., Mennini, T. and Di Chiara, G. (1988) *Neuroscience*, **27**, 865.
58. Starke, K., Gothert, M. and Kilbinger, H. (1989) *Physiol. Rev.*, **69**, 864.
59. Wolf, M. E. and Roth, R. H. (1990) *Ann. N. Y. Acad. Sci.*, **604**, 323.
60. Chesi, A. J. R., Feasey-Truger, K. J., Alzheimer, C. and ten Bruggencate, G. (1995) *Eur. J. Neurosci.*, **7**, 2450.
61. Kreiss, D. S., Bergstrom, D. A., Gonzalez, A. M., Huang, K. X., Sibley, D. R. and Walters, J. R. (1995) *Eur. J. Pharmacol.*, **277**, 209.
62. Lejeune, F. and Millan, M. J. (1995) *Eur. J. Pharmacol.*, **275**, R7.
63. Meller, E., Bohmaker, K., Goldstein, M. and Basham, D. A. (1993) *Eur. J. Pharmacol.*, **249**, R5.
64. Nissbrandt, H., Ekman, A., Eriksson, E. and Heilig, M. (1995) *Neuroreport*, **6**, 573.
65. Tang, L., Todd, R. D. and O'Malley, K. L. (1994) *J. Pharmacol. Exp. Ther.*, **270**, 475.
66. Koeltzow, T. E., Xu, M., Cooper, D. C., Hu, X.-T., Tonegawa, S., Wolf, M. E. and White, F. J. (1998) *J. Neurosci.*, **18**, 2231.
67. Diaz, J., Levesque, D., Lammers, C. H., Griffon, N., Martres, M.-P., Schwartz, J.-C. and Sokoloff, P. (1995) *Neuroscience*, **65**, 731.
68. Murray, A. M., Ryoo, H. L., Gurevich, E. and Joyce, J. N. (1994) *Proc. Natl Acad. Sci. USA*, **91**, 11271.
69. Bouthenet, M.-L., Souil, E., Martres, M.-P., Sokoloff, P., Giros, B. and Schwartz, J.-C. (1991) *Brain Res.*, **564**, 203.

70. Mengod, G., Villaro, M. T., Landwehrmeyer, G. B., Martinez-Mir, M. I., Niznik, H. B., Sunahara, R. K., Seeman, P., O'Dowd, B. F., Probst, A. and Palacios, J. M. (1992) *Neurochem. Intl*, **20** (*Suppl.*), 33S.
71. Bancroft, G. N., Morgan, K. A., Flietstra, R. J. and Levant, B. (1998) *Neuropsychopharmacology*, **18**, 305.
72. Griffon, N., Diaz, J., Levesque, D., Sautel, F., Schwartz, J.-C., Sokoloff, P., Simon, P., Constentin, J., Garrido, F., Mann, A. and Wermuth, C. (1995) *Clin. Neuropharmacol.*, **18**, *Suppl. 1*, S130.
73. Piercey, M. F., Hoffman, W. E., Smith, M. W. and Hyslop, D. K. (1996) *Eur. J. Pharmacol.*, **312**, 35.
74. DeWald, H. A., Heffner, T. G., Jaen, J. C., Lustgarten, D. M., Meltzer, L. T., Pugsley, T. A. and Wise, L. D. (1990) *J. Med. Chem.*, **33**, 445.
75. Pugsley, T. A., Davis, M. D., Akunne, H. C., MacKenzie, R. G., Shih, Y. H., Damsma, G., Wikstrom, H., Whetzel, S. Z., Georgic, L. M., Cooke, L. W., Demattos, S. B., Corbin, A. E., Glase, S. A., Wise, L. D., Djikstra, D. and Heffner, T. G. (1995) *J. Pharmacol. Exp. Ther.*, **275**, 1355.
76. Sautel, F., Griffon, N., Sokoloff, S., Schwartz, J. H., Launay, C., Simon, P., Constentin, J., Schoenfelder, A., Garrido, F., Mann, A. and Wermuth, C. G. (1995) *J. Pharmacol. Exp. Ther.*, **275**, 1239.
77. Whetzel, S. Z., Shih, Y. H., Georgic, L. M., Akunne, H. C. and Pugsley, T. A. (1997) *J. Neurochem.*, **69**, 2363.
78. Klewen, M. S. and Koek, W. (1997) *Eur. J. Pharmacol.*, **321**, 1.
79. Bowery, B. J., Razzaque, Z., Emms, F., Patel, S., Freedman, S., Bristow, L., Kulagowski, J. and Seabrook, G. R. (1996) *Brit. J. Pharmacol.*, **119**, 1491.
80. Blanchet, P. J., Grondin, R., Bedard, P. J., Shiosaki, K. and Britton, D. R. (1996) *Eur. J. Pharmacol.*, **309**, 13.
81. Loschmann, P. A., Smith, L. A., Lange, K. W., Jahnig, P., Jenner, P. and Marsden, C. D. (1992) *Psychopharmacology*, **109**, 49.
82. Deveney, A. M. and Waddington, J. L. (1995) *Brit. J. Pharmacol.*, **116**, 2120.
83. Waddington, J. L., Deveney, A. M., Clifford, J., Tighe, O., Croke, D. T., Sibley, D. R. and Drago, J. (1998) *Adv. Pharmacol.*, **42**, 514.
84. Zhang, M., Ouagazzal, A.-M. and Creese, I. Unpublished observations.
85. Boss, R., Cools, A. R. and Ogren, S. (1988) *Psychopharmacology*, **95**, 447.
86. Hillegaart, V. and Ahlenius, S. (1987) *Pharmacol. Toxicol.*, **60**, 350.
87. Mogenson, G. J. and Yang, C. R. (1991) *Adv. Exp. Med. Biol.*, **295**, 265.
88. Xu, M., Moratalla, R., Gold, L. H., Hiroi, N., Koob, G. F., Moratalla, R., Graybiel, A. M. and Tonegawa, S. (1994) *Cell*, **79**, 729.
89. Xu, M., Hu, X.-T., Cooper, D. C., Moratalla, R., Graybiel, A. M., White, F. J. and Tonegawa, S. (1994) *Cell*, **79**, 945.
90. Zhou, L.-W., Zhang, S.-P., Qin, Z.-H. and Weiss, B. (1994) *J. Pharmacol. Exp. Ther.*, **268**, 1015.
91. Ouagazzal, A., Nieoullon, A. and Amalric, M. (1993) *Psychopharmacology*, **111**, 427.
92. Baik, J. H., Picetti, R., Saiardi, A., Thiriet, G., Dierich, A. Depaulis, A., Le Meur, M. and Borrelli, E. (1995) *Nature*, **377**, 424.
93. Accili, D., Fishburn, C. S., Drago, J., Steiner, H., Lachowicz, J. E., Park, B. H., Gauda, E. B., Lee, E. J., Cool, M. H., Sibley, D. R., Gerfen, C. R., Westphal, H. and Fuchs, S. (1996) *Proc. Natl Acad. Sci. USA*, **93**, 1945.

94. Xu, M., Koeltzow, T. E., Santiago, G. T., Moratalla, R., Cooper, D. C., Hu, X.-T., White, N. M., Graybiel, A. M., White, F. J. and Tonegawa, S. (1997) *Neuron*, **19**, 837.
95. Kling-Petersen, T., Ljung, E. and Svensson, K. (1995) *J. Neural Transm.*, **102**, 209.
96. Waters, N., Svensson, K., Haadsma-Svensson, S. R., Smith, M. W. and Carlsson, A. (1993) *J. Neural Transm.*, **94**, 11.
97. Tepper, J. M, Damlama, M. and Trent, F. (1994) *Neuroscience*, **60**, 469.
98. Weiss-Wunder, L. T. and Chesselet, M. F. (1992) *Neuroscience*, **49**, 297.

7

Antisense mapping: exploring the functional significance of alternative splicing

GAVRIL W. PASTERNAK

1. Introduction

Antisense approaches have become widely used to explore the functional significance of various proteins, particularly within the central nervous system (CNS). Many of the advantages of antisense paradigms have been well established, as described throughout this volume. Unlike knockout strategies, they are not restricted to mice and can be employed with any number of species. Within the CNS, specific brain regions can be targeted by microinjection techniques. Equally important, the ability to use adult animals eliminates potential compensatory developmental changes which have been encountered in knockout animals. On the practical side, antisense studies are inexpensive and can be conducted quickly and easily.

Antisense mapping extends the utility of traditional antisense methodologies and provides a novel approach capable of defining the functional significance of alternative splicing (1). It is based upon our observation that short antisense probes (~20 bases) targeting sequences anywhere along an mRNA can down-regulate the message equally well (2); however, care must be taken in their design. This ability to direct antisense probes against individual exons permits the functional examination of splice variants derived from a single gene, which was not previously possible. This ability to target all along the length of an mRNA molecule has also enabled investigators to assess the functional relevance of partial cDNA fragments before obtaining a full clone. This chapter will review the use of antisense mapping in examining opioid function within the nervous system.

2. Antisense mapping of DOR-1, a delta opioid receptor

Soon after the delta opioid receptor, DOR-1, was cloned (3,4), we examined the relevance of this receptor in delta analgesia using antisense approaches.

To validate the model, we explored the ability of antisense probes to down-regulate delta receptor binding in NG108 cells, which express the receptor naturally. As anticipated, we found that antisense oligodeoxynucleotides (ODNs) effectively lowered delta receptor binding while a mismatch control was inactive (*Figure 1a*). Many investigators believed that antisense probes would only work near the initiation site. However, we found that antisense ODNs could be effective regardless of where along the mRNA they were targeted (2). Five different antisense ODNs targeting all three exons of DOR-1 mRNA lowered delta opioid binding equally well, even when directed against a sequence in the 3′-non-coding region (*Figure 1a*). We obtained similar results *in vivo* (2,5). [D-Pen^2,D-Pen^5]enkephalin (DPDPE) is an effective analgesic when given spinally in mice. Binding studies and its sensitivity to various opioid antagonists have confirmed its selectivity towards delta opioid receptors (6,7). Antisense probes targeting each of the three DOR-1 exons reduce spinal DPDPE analgesia (*Figure 1b*), confirming that this response is mediated through DOR-1.

The utility of antisense mapping also depends upon the ability of the antisense probes to down-regulate only mature mRNA. We have also examined a number of intron sequences in a number of cDNAs. None of them has been effective. This observation contrasts greatly with our experience using probes targeting exon sequences in which almost all probes are active in at least one functional model. This would suggest that the antisense ODNs may be acting on mature mRNA, enabling the selective down-regulation of individual splice variants of a single gene.

3. Antisense mapping of MOR-1, a mu opioid receptor

We employed a similar approach towards MOR-1, which encodes a mu opioid receptor. Our initial studies were limited to the rat since this was the species from which MOR-1 was initially cloned (8,9). Microinjecting an antisense ODN targeting exon 1 directly into the periaqueductal gray effectively down-regulated morphine analgesia (10). After cloning the murine homolog of MOR-1, we then confirmed the importance of MOR-1 in morphine analgesia in mice (11). Three different antisense probes targeting exon 1 blocked morphine analgesia, a result similar to that seen in rats. However, three additional antisense probes based upon exon 2 were all inactive. We then examined the effects of these antisense treatments on the actions of a very potent morphine metabolite, morphine-6β-glucuronide (M6G) (7). Evidence from other pharmacological paradigms implied that M6G acted through a different receptor from morphine (12). Antisense studies supported this distinction between the two opioids. In contrast to morphine, none of the three exon 1 antisense probes significantly lowered M6G analgesia. More surprisingly, the three antisense ODNs targeting exon 2, which were inactive against mor-

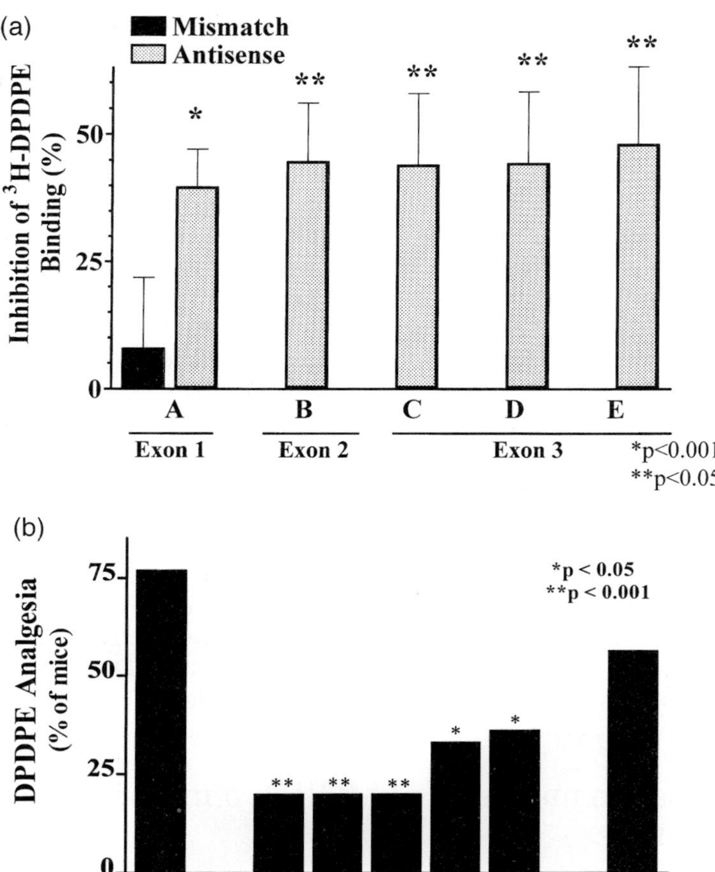

Figure 1. Antisense mapping of DOR-1. (a) NG108 cells, which normally express delta receptors, were treated with antisense oligodeoxynucleotides targeting the indicated exon. Cells were harvested and [^{3}H]DPDPE binding determined. All antisense probes reduced binding to a similar extent and the mismatch control was inactive. Adapted from reference 2. (b) Groups of mice received the indicated antisense (5 μg) on days 1, 3 and 5 and DPDPE analgesia was assessed on day 6. Analgesia was defined quantally as a doubling or greater increase in tailflick latency from baseline values. Adapted from reference 2.

phine, effectively lowered M6G analgesia (*Figure 2*). Returning to the rat, we saw the same distinction between morphine and M6G (13). Again, antisense ODNs based upon exon 1 effectively blocked morphine but not M6G analgesia, while additional antisense probes based upon exon 2 lowered only M6G analgesia. Similarly, exon 3 and 4 probes differentially blocked either

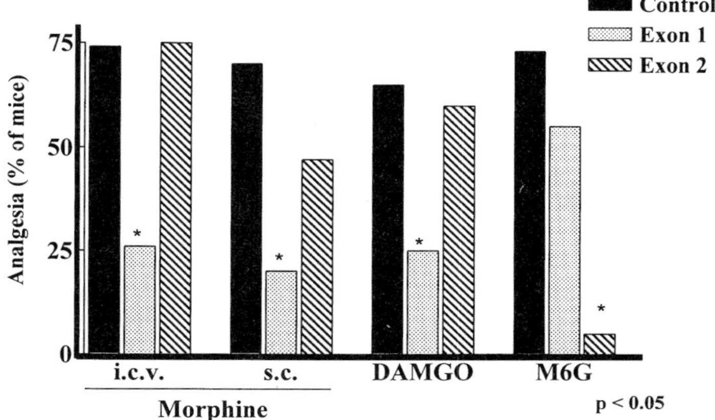

Figure 2. Antisense mapping of MOR-1. Groups of mice received the indicated antisense (5 μg) on days 1, 3 and 5 and morphine or M6G analgesia assessed on day 6 as described in the legend to *Figure 1*. Adapted from reference 11.

morphine or M6G. Similar results have been obtained in a number of other opioid actions (14).

The only factor that influenced the selectivity of the antisense for either morphine or M6G analgesia was the exon being targeted. In the mouse at least three different antisense probes from exon 1 were active against only morphine while another three antisense ODNs based upon exon 2 blocked only M6G. These results strongly implicated MOR-1 in the actions of both morphine and M6G. The importance of MOR-1 in their actions has now been confirmed in animals in which the MOR-1 gene has been disrupted (15–19). However, the differential activity of the probes against only one of the two drugs implied that morphine and M6G acted through different receptors. One explanation for these divergent results is that the two receptors will turn out to be splice variants of MOR-1. Evidence has been emerging suggesting extensive alternative splicing of MOR-1. Soon after the initial report, two variants were reported (20,21). More recently, we uncovered three new splice variants derived from combinations of four new exons within the MOR-1 gene, which is now known to extend for at least 200 kb (22). Although these variants are probably not the morphine and M6G receptors predicted from the antisense mapping studies, it will be interesting to see if additional MOR-1 splice variants corresponding to these receptors will be cloned.

4. Antisense mapping of neuronal nitric oxide synthase

Nitric oxide (NO) is one of the most important transmitters in the CNS and is generated as needed from arginine by the enzyme nitric oxide synthase

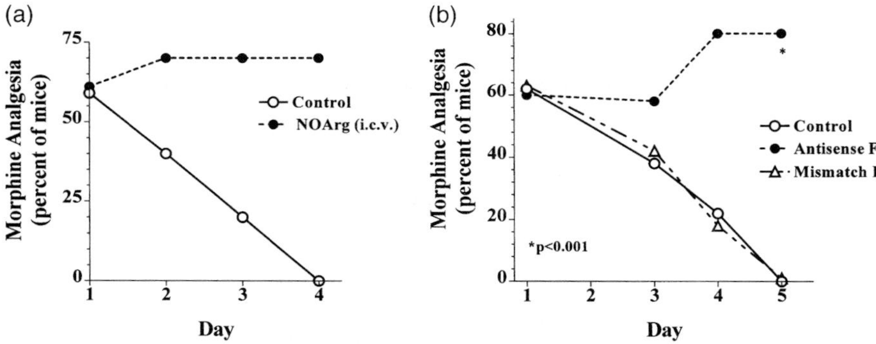

Figure 3. Blockade of morphine tolerance by nitroarginine and an nNOS antisense. (a) Groups of mice received daily morphine injections (5 mg/kg, subcutaneously (s.c.)) alone or in conjuction with nitroarginine (intracerebroventricularly (i.c.v.)). (b) Groups of mice received daily morphine injections (5 mg/kg, s.c.) alone or in conjunction with either antisense F or its mismatch control. Adapted from reference 25.

(23,24). Within the brain, NO has been implicated in many actions, including the production of opioid tolerance (25–27). Tolerance is manifested as a diminished response to a fixed dose of drug or the need to increase the dose to maintain an effect. Pharmacologically, it is possible to dissociate morphine analgesia from tolerance. Although NMDA receptor antagonists had no effect upon morphine analgesia, they blocked morphine tolerance without interfering with analgesia (28,29). NMDA receptors have been associated with NO in many systems. Work from our laboratory demonstrated a similar association with morphine tolerance, with the nitric oxide synthase (NOS) inhibitor nitroarginine blocking morphine tolerance (26,27). To determine which NOS isoform was responsible for this action, we employed an antisense approach (25).

First, we simply wanted to determine whether neuronal NOS (nNOS), the predominant isoform in the brain, mediated the actions of NO on tolerance. An antisense probe targeting the mRNA encoding nNOS prevented morphine tolerance as effectively as the enzyme inhibitor while its mismatch control was ineffective (*Figure 3*). In contrast, an antisense ODN based upon the inducible isoform of NOS (iNOS), which is encoded by a different gene, was inactive. Thus, we were able to establish the importance of nNOS in producing morphine tolerance.

nNOS has a number of splice variants. In addition to the major isoform of nNOS, nNOS-1, another one (nNOS-2) is present at far lower abundance; in the latter isoform, exons 9 and 10 are spliced out (*Figure 4*) (30,31). We explored the potential role of these two splice variants by antisense mapping. To down-regulate both nNOS-1 and nNOS-2, we designed antisense probes based upon exons common to both isoforms. By targeting exons in nNOS-1 which were not present in nNOS-2, we hoped to selectively lower nNOS-1

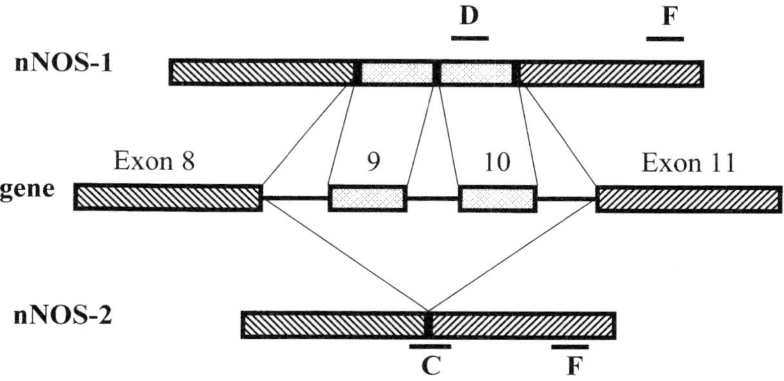

Figure 4. Schematic of nNOS-1 and nNOS-2. Adapted from reference 25.

mRNA. The biggest challenge was selectively down-regulating nNOS-2 since all the sequences in this mRNA are also present in nNOS-1. The only unique aspect of this mRNA is the splice site between exons 8 and 11. Therefore, we designed an antisense ODN spanning this splice site. The probe had 26 bases, with 14 bases targeting exon 8 and 12 bases targeting exon 11. Theoretically, the entire probe could bind to the nNOS-2 mRNA and down-regulate it. However, binding of the probe to the nNOS-1 mRNA would be limited to at most 14 bases in exon 8 or 12 bases in exon 11, sequences we predicted would be too short for antisense activity. Thus, we anticipated that this probe would selectively lower nNOS-2.

We tested this approach by first determining the effects of antisense treatment on mRNA levels using RT-PCR (*Figure 5*). As expected, antisense F, which targeted both isoforms, lowered the levels of both while antisense D selectively lowered only nNOS-1 mRNA levels (*Figure 5*). Antisense C selectively lowered only nNOS-2 mRNA levels, confirming our predictions. Thus, antisense approaches can selectively lower each of the splice variants.

The functional roles of these two splice variants were markedly different. First, we examined the effects of the antisense ODN on the analgesic activity of single morphine doses. Given intrathecally, the nNOS-1 selective probe, antisense D, had no effect upon morphine analgesia acutely (*Figure 6*). In contrast, antisense C, which targeted nNOS-2, markedly lowered morphine's analgesic response. Thus, nNOS-2 facilitates morphine analgesia since its down-regulation impaired morphine's response. A different picture emerged when we examined morphine tolerance. Here, intrathecal antisense D clearly prevented the development of morphine tolerance (*Figure 7*). We observed a similar result supraspinally with a series of antisense probes targeting nNOS-1 (25). Antisense C could not be examined in the tolerance model because of its direct actions on morphine analgesia.

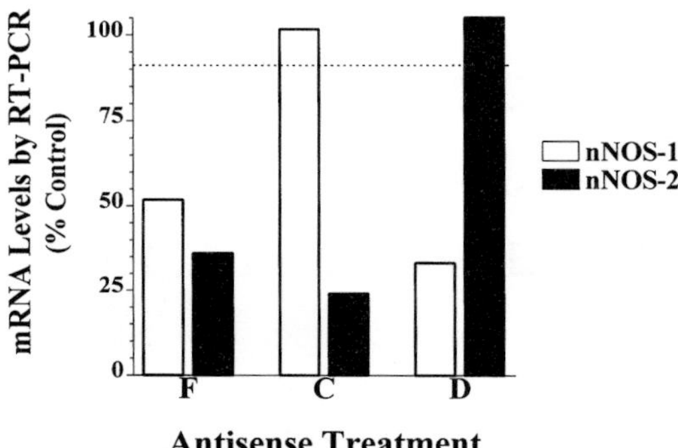

Figure 5. Down-regulation of nNOS mRNA by nNOS-1 and nNOS-2 antisense probes. Mice were treated with antisense probes C, D or F, as shown above. Antisense F is common to both isoforms, antisense D is selective for nNOS-1 and antisense C is selective for nNOS-2. Levels of mRNA for the two isoforms were determined using RT-PCR. Adapted from reference 25.

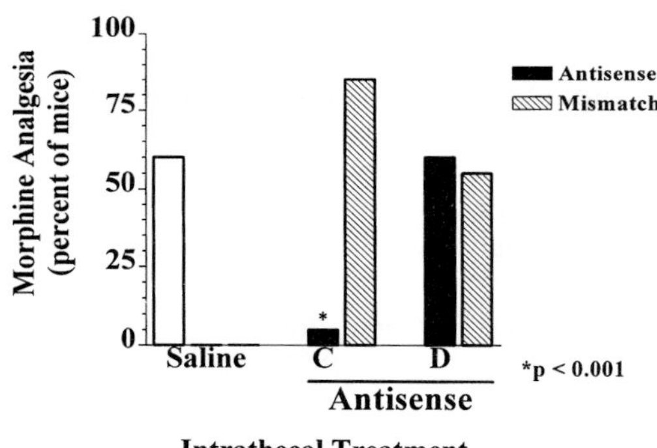

Figure 6. Effects of nNOS antisense on acute morphine analgesia. Groups of mice were treated with either saline or the indicated antisense intrathecally over 5 days and morphine analgesia (5 mg/kg, s.c.) determined on day 6. Adapted from reference 25.

These results clearly indicate that these two nNOS isoforms play opposing roles in opioid function. nNOS-2 facilitates the analgesic action of morphine while nNOS-1 acts to diminish morphine's actions. These insights into the actions of NO and opioid function would not have been possible without antisense mapping. None of the various enzyme inhibitors can differentiate between these two isoforms. Even knockout approaches are probably too coarse for the subtle molecular differences between the two proteins.

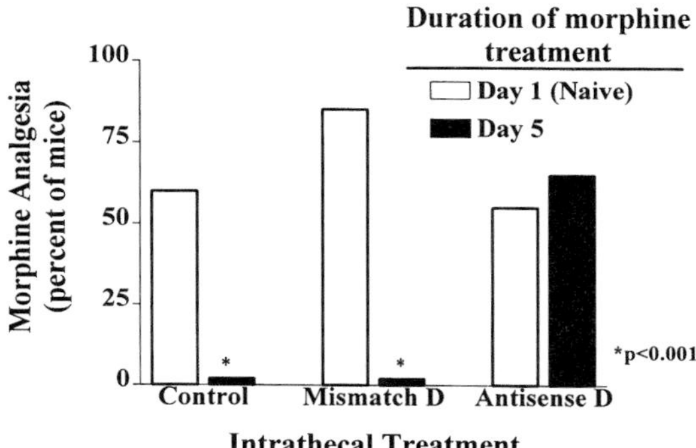

Figure 7. Effects of nNOS antisense on morphine tolerance. Groups of mice were treated with either saline or the indicated antisense intrathecally over 5 days. The mice then received daily injections of morphine analgesia (5 mg/kg, s.c.) and analgesia was determined on the first and fifth days of morphine treatment. Adapted from reference 25.

5. Conclusion

Antisense techniques provide an effective approach towards defining the functional role of proteins. Antisense ODNs are not always active, but careful design of the probes can greatly enhance the chances of success. Designing probes requires attention to the GC content and the secondary structure of the mRNA. However, these issues are independent of the location along the length of the mRNA. As we have shown, all regions all along the mRNA are equally susceptible to antisense probes. This provides the ability to target individual exons and address the functional significance of alternative splicing, a major advantage over knockout models. It also enables investigators to assess the functional significance of partial cDNA sequences before obtaining a full-length clone, as we have done with a member of the opioid receptor family (32,33). Thus, antisense mapping can provide valuable insights in molecular characterization of function.

References

1. Pasternak, G. W. and Standifer, K. M. (1995) *Trends Pharmacol. Sci.*, **16**, 344.
2. Standifer, K. M., Chien, C.-C., Wahlestedt, C., Brown, G. P. and Pasternak, G. W. (1994) *Neuron*, **12**, 805.
3. Kieffer, B. L., Befort, K., Gaveriaux-Ruff, C. and Hirth, C.G. (1992) *Proc. Natl Acad. Sci. USA*, **89**, 12048.
4. Evans, C. J., Keith, D. E., Jr, Morrison, H., Magendzo, K. and Edwards, R. H. (1992) *Science*, **258**, 1952.
5. Rossi, G. C., Su, W., Leventhal, L., Su, H. and Pasternak, G. W. (1997) *Brain Res.*, **753**, 176.

6. Pasternak, G. W. (1993) *Clin. Neuropharmacol.*, **16**, 1.
7. Reisine, T. and Pasternak, G. W. (1996) In Hardman, J. G. and Limbird, L. E. (Eds), *Goodman & Gilman's The Pharmacological Basis of Therapeutics*, pp. 521–556. McGraw-Hill, New York.
8. Wang, J. B., Imai, Y., Eppler, C. M., Gregor, P., Spivak, C. E., and Uhl, G. R. (1993) *Proc. Natl Acad. Sci. USA*, **90**, 10230.
9. Chen, Y., Mestek, A., Liu, J., Hurley, J. A. and Yu, L. (1993) *Mol. Pharmacol.*, **44**, 8.
10. Rossi, G. C., Pan, Y.-X., Cheng, J. and Pasternak, G. W. (1994) *Life Sci.*, **54**, PL375.
11. Rossi, G. C., Pan, Y.-X., Brown, G. P. and Pasternak, G. W. (1995) *FEBS Lett.*, **369**, 192.
12. Rossi, G. C., Brown, G. P., Leventhal, L., Yang, K. and Pasternak, G. W. (1996) *Neurosci. Lett.*, **216**, 1.
13. Rossi, G. C., Leventhal, L., Pan, Y. X., Cole, J., Su, W., Bodnar, R. J. and Pasternak, G. W. (1997) *J. Pharmacol. Exp. Ther.*, **281**, 109.
14. Leventhal, L., Bodnar, R. J., Cole, J. L., Rossi, G. C., Pan, Y.-X. and Pasternak, G. W. (1996) *Brain Res.*, **719**, 78.
15. Matthes, H. W. D., Maldonado, R., Simonin, F., Valverde, O., Slowe, S., Kitchen, I., Befort, K., Dierich, A., Le Meur, M., Dollé, P., Tzavara, E., Hanoune, J., Roques, B. P. and Kieffer, B. L. (1996) *Nature*, **383**, 819.
16. Tian, M., Broxmeyer, H. E., Fan, Y., Lai, Z., Zhang, S., Aronica, S., Cooper, S., Bigsby, R. M., Steinmetz, R., Engle, S. J., Mestek, A., Pollock, J. D., Lehman, M. N., Jansen, H. T., Ying, M., Stambrook, P. J., Tischfield, J. A. and Yu, L. (1997) *J. Exp. Med.*, **185**, 1517.
17. Loh, H. H., Liu, H. C., Cavalli, A., Yang, W. L., Chen, Y. F. and Wei, L. N. (1998) *Mol. Brain Res.*, **54**, 321.
18. Roy, S., Liu, H. C. and Loh, H. H. (1998) *Mol. Brain Res.*, **56**, 281.
19. Schuller, A. G. P., King, M. A., Zhang, J., Boland, E., Chang, A., Czick, M. E., Unterwald, E., Pasternak, G. W. and Pintar, J. E. (1999) *Nature Neurosci*, **2**, 151.
20. Bare, L. A., Mansson, E. and Yang, D. (1994) *FEBS Lett.*, **354**, 213.
21. Zimprich, A., Simon, T. and Hollt, V. (1995) *FEBS Lett.*, **359**, 142.
22. Pan, Y.-X., Xu, J., Boland, E., Abbadie, C., Chang, A., Zuckerman, A., Rossi, G. C. and Pasternak, G. W. (1999) *Mol. Pharmacol* (in press).
23. Snyder, S. H. and Bredt, D. S. (1992) *Sci. Amer.*, **266**, 68.
24. Zhang, J. and Snyder, S. H. (1995) *Annu. Rev. Pharmacol. Toxicol.*, **35**, 213.
25. Kolesnikov, Y. A., Pan, Y. X., Babey, A. M., Jain, S., Wilson, R. and Pasternak, G. W. (1997) *Proc. Natl Acad. Sci. USA*, **94**, 8220.
26. Kolesnikov, Y. A., Pick, C. G., Ciszewska, G. and Pasternak, G. W. (1993) *Proc. Natl Acad. Sci. USA*, **90**, 5162.
27. Kolesnikov, Y. A., Pick, C. G. and Pasternak, G. W. (1992) *Eur. J. Pharmacol.*, **221**, 339.
28. Pasternak, G. W., Kolesnikov, Y. A. and Babey, A. M. (1995) *Neuropsychopharmacology*, **13**, 309.
29. Trujillo, K. A. and Akil, H. (1991) *Science*, **251**, 85.
30. Ogura, T., Yokoyama, T., Fujisawa, H., Kurashima, Y. and Esumi, H. (1993) *Biochem. Biophys. Res. Commun.*, **193**, 1014.
31. Hall, A. V., Antoniou, H., Wang, Y., Cheung, A. H., Arbus, A. M., Olson, S. L., Lu, W. C., Kau, C.-L. and Marsden, P. A. (1994) *J. Biol. Chem.*, **269**, 33082.

32. Pan, Y.-X., Cheng, J., Xu, J. and Pasternak, G. W. (1994) *Regul. Peptides*, **54**, 217.
33. Pan, Y.-X., Cheng, J., Xu, J., Rossi, G. C., Jacobson, E., Ryan-Moro, J., Brooks, A. I., Dean, G. E., Standifer, K. M. and Pasternak, G. W. (1995) *Mol. Pharmacol.*, **47**, 1180.

8

Medicinal chemistry of antisense oligonucleotides

SUDHIR AGRAWAL and EKAMBAR R. KANDIMALLA

1. Introduction

The demonstration in 1978 by Zamecnik and Stephenson that Rous sarcoma virus (RSV) could be inhibited by oligodeoxynucleotides that were complementary to its mRNA (1,2) has become the basis for antisense therapeutics (reviewed in 3). The field of antisense therapeutics has progressed tremendously in the last decade (4–11). The principle underlying antisense therapeutics is simple and rational. An exogenously supplied antisense oligodeoxynucleotide complementary to a portion of a known mRNA sequence binds to the target mRNA in a sequence-specific manner and forms an RNA–oligonucleotide duplex through Watson–Crick base pairing, which prevents translation of the targeted mRNA into protein.

In principle, the antisense approach should allow the design of drugs to target and specifically inhibit expression of any gene whose sequence and function is known. Antisense oligonucleotides inhibit gene expression in a wide variety of cell culture systems and animal models for a range of disease targets, including cancers, viral infections, inflammatory diseases and central nervous system (CNS) diseases (4–11). In this chapter, we review the progress we have made in understanding the impact of chemical modification of oligonucleotides on biological activity, more specifically biophysical and biochemical properties, delivery and pharmacokinetic and safety profiles.

2. Desirable properties of effective antisense oligonucleotides

In the last decade numerous studies have shown the utility of antisense technology in cell-free systems, cell cultures and animal models (4–11). Based on the studies carried out to date, it has become evident that an antisense agent should possess the following combination of properties to be an effective inhibitor of translation:

- solubility in aqueous medium and stability against cellular nucleases
- ability to cross the cellular membrane (cell uptake)
- high binding affinity and specificity towards the target mRNA
- RNase H activation upon binding to the target

'Natural' phosphodiester oligodeoxynucleotides (PO-ONs) were used extensively in earlier studies. PO-ONs exhibit high affinity and specificity towards target mRNA, are taken up by cells efficiently and activate RNase H upon binding to the target mRNA. However, they are rapidly degraded by intracellular and extracellular nucleases *in vivo* (12). Hence, it was necessary to develop nuclease-resistant chemical modifications of PO-ONs that could meet all the requirements mentioned above.

3. Choice of chemical modifications

A number of oligonucleotides, in which natural phosphodiester internucleotide linkages were replaced with modified linkages, have been synthesized and studied for their use as antisense agents. These modified oligonucleotide analogs include phosphorothioates, methylphosphonates, methylphosphonothioates, *S*-methylphosphorothioates, phosphoramidates, phosphorodithioates, methylphosphotriesters, methylphosphothiotriesters, carbamates, formacetal, MMI [Methyleneoxyl (Methylimino)] and *N*3′-*P*5′-phosphoramidates and α-oligonucleotides (reviewed in 13,14). Analogs of oligoribonucleotides, including oligoribonucleotide phosphorothioates (15) and 2′-*O*-alkyl (e.g., methyl, ethyl, propyl, methoxyethyl, fluoro and allyl) phosphorothioates (16–18), methylphosphonates (19,20), and methylphosphonothioates, have also been studied (*Figure 1*). One modification of the nucleic acid backbone, peptide nucleic acid (PNA), is worth mentioning, although its use as an antisense agent is limited because of its poor solubility and cellular uptake (21). Some of these oligonucleotide analogs have a higher affinity for the target RNA compared with their natural counterparts, while others have lower affinity (22). Most of the modified analogs are more stable towards nucleases. Of all the modifications studied, only phosphorothioate and phosphorodithioate (with lower efficiency) analogs activate RNase H, as do PO-ONs. Phosphorothioate oligodeoxynucleotides (PS-ONs), which retain all the desirable properties as antisense agents, have been extensively studied, and are presently being evaluated for their potential in human clinical trials.

In addition to backbone and sugar modifications, modifications of the heterocyclic bases have also been studied in the course of antisense oligonucleotide development (reviewed in 14). Incorporation of modified

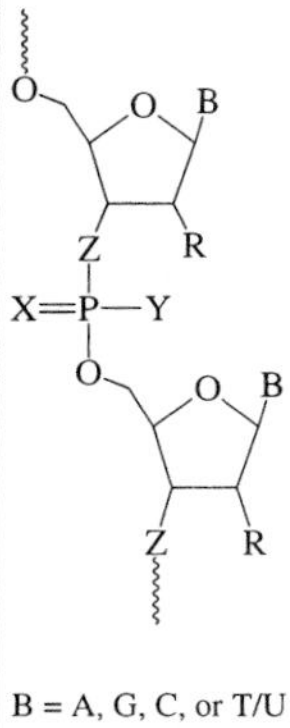

B = A, G, C, or T/U

	X	Y	Z	R
Phosphodiester	O	O^-	O	H; OCH_3; $OCH_2CH_2CH_3$; $CH_2CH_2OCH_3$; $(CH_2CH_2O)_3CH_3$; $CH_2CH(CH_3)OCH_3$; F
Phosphorothioate	O	S^-	O	H; OCH_3; $OCH_2CH_2CH_3$; $CH_2CH_2OCH_3$; $(CH_2CH_2O)_3CH_3$; $CH_2CH(CH_3)OCH_3$; F
Methylphosphonate	O	CH_3	O	H; OCH_3
Methylphosphonothioate	S	CH_3	O	H; OCH_3
Phosphorodithioate	S	S^-	O	H
Phosphoramidate	O	NH_2	O	H
N3'-P5'-Phosphoramidate	O	O^-	NH	H
Phosphotriester	O	OR	O	H
Phosphothiotriester	S	OR	O	H

Figure 1. 'Natural' phosphodiester oligonucleotides (PO-ONs) and some backbone modifications. Phosphorothioate modification is extensively used for antisense applications and several PS-ONs are currently being evaluated for their potential in human clinical trials.

nucleobases may enhance binding affinity. One such modification that has been studied extensively for antisense oligonucleotide development is 5-propyne substitution on 2′-deoxyuridine and deoxycytidine (23). While *in vitro* experiments suggested increased binding affinity to target, cell culture experiments showed that these modifications reduced antisense efficacy unless the oligonucleotides were microinjected (24). However, *in vivo* studies have shown that oligonucleotides containing 5-propyne-substituted heterocyclic bases are more toxic than those containing natural heterocyclic bases (25). Other substitutions, such as 5-methylcytosine, do not seem to be toxic.

4. PS-ONs

In a PS-ON, one of the non-bridging oxygens of the internucleotide PO linkage is replaced with a sulfur (*Figure 1*). This makes PS-ONs more stable against nucleases than PO-ONs both *in vitro* and *in vivo*, and activates RNase H (4). A PS-ON, however, has lower affinity for the target RNA than does the natural PO-ON. Introduction of the sulfur atom results in chirality at the phosphorus center and automated chemical synthesis leads to a mixture of [*Rp*] and [*Sp*] diastereomers at each internucleotide linkage. Protocols have been established to synthesize and purify PS-ONs (*Figure 2*) for antisense experiments (26). The purity of the PS-ON greatly affects the outcome of the experiments.

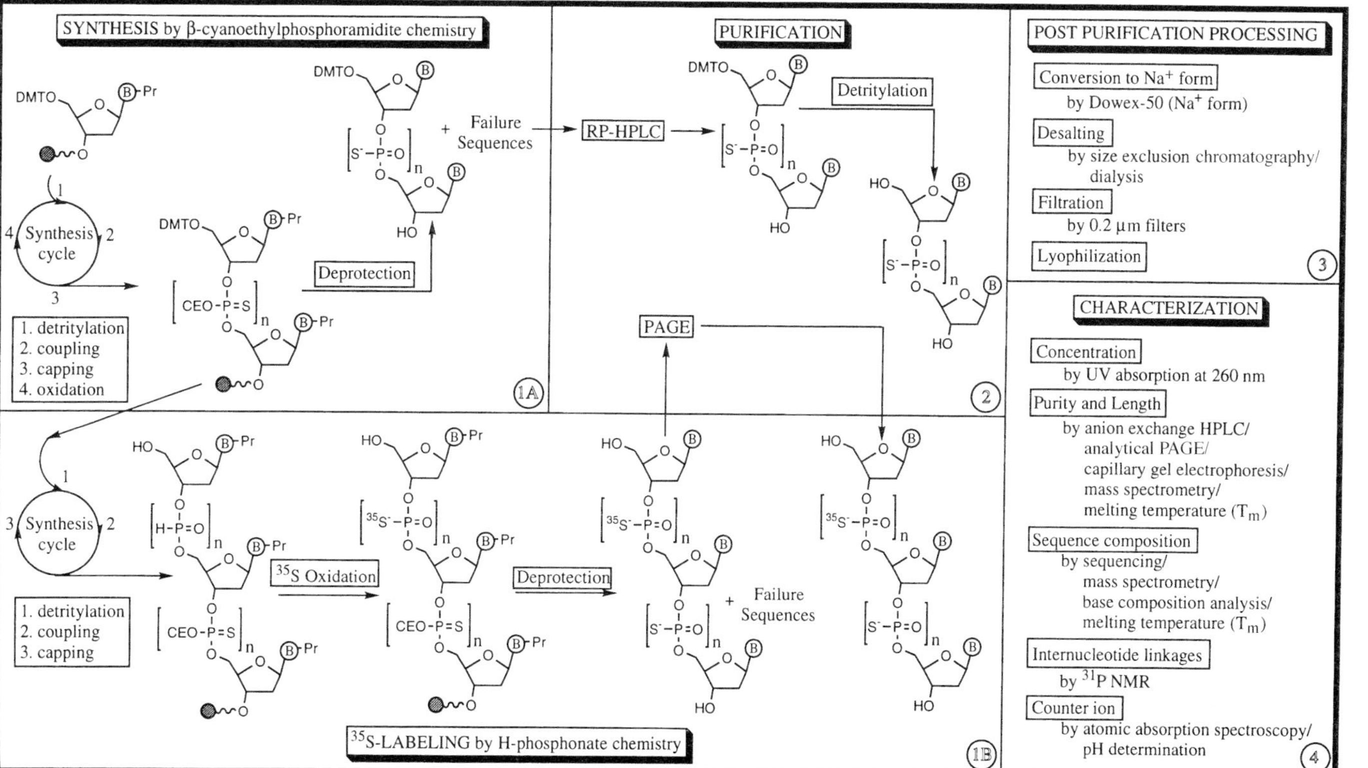

Figure 2. Solid-phase synthetic schemes for the preparation of oligonucleotides (1A) and ^{35}S-labeling of PS-ONs (1B), purification (2), subsequent processing steps (3) and methods of characterization (4) for PS-ONs.

4.1 Synthesis

In general, solid-phase synthesis technology in combination with phosphoramidite, phosphotriester or *H*-phosphonate chemistry is used for automated synthesis of PS-ONs (27,28). Essentially, there are three steps in the solid-phase oligonucleotide synthesis:

(1) attachment of the first nucleoside to the solid support through the 3′-hydroxyl group;
(2) synthesis of the required length and sequence of the oligonucleotide on the solid support from the 3′ end to the 5′ end; and
(3) deprotection and cleavage of the oligonucleotide from the solid support (*Figure 2*).

Each nucleoside addition cycles through:

(1) removal of the acid-labile dimethoxytrityl (DMT) group at the 5′ end;
(2) coupling of the 3′ end of the incoming nucleoside to the 5′ end of the nucleoside on the solid support;
(3) capping the unreacted sites on the solid support; and
(4) appropriate washing and oxidation (*Figure 2*).

For the synthesis of PS-ONs, β-cyanoethylphosphoramidite chemistry is generally utilized, and 3*H*,1,2-benzodithiazole-3*H*-one-1,1-dioxide (29) is used for oxidation. In our laboratory, we synthesize oligonucleotides with the DMT group intact at the 5′ end for convenient purification on reversed-phase high performance liquid chromatography (HPLC).

4.2 Purification

Purification of the oligonucleotide is essential to separate failure sequences from the full-length oligonucleotide. There are a number of methods reported for purification of PS-ONs, including reversed-phase and anion-exchange HPLC techniques. A consistently pure oligonucleotide is required to obtain reproducible biological data. Recently, it has been concluded that the differences in antisense activity observed with the same PS-ON sequence in different laboratories could result from differing levels of purity of the oligonucleotides used (30). A reversed-phase HPLC method can be used to purify small (1 mg) to large (5 g) amounts of crude PS-ON containing a 5′-DMT group (31).

Following purification, solvents are evaporated to dryness and the oligonucleotide is treated with 80% acetic acid to cleave the 5′-DMT group. The purified and deprotected oligonucleotide is converted to its Na^+ form by passing it through Dowex-50 (Na^+ form) column. The excess salt present in the oligonucleotide should be removed before characterization and use of the oligonucleotide in further studies. Desalting of an oligonucleotide is carried out by size exclusion chromatography using Sephadex G15 or G25. Alternatively, the oligonucleotide can be extensively dialyzed against double-distilled water using an appropriate molecular weight cut-off dialysis bag. The oligonucleotide solution should be filtered through a 0.2 μm filter to obtain a particle-free sterile solution before lyophilization. The lyophilization step also removes some of the evaporable impurities from the oligonucleotide.

4.3 Characterization

It is important to characterize oligonucleotides, in terms of their purity, base composition, sequence and backbone integrity, before using them for other studies. A number of methods (*Figure 2*) are routinely used to characterize oligonucleotides (31,32). Measurement of UV absorbance at 260 nm is the most convenient method for determining oligonucleotide content. The length of oligonucleotides can be verified by anion-exchange HPLC, capillary gel electrophoresis (CGE) or polyacrylamide slab gel electrophoresis (PAGE), mass spectrometry, and/or measuring the melting temperature (T_m; a biophysical measure of target-binding affinity) with a complementary DNA or RNA strand at 260 nm using a UV spectrophotometer. Sequence integrity is determined by sequencing, mass spectrometry, measuring T_m or base composition analysis. Atomic absorption spectrometry or pH determination are utilized for determining counterions. The nature of internucleotide linkages is examined by ^{31}P-NMR spectroscopy.

4.4 Radiolabeling

A number of radioactive isotopes, including ^{35}S, ^{3}H, ^{14}C, ^{32}P and ^{33}P, can be used to label oligonucleotides. The isotopes used for internal labeling (^{35}S, ^{3}H or ^{14}C) have a longer half-life than those used for end-labeling (^{32}P and ^{33}P). For PS-ONs, ^{35}S is the most appropriate isotope to use for labeling because it is more easily incorporated either uniformly or site-specifically than is ^{3}H or ^{14}C (33). Uniform and site-specific ^{35}S labeling of PS-ONs can both be achieved using phosphoramidite or *H*-phosphonate chemistries. Detailed protocols for various radiolabeling methods have been published recently (33). For *in vivo* studies, internally labeled oligonucleotides give more consistent results than end-labeled oligonucleotides, as removal of labeled phosphate by phosphatases may give confusing results.

5. Factors that influence antisense activity

5.1 Target site

In addition to choosing an appropriate chemical modification, selection of a suitable target site on mRNA is essential for identifying an effective antisense molecule with biological activity. In principle, an oligonucleotide of 15–20 bases length is sufficient to specifically recognize a unique sequence on the mRNA target. Empirical selection of a suitable site is very difficult, however, because there are no defined guidelines. There are currently no reliable methodologies available to predict local secondary structures adopted by single-stranded RNAs. It is considered best, therefore, to screen a number of oligonucleotides that encompass different regions on mRNA, including initiation codon sites, splice acceptor or donor sites, 5′- or 3′-untranslated regions, etc., to identify a set of optimal target sites.

5.2 Base composition and sequence of antisense oligonucleotide

5.2.1 Inter- and intra-molecular interactions

The antisense activity of oligonucleotides depends not only on their length, chemical modification and target site, but also on their base composition and sequence. The affinity of an oligonucleotide for its target RNA depends on its base composition (22,34,35). The sequence of each oligonucleotide selected should be verified thoroughly for possible self-complementary structures, such as partial duplexes, hairpins and other unconventional structures. Any commercially available software can be used to search for the formation of conventional structures involving Watson–Crick base pairing. Examination of the oligonucleotide alone on non-denaturing polyacrylamide gels, measurement of T_m and circular dichroism spectroscopy under appropriate physiological conditions can also reveal the formation of secondary structures by antisense oligonucleotides. If a selected antisense oligonucleotide forms such structures, it would be difficult to distinguish sequence-specific antisense effects from those of sequence-dependent and -independent non-antisense effects.

5.2.2 G-rich sequences: tetrameric structures

Oligonucleotides containing four or more contiguous Gs form four-stranded, or tetraplex, structures (36–39). This phenomenon has been observed with both oligodeoxyribonucleotides and oligoribonucleotides (including 2′-*O*-substituted analogs). This hyperstructure formation depends on flanking sequences, concentrations of oligonucleotide and salt, and the nature of the cation present in the solution (*Figure 3*) (36–39). These tetrameric structures have an overall higher charge density (polyanionic nature) than oligonucleotides that do not contain contiguous Gs, which affects their cellular uptake, tissue distribution, stability towards nucleases, pharmacokinetics and *in vivo* tissue disposition (39,40). Oligonucleotides containing G-rich sequences, with the potential to form hyperstructures, are known to have increased side effects, such as prolongation of aPTT (activated partial thromboplastin time) and inhibition of complement lysis (39), as a result of the increased charge density. Even PO-ONs containing few phosphorothioate linkages have been

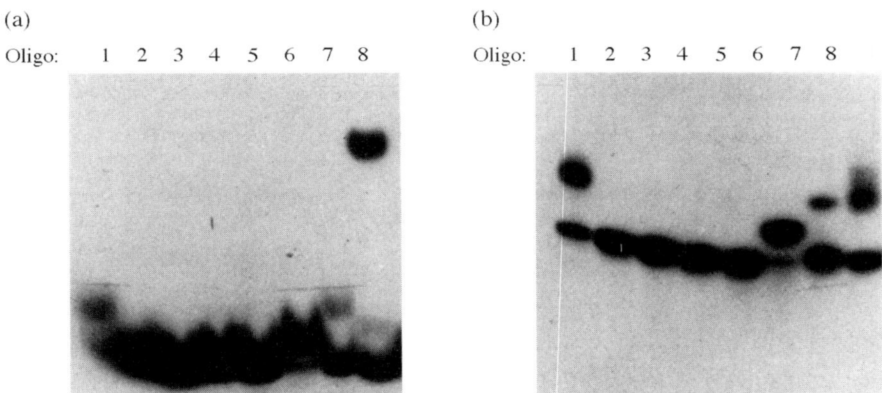

Figure 3. Characterization of hyper-structure formation by G-rich PS-ONs on 10% non-denaturing polyacrylamide gel (a) and 20% denaturing urea polyacrylamide gel (b). The sequences of the oligonucleotides (in both panels) were as follows: lane 1, 5′-TGTTTAAATCTTGTGGGG; lane 2, 5′-GTGTTTAAATCTTGTGGG; lane 3, 5′-GGTGTTTA-AATCTTCTGG; lane 4, 5′-TGGTGTTTAAATCTTGTG; lane 5, 5′-ATGGTGTTTAAATCTTGT; lane 6, 5′-GGGTGTTTAAATCTTGTGGG; lane 7, 5′-GGGGTGGCTCCTTCTGAT; lane 8, 5′-ATCTTGCGGGGTGGCTCC. The PS-ONs that have at least four contiguous Gs (lanes 1 and 6–8) move more slowly on non-denaturing gel. Panel b suggests that these oligonucleotides (in lanes 1 and 6–8) tend to form structures that cannot be disrupted even on denaturing gels (reproduced, with permission, from reference 39).

shown to have these effects in cynomolgus monkeys (41). In addition, G-rich oligonucleotides have a number of sequence-dependent and sequence-independent biological effects (42–46). Studies with oligonucleotides containing dG sequences indicate that G-rich motifs can directly stimulate B cells and enhance the activity of immunostimulatory CpG motifs (47), or, in some cases, block cytokine expression (48).

5.2.3 CpG motifs

Oligonucleotides containing CpG motifs induce cell proliferation and immune responses *in vitro* (49–53). In mice injected with a single dose of a PS-ON containing CpG motifs, increased expression of cytokines (49–51) and chemokines (50) occurs (*Figure 4*). Some PS-ONs have anti-inflammatory (54), antiviral (55), anticancer (56) or antimicrobial (57) activities, which are due not to antisense mechanisms, but to sequence-dependent, non-antisense mechanisms. The presence of CpG motifs is a major factor contributing to non-antisense-mediated PS-ON activity, and such PS-ONs probably induce one or more cytokines in these systems. We have shown that PS-ONs containing appropriate CpG motifs are more toxic than PS-ONs without CpG motifs (50). These effects are alleviated when the CpG motifs are modified.

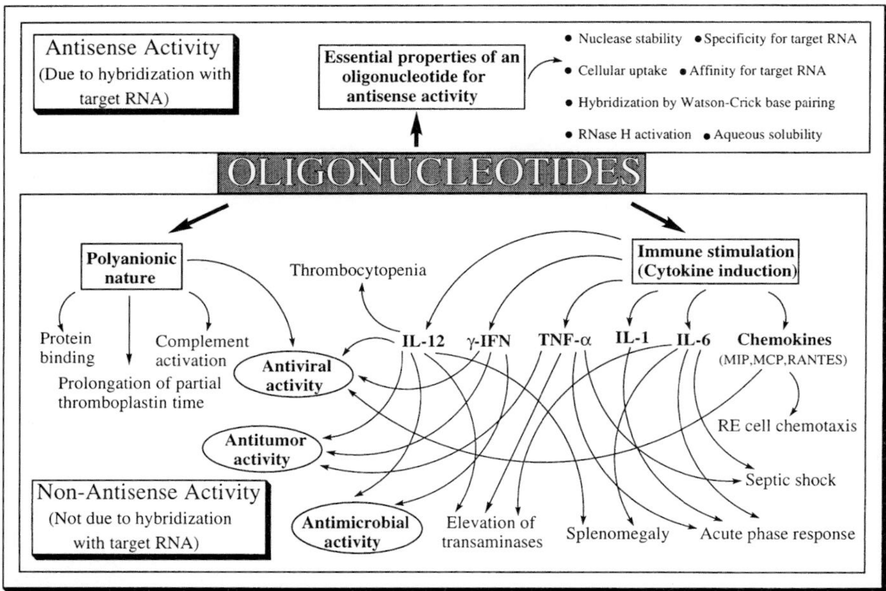

Figure 4. The two sides of antisense oligonucleotides. Although designed to hybridize specifically to target RNA (desirable properties of antisense oligonucleotides are shown in the upper panel), PS-ONs can interact with intracellular and extracellular proteins by virtue of their polyanionic nature in a sequence-independent but length-dependent manner, causing side effects (lower panel). In addition, PS-ONs with certain sequences and structures, such as CpG dinucleotide motifs, palindromes and/or contiguous Gs (sequence-dependent but length-independent), can be immune-stimulatory and induce production of various cytokines and chemokines as shown in lower panel. These cytokines or chemokines, in turn, may be toxic (causing, for example, thrombocytopenia, elevation of transaminases and acute phase response) or have antiviral, antitumor and antimicrobial activities (lower panel). At times the effects shown in the lower panel overlap with those of antisense activities (upper panel) of some PS-ONs. If proper design principles and control PS-ONs are not used, it would be difficult to distinguish the antisense effects (resulting from the properties shown in the top panel) from those of non-antisense effects (shown in the lower panel) (adapted from reference 122).

Non-antisense-mediated biological activity and side effects produced by the presence of CpG motifs can be minimized by substituting 5-methylcytosine for cytosine, introducing a non-ionic internucleotide linkage (methylphosphonate) between C and G, or replacing d(CpG) dinucleotide repeats with 2′-*O*-methylribonucleoside CpG repeats (52). Oligonucleotides containing certain palindromic sequences (e.g. 5′-GACGTC, 5′-AGCGCT or 5′-AACGTT) may also show both sequence-dependent and sequence-independent cellular effects, such as immune response (53), natural killer cell activity (58) and interferon production (59).

5.3 Delivery of oligonucleotides

5.3.1 In cell cultures

For antisense oligonucleotides to be effective, they must be taken up by cells. Cellular uptake of oligonucleotides is a complex process and the mechanism by which it occurs is not yet understood in detail. Studies to date have revealed that cellular uptake of oligonucleotides depends on several factors, such as cell type, the stage of cell cycle, concentration of serum in the medium, length, chemical modification and structure of the oligonucleotide, temperature and incubation time (6–10). The intracellular distribution of the oligonucleotide is also dependent on cell type (60). In addition, antisense activity of an oligonucleotide in cell cultures may also be affected by binding of the oligonucleotide to cellular proteins, enzymes, cell-surface receptors and serum proteins. Nonetheless, antisense oligonucleotides have shown activity against a number of disease targets, including cancers and viruses, in a variety of cell culture systems (3–9).

Use of lipophilic carriers (61) can improve the effectiveness of antisense oligonucleotides in cell cultures. Cationic lipids such as lipofectin can cause non-specific cytotoxic effects if used alone or together with antisense oligonucleotides (62). When using these carriers, it is important to maintain the lipid carrier:oligonucleotide ratio, as excess lipid carrier can cause toxicity. There is continued interest in developing less toxic and more effective lipid agents for antisense drug delivery (63). Use of lipid carrier does complicate evaluation of results as different oligonucleotide sequences or modifications may form complexes with lipids which might affect biological activity. For *in vivo* applications, significant cellular uptake is achieved without the use of any carrier.

5.3.2 *In vivo* disposition and metabolism

Pharmacokinetics, tissue distribution and *in vivo* stability of several PS-ONs of different lengths and sequences have been studied in mice, rats, monkeys and humans (64–67). PS-ONs have been administered intravenously, intraperitoneally, subcutaneously, intradermally, intratracheally and intraocularly.

PS-ONs are rapidly distributed from plasma following intravenous (i.v.) administration, with a distribution half-life of <1 h. Plasma clearance is biphasic, with a terminal elimination half-life ranging from 40–60 h, based on radioactivity levels (68,69). Other modes of administration (intraperitoneal, subcutaneous and intradermal) resulted in lower peak plasma concentrations, but similar tissue distributions as with i.v. administration (68–73).

In general, PS-ONs are distributed to a wide range of tissues, including liver, kidneys, heart, lungs and spleen, within minutes after administration (74–78). The greatest accumulation of PS-ON occurs in liver and kidney, followed by spleen and bone marrow. The least is found in brain. These pharmacokinetic studies provide valuable information about tissue disposition, but fail to provide details of specific cell uptake of oligonucleotides in various organs.

A number of reports have recently appeared in which cellular uptake has been studied *in vivo*. In kidneys, PS-ONs are taken up primarily by proximal tubular cells (79). In liver, cellular uptake is facilitated by scavenger receptors on endothelial cells (80). In our studies, we have used flow cytometry and have analyzed blood samples and tissue homogenates following i.v. administration of fluorescently tagged PS-ONs to rats and have shown high concentrations of these oligonucleotides in liver and kidneys, intermediate concentrations in spleen and bone marrow and very low concentrations in peripheral blood mononuclear cells (PBMCs). Four hours after administration, the oligonucleotide is distributed to PBMCs, spleen lymphocytes and bone marrow cells in the order: monocytes/macrophages > B cells > T cells (81).

Analysis of PS-ON samples extracted from plasma and various tissues by HPLC, PAGE and CGE revealed the presence of intact PS-ON for up to 24 h, along with shorter metabolites (68–70). The rate and pattern of degradation of PS-ONs in plasma and tissues are dependent on time and type of the tissue (68). Examination of the degradation patterns suggests that PS-ONs are digested primarily from the 3′ end, but also from the 5′ end (69,82–85).

5.3.3 Oligonucleotide delivery to brain

The applicability of antisense therapeutics to CNS diseases depends on delivery of oligonucleotides to the CNS. Systemically administered oligonucleotides do not penetrate the CNS well (12), limiting the applicability of antisense technology to CNS diseases (86–88). Oligonucleotides are taken up efficiently by cells in the CNS if administered directly to cerebrospinal fluid. A high-flow microinfusion technique has recently been used to deliver antisense oligonucleotides directly into rat brain parenchyma (86,88). A much higher concentration of oligonucleotides than that required to show efficacy in cell culture systems has been delivered to the brain by this technique (86). Within a short period after infusion, oligonucleotide was distributed throughout the brain from parenchymal cells to white matter to gray matter (*Figure 5*) and most of the oligonucleotide was found intact up to 48 h after infusion. The possible delivery of oligonucleotides to the brain using this microinfusion technique raises hopes for the wide applicability of antisense oligonucleotides to CNS diseases in the near future.

5.4 Excretion of oligonucleotides

PS-ONs are eliminated primarily in urine, with about 40% excreted within 48 h of administration (69). A smaller amount of PS-ON is excreted in feces and bile. The majority of the PS-ON excreted through urine is in the form of shorter metabolites.

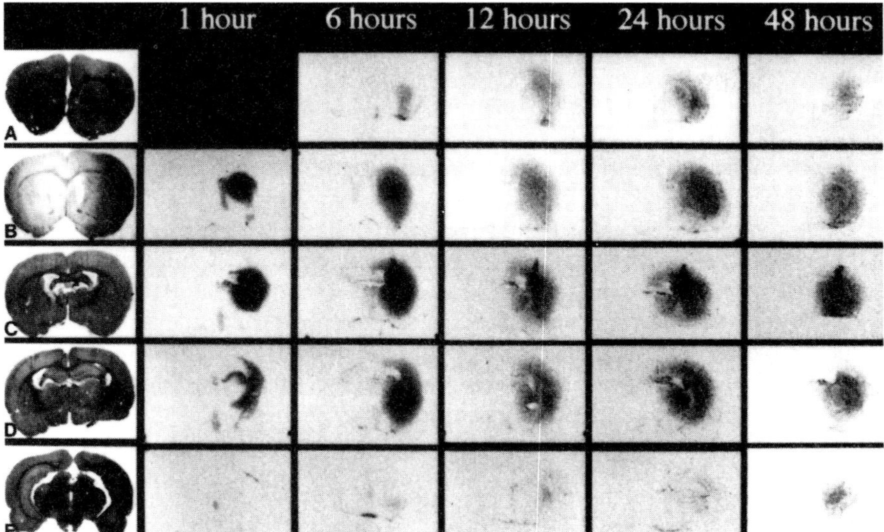

Figure 5. Representative coronal sections and autoradiograms showing distribution of ^{35}S-labeled MBO after high-flow microinfusion into rat brain. On the left are representative coronal sections. Rows A–E are arranged in an anterior-to-posterior orientation. See reference 86 for details (reproduced, with permission from the author, from reference 86).

5.5 Safety of PS-ONs

5.5.1 In mice and rats

In general, PS-ONs are well tolerated, with an LD_{50} of 500 mg/kg in mice and rats following i.v. administration. Subchronic or chronic administration of PS-ONs has side effects, including splenomegaly, thrombocytopenia and elevation of serum transaminases (alanine aminotransferase (ALT) and aspartate aminotransferase (AST)) (4). Histopathology revealed multiorgan mononuclear infiltration (pronounced in kidney and liver), RE (Reticulo Endothelial) cell and lymphoid hyperplasia, and renal tubule degeneration/necrosis. The severity of the side effects depends on the dose, frequency and duration of administration (4,50,64,89–91). A review of the toxicity of PS-ONs of varying sequences in mice and rats shows that the general toxicity profiles of PS-ONs are similar. The severity of toxicity is largely dependent on the sequence of PS-ON administered (4,50,64,89–91).

5.5.2 In monkeys

The toxicological profile of PS-ON in monkeys differs from that observed in rats and mice. High-dose ($\geq$5 mg/kg) i.v. bolus administration of PS-ONs to Rhesus monkeys produced dose-dependent hemodynamic effects, such as acute changes in blood pressure and heart rate, with decreased serum hemolytic complement and increased levels of circulating complement fragment C5a in blood, and prolongation of partial thromboplastin time (92). The severity of the acute toxicity of PS-ON in monkeys correlates with the peak plasma concentration. These effects are rapidly resolved, however, and can be kept under control by slow i.v. infusion of PS-ONs. These effects are sequence-independent and thought to be related to the polyanionic nature of the PS-ONs, since similar effects have also been reported for other polyanionic compounds, such as dextran sulfate, heparin sulfate and cyclodextrin sulfate (93). Our *in vitro* studies on prolongation of aPTT and inhibition of complement lysis revealed that these effects are dependent on the dose, length and backbone chemistry of the oligonucleotide, but independent of the sequence (other than G-rich sequences) (94,95). In addition to slow i.v. infusion, our *in vitro* studies suggest that the use of polycationic substances such as protamine may minimize these effects (95).

5.5.3 In humans

In humans, the major side effects observed with PS-ONs include transient prolongation of aPTT, thrombocytopenia and elevation of serum ALT and AST (96,97). These effects were transient and dependent on the frequency and duration of the administration.

5.5.4 Interaction with proteins

Oligonucleotides interact with molecules other than their desired targets (mRNA), such as proteins. These interactions could be highly sequence-specific, as in the case of oligonucleotide aptamers (46,98). In some cases, oligonucleotides interact with a number of proteins in a sequence-independent manner (99,100). In general, it has been observed that the latter type of interactions are more pronounced with PS-ONs than with PO-ONs of the same sequence, suggesting that sulfur substitution for one of the non-bridging oxygens on internucleotide phosphorus is responsible for these interactions (95,101,102). The sequence-independent side effects observed in monkeys could be related to the ability of PS-ONs to interact with one or more of the proteins involved in the clotting cascade and complement pathway (95,103,104). PS-ONs interact with a number of human serum proteins, including albumin, γ-globulins and fibrinogen. Our studies showed that the affinity of PS-ONs for human serum proteins is in the order fibrinogen > γ-globulins > albumin (Kandimalla and Agrawal, unpublished results). A recent study showed that these effects are not only dependent on the phosphorothioate linkage, but also on the nature of the nucleoside sugar moiety (105). In addition, the interaction of PS-ONs to proteins can be affected by the presence of cationic agents or drugs such as aspirin, sulfa drugs, etc. (101,102).

6. Beyond phosphorothioate oligonucleotides

A number of PS-ONs are currently in the clinical evaluation stage for the treatment of viral infections, cancers and inflammatory diseases. While the preliminary indications of activity observed in clinical trials are exciting, detailed studies are needed to understand fully the therapeutic potential of PS-ONs.

While PS-ONs have yielded very promising results, there are certain drawbacks that should be addressed in the new generation of antisense oligonucleotides. In *Figure 4* (upper panel), we have attempted to summarize the desirable properties of antisense oligonucleotides needed to obtain efficient biological activity. Experience with PS-ONs suggest that they may exhibit properties shown in the lower panel of *Figure 4*, which are largely dependent on the sequence and length, that may interfere with observed biological activity and mechanism of action and may also cause toxicity. In order to reduce polyanionic-related effects, efforts have been made to reduce the number of phosphorothioate linkages in a PS-ON by replacing them with phosphodiester linkages in the center. The resulting oligonucleotide with phosphorothioate linkages at both the ends and phosphodiester linkages in the middle were stable to nucleases *in vitro*, but were very unstable *in vivo*, suggesting that even the internal PO-ON segments are highly susceptible to nuclease degradation (106).

Lessons have been learned by studying a number of other modifications of oligonucleotides, which provide some of the desirable properties, but still lack others. For example, oligonucleotides containing methylphosphonate linkages are non-ionic and resistant towards nucleases, but have a lower affinity for target RNA and do not activate RNase H. Similarly 2′-*O*-alkyl-oligoribonucleotides have a higher affinity for target RNA than PS-ONs and are stable towards nucleases, but do not activate RNase H. Because of their increased duplex stability, 2′-*O*-alkyl-oligoribonucleotides have been employed as antisense agents to inhibit aberrant splicing (107) or translation by hybridization arrest mechanism (108).

7. Mixed-backbone oligonucleotides

When designing the new generation of oligonucleotides, we must consider not only how to maximize desirable properties but also how to minimize non-desirable properties (e.g. polyanionic and immune-stimulatory effects) by use of chemical modifications. We have combined the advantages of PS-ONs and other modifications so that the resulting oligonucleotide analogs will have all desirable properties, and at the same time minimize some of the disadvantages associated with PS-ONs. These oligonucleotides are referred here as ‘mixed-backbone oligonucleotides’ (MBOs).

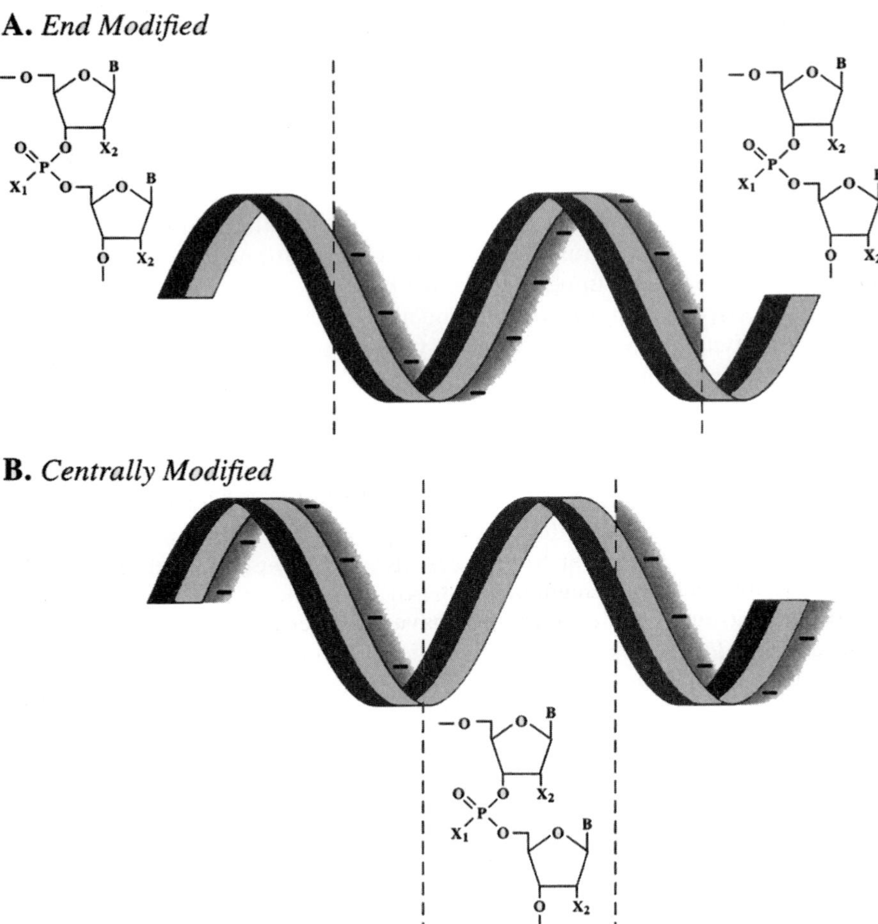

Figure 6. Schematic representation of mixed backbone oligonucleotides. (a) End-modified MBOs and (b) centrally modified MBOs. 2′-*O*-Methylribonucleotides: X_1 and X_2 are S^- and OCH_3, respectively; methylphosphonate: X_1 and X_2 are CH_3 and H, respectively. The advantage of MBOs is that, while they retain the desirable property of PS-ONs (RNase H activation), the side effects inherent in PS-ONs can be minimized. The placement of methylphosphonate linkages at the ends reduces the overall polyanion-related side effects, and increases the *in vivo* stability by protecting both ends of the oligonucleotide from digestion. Similarly, placement of 2′-*O*-methylribonucleotide segments provides increased affinity for the target m-RNA and *in vivo* stability. Placement of modified segments in the center of the PS-ON makes it possible to modulate the rate of degradation, the nature of metabolites being generated *in vivo*, and the elimination of metabolites. Oligonucleotides that are more resistant to nucleases have two advantages: their longer duration of action will mean that less frequent dosing is required, and the presence of fewer degradation metabolites will decrease the possible side effects from such metabolites.

MBOs have certain PS-ON regions and certain modified oligonucleotide regions which can be either oligodeoxynucleotides or oligoribonucleotides. MBOs can be divided into two classes based on the location of the modification in the sequence: end-modified MBOs and centrally modified MBOs. In the former, segments of the modified oligonucleotides are placed at the 3′ end or at both the 3′ and 5′ ends of the PS-ON, while in the latter, the segment of the modified oligonucleotide is placed in the center of the PS-ON (*Figure 6*).

7.1 End-modified MBOs

Most of the early studies were carried out with 3′-end-modified oligonucleotides (82,83,109), but MBOs containing modifications at both the 3′ and the 5′ end have recently been used extensively. There are two reasons for incorporating modifications at both ends:

(1) Although PS-ONs are primarily digested from the 3′ end by exonucleases, a significant amount of oligonucleotide is also degraded from the 5′ end in tissues (84).

(2) *In vitro* studies of *Escherichia coli* RNase H and MBOs containing 2′-*O*-methylribonucleotide segments at both ends or only at one end suggest that MBOs modified at both ends have a higher affinity for target RNA and higher RNase H cleavage selectivity (110,111) (*Figure 7*).

A number of modifications have been incorporated at the ends of PS-ONs in order to improve metabolic stability, pharmacokinetics and safety profiles. These are discussed in the following sections.

7.1.1 End-modified MBOs containing segments of 2′-*O*-alkylribonucleotide (with phosphodiester linkages) and PS-ONs

2′-*O*-Alkyl oligoribonucleotides have higher affinity for target RNA than PS-ONs and better nuclease resistance than PO-ONs *in vitro* (17,112). A number of MBOs containing segments of 2′-*O*-alkyloligoribonucleotides (fluoro, methyl, ethyl, propyl, butyl, pentyl, nonyl, allyl, aminopropyl and benzyl) at the 3′ and 5′ ends have shown increased affinity for target RNA (17,111,112), are substrates for RNase H activity and also have shown biological activity comparable to or higher than that of PS-ONs (112–114). However, the metabolic stability of these MBOs *in vivo* is less than that of PS-ONs (114,115). In addition, significant differences in the *in vivo* disposition of these MBOs have been observed, most probably because of their lower binding to serum proteins than PS-ONs (114,115). The MBOs containing 2′-*O*-alkylribonucleotide (phosphodiester linkages) segments had less of an effect on prolongation of aPTT and hemolytic complement activation than did PS-ONs (112–114).

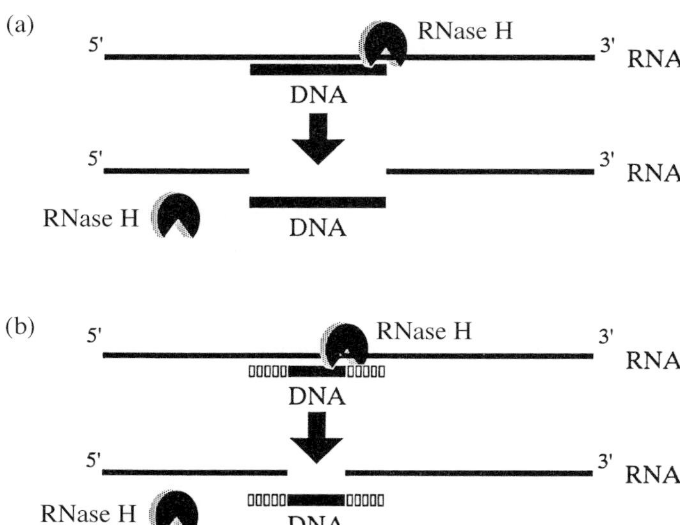

Figure 7. Schematic representation of RNase H cleavage pattern of the RNA target strand in the presence of (a) a PS-ON and (b) an MBO with both ends modified. The initial cleavage of target RNA by RNase H is at the heteroduplex site towards the 5′-terminus of the antisense oligonucleotide. Modification at both the ends confines RNase H cleavage to the center of the target site, increasing the cleavage specificity compared with PS-ON (111). In contrast, modification in the middle of the PS-ON results in RNase H cleavage of target RNA on both sides of the modification, resulting in greater specificity of RNase H cleavage and higher RNase H hydrolysis rate of the target RNA (114) (not shown in figure).

7.1.2. End-modified MBOs containing segments of 2[pri}-*O*-methyloligoribonucleotides with phosphorothioate linkages and PS-ONs

To increase the nuclease stability of 2′-*O*-methylribonucleotides with phosphodiester linkages in MBOs (as discussed above), we have replaced phosphodiester linkages with phosophorothioate linkages. Segments of 2′-*O*-methyloligoribonucleotides with phosphorothioate linkages provide increased stability against nucleases both *in vitro* and *in vivo*, bind to target RNA with higher affinity and have greater biological activity than PS-ONs (17,116,117)

Pharmacokinetic studies have shown that there are no significant differences in plasma clearance or tissue distribution between these MBOs and PS-ONs (118). These MBOs were distributed rapidly to organs and retained in various tissues, because of their longer *in vivo* stability (118). The increased metabolic stability of MBOs may mean that less frequent dosing would be needed in order to maintain the biological effect. In addition, the increased metabolic stability of MBOs has been useful in exploring oral delivery of oligonucleotides (see Section 8). Urinary excretion was the major pathway of elimination, as for PS-ON.

MBOs containing 2′-*O*-methylribonucleotide (with phosphorothioate linkages) segments have good safety profiles (50). As discussed in the previous sections, however, the toxicity of a given PS-ON depends on whether certain sequence motifs are present, and if these motifs are not appropriately modified, the MBO may be more toxic (89). The *in vitro* studies showed that this MBO affected the prolongation of aPTT and inhibition of complement lysis less than PS-ON (94,95).

7.1.3 End-modified MBOs containing segments of 2′,5′-oligoribonucleotides

Incorporation of segments of 2′,5′-oligoribonucleotide with phosphodiester as well as phosphorothioate linkages at both ends of a PS-ON has been reported (119). These MBOs were more stable to serum nucleases *in vitro* and had a higher binding affinity for target RNA than did the target DNA.

MBOs containing 2′,5′-ribonucleotide segments showed lower or negligible effects on prolongation of aPTT, inhibition of complement lysis and lymphocyte proliferation, with anti-HIV-1 activity comparable to that of PS-ON in cell cultures (119). These MBOs are being studied *in vivo*.

7.1.4 End-modified MBOs containing non-ionic segments

In an effort to design antisense molecules with reduced phosphorothioate linkages, we have incorporated segments containing methylphosphonate linkages (non-ionic) at the 3′ and/or 5′ end (110,120).

In general, MBOs containing segments of methylphosphonate linkages form duplexes with the target RNA that have lower T_ms than duplexes of a PS-ON and its complementary RNA target strand. The rate of RNase H hydrolysis of the RNA target strand is unaffected when the methylphosphonate segment is at the 3′ end but is slower when this segment is at the 5′ end of the MBO (120). These results are consistent with those observed with end-modified MBOs containing 2′-*O*-methylribonucleotide segments (111).

The *in vivo* disposition and stability of MBOs containing methylphosphonate segments are similar to those observed with MBOs containing 2′-*O*-methyloligoribonucleotide segments (121).

The side effects of end-modified MBOs containing non-ionic segments are lower than those seen with PS-ON or are negligible, and include lymphocyte proliferation (52), prolongation of aPTT and inhibition of complement lysis (94,95). In a comparative toxicological study in rats, this MBO also showed low toxicity relative to a PS-ON (89). These results suggest that reduction in total anionic charge or phosphorothioate content of oligonucleotide reduces several of the side effects observed with PS-ONs.

7.2 Centrally modified MBOs

Compared with PS-ONs, MBOs containing end modifications are more stable to nucleases *in vivo* and show reduced side effects; they have desirable pharmacokinetic properties and are being evaluated for their potential in human clinical trials (122). In continuation of our efforts to understand further the parameters that govern biological activity, *in vivo* stability and safety profiles of antisense oligonucleotides, we have designed MBOs containing modified segments in the center. The aim of this modification was not to improve the metabolic stability of PS-ON, but to:

(1) reduce the length of contiguous PS-ON linkages, thereby reducing polyanion-related side effects,
(2) modulate mitogen-related effects,
(3) control the rate of *in vivo* metabolism and the nature of metabolites generated, and
(4) improve binding affinity to RNA target and RNase H activity (*Figure 7*).

7.2.1 MBOs containing 2′-*O*-methylribonucleotide segments in the center

The synthesis, biophysical characterization, pharmacokinetic properties and toxicity of MBOs with centrally placed 2′-*O*-methylribonucleotide segments have been reported recently (114). In general, such MBOs have higher affinity for target RNA and greater RNase H hydrolysis rates than PS-ONs. The *in vitro* degradation profiles of centrally modified MBOs differ from those of PS-ON: they produce a ladder until the nuclease encounters the central modification, and then the degradation slows down as a result of the presence of 2′-*O*-methyl modification with phosphorothioate linkages. MBOs with this modification have higher anti-HIV-1 activity in cell cultures compared with PS-ON (114).

The *in vivo* degradation profiles of centrally modified MBOs are distinctive: whereas PS-ONs show a continuous degradation ladder, centrally modified MBOs show initial degradation of the PS-ON segment from the 3′ end and then no further degradation when the nucleases encounter the central 2′-*O*-methyl modification with phosphorothioate linkages (114). Pharmacokinetic studies in rats have shown that, following i.v. administration, this type of MBO has a plasma clearance similar to that of PS-ONs. Centrally modified MBOs are distributed to all tissues, as for PS-ONs. Urinary excretion is the major pathway of elimination (114).

This type of MBO has less of an effect on prolongation of aPTT, inhibition of complement lysis and lymphocyte proliferation than PS-ONs (114). *In vivo* safety studies in rats have shown that MBOs produced lower levels of thrombocytopenia and insignificant elevation of serum ALT and AST than did PS-ONs. Similarly, histopathology of kidneys revealed less renal tubule degeneration with centrally modified MBOs than PS-ONs (114).

7.2.2 MBOs containing methylphosphonate (non-ionic) linkages in the center

This modification makes it possible to reduce not only the length of contiguous PS-ON linkages, but also the overall negative charge or total phosphorothioate content of the molecule. Although these MBOs have slightly lower binding affinity for the target RNA than PS-ONs, the rate of RNase H cleavage of RNA is enhanced. The pattern and rate of nuclease degradation *in vitro* are similar to those of MBOs containing a central 2′-*O*-methyl modification with phosphorothioate linkages, but with higher resistance to nuclease action. In cell cultures these MBOs showed anti-HIV-1 activity similar to that of PS-ON (114).

Plasma clearance of this type of MBO in rats following i.v. administration was similar to that of PS-ONs. This MBO was digested in plasma and tissues from the 3′ end and no degradation products were noted in the methylphosphonate segment. This MBO was also distributed widely to all major tissues, and was present in higher concentrations in kidney and in lower concentrations in liver than PS-ON. MBOs containing central non-ionic methylphosphonate linkages were eliminated faster than those containing a central 2′-*O*-methylribonucleotide segment and PS-ONs (114).

The effects of these MBOs on complement and coagulation parameters *in vitro* are less than those of PS-ONs or are negligible. These MBOs also have significantly less effect on lymphocyte proliferation than PS-ONs. In rats, this type of MBO produced significantly less thrombocytopenia and elevation of serum AST and ALT than PS-ONs. Histopathalogy revealed reduced renal tubular degeneration in kidneys of animals receiving this type of MBO than PS-ONs or MBOs containing a central 2′-*O*-methylribonucleotide segment with phosphorothioate linkages in the middle (114).

8. Oral and colorectal delivery of MBOs

The increased stability of MBOs *in vivo* against nucleases compared with PS-ONs allows their delivery by oral (123) or colorectal (124) administration. While studying the pharmacokinetic properties of PS-ONs and end-modified MBOs containing 2′-*O*-methylribonucleotide segments with phosphorothioate linkages in rats following i.v. administration, we observed high levels of oligonucleotide-associated radioactivity in gastrointestinal tissues and their contents (118). Both intact and degraded oligonucleotides were present in the material extracted from these tissues and their contents. In particular, a higher percentage of intact material was found in the case of end-modified MBOs. The fact that insignificant amounts of oligonucleotide-associated radioactivity are found in feces suggests enterohepatic circulation and reabsorption of the oligonucleotides from the intestinal tract, and prompted us to explore the possibility of oral delivery of PS-ONs.

PS-ONs remain intact in the stomach but are degraded in the intestine when administered orally to rats. End-modified MBOs, in contrast, show good *in vivo* stability in the stomach, small intestine and large intestine (123), and intact and degraded forms of MBO are found in plasma and various tissues, suggesting oral absorption. More detailed studies are required, however, to elucidate the site of absorption, impact of chemical modifications of the oligonucleotide, and impact of formulation and delivery vehicle on oligonucleotide absorption following oral administration.

9. Other important modifications

9.1 Oligonucleotides containing a 3′-hairpin structure or self-stabilized oligonucleotides

In order to stabilize oligonucleotides against 3′-exonucleases, a short PS-ON segment complementary to six to eight bases at the 3′ end has been added, so that the resulting PS-ON forms a hairpin structure at the 3′ end. The biophysical and biochemical properties of self-stabilized PS-ONs have been studied (125), as have the pharmacokinetic (126) and safety profiles in rats (89). Self-stabilized PS-ONs have plasma clearance and tissue distribution profiles similar to those of PS-ONs, with significant metabolic stability *in vivo* as a result of the 3′-hairpin structure (126). In toxicity studies in rats, a self-stabilized PS-ON was significantly less toxic than a PS-ON, although it was eight nucleotides longer than the PS-ON (89). However, the effects of a self-stabilized PS-ON on prolongation of aPTT, complement activation (94,95) and lymphocyte proliferation (52) were similar to that of a PS-ON. The low *in vivo* toxicity of a self-stabilized PS-ON in rats could result from some part of the sequence being masked by formation of a duplex structure.

9.2 3′–3′-Linked oligonucleotides

One of the major problems associated with development of antiviral drugs is the rapidity with which mutations occur in the viral genome. It will be necessary to develop strategies to target more than one site at a time, so that if one target site acquires a mutation, the other site is still vulnerable to antisense attack, and the virus is completely eradicated. We have reported such a strategy, in which two oligonucleotides can be attached through a phosphodiester or other modified linkage of their free 3′-OH groups. This provides the additional advantage of protecting the oligonucleotides from 3′-exonucleases *in vivo* (127). In addition, these oligonucleotides can target two different mRNAs at the same time.

9.3 Pro- or bio-reversible oligonucleotide analogs

To improve cellular uptake and avoid unwanted association of PS-ONs with cellular proteins due to backbone negative charge, we have synthesized and studied PS-ONs that have been derivatized by attaching an acyloxyalkyl group to the backbone sulfur moiety (128). The pendent group attached to the sulfur atom masks the negative charge of the derivatized PS-ON, thus making it more lipophilic and facilitating its uptake. After internalization of the derivatized PS-ON, intracellular esterases act upon the pendent group, generating the unmasked parent PS-ON. By choosing an appropriate pendent ester group, it would be possible to design pro-oligonucleotides for sustained release, oral bio-availability and site-specific targeting. Protocols have recently been developed for the synthesis of a variety of pro-oligonucleotide derivatives and *in vivo* studies are being performed (129,130,131).

9.4 Stereoregular PS-ONs

Substitution of sulfur for a non-bridging oxygen on phosphorus introduces chirality at the phosphorus center, resulting in [*Rp*] and [*Sp*] diastereomers. PS-ONs are obtained as a mixture of 2^n diastereomers (where *n* is the number of phosphorothioate internucleoside linkages) on an automated DNA synthesizer using β-cyanoethylphosphoramidite chemistry. There are no methods available to separate such diastereomeric mixtures. Even if it were possible to purify such a mixture, the yield of the stereoregular PS-ON obtained from this mixture would be very low. Our previous studies comparing an enzyme-synthesized stereoregular [*Rp*] PS-ON with a diastereomeric mixture of PS-ONs suggested stereochemistry-dependent biophysical and biochemical properties (132). Stereoregular [Rp] PS-ON binds to the RNA target with higher affinity, activates RNase H better and is more susceptible to 3′-exonuclease digestion than stereoregular [*Sp*] PS-ON and diastereomeric mixtures of PS-ONs (132–134). In addition, certain polymerases and nucleases interact with and act upon PS-ONs in a diastereomer-selective fashion (135). Pharmacokinetic and safety profiles of stereoregular PS-ONs have not been studied, because there are no convenient synthetic methods for preparing diastereomerically pure PS-ONs in the quantities required for these studies. We have recently established methods for synthesizing stereoenriched [*Rp*] and [*Sp*] PS-dimers on a solid support using nucleoside bicyclic oxazaphospholidines as synthons (*Figure 8*) (136). Using this method, we have obtained stereo-enriched PS-ONs for detailed studies, which are presently ongoing.

10. Conclusions and future perspectives

Phosphorothioate modification has proven to be the most suitable chemical modification for development of antisense therapeutics. PS-ONs have

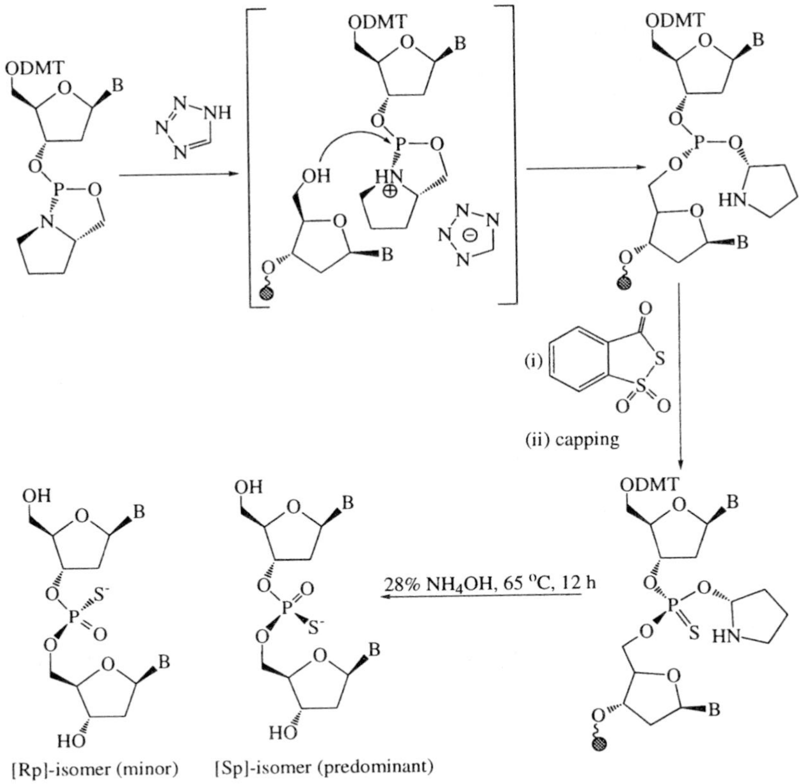

Figure 8. Scheme for the synthesis of stereoregular PS-dimers (reproduced, with permission, from reference 136).

favorable pharmacokinetic and safety profiles, but they can have non-antisense-mediated effects as well as the desired antisense effects. Several of these non-antisense-mediated effects are related not to the polyanionic nature of the phosphorothioate backbone, but to the sequence, base composition and secondary structures of the oligonucleotides. There have been several reports of how sequence-dependent effects can be overcome (4,52,81,95,105,122), non-antisense side effects reduced and antisense activity enhanced. Several of the second-generation MBOs have improved pharmacokinetic and safety profiles *in vitro* and *in vivo*. MBOs provide a way to modulate biological, pharmacodynamic and safety profiles. The advantage of MBOs is that, while they retain the RNase H-activating property of PS-ONs, the side effects inherent to PS-ONs can be minimized. The properties of a PS-ON depend critically on the position of the modified oligodeoxyribonucleotide or oligoribonucleotide segment. By changing the alkyl group at the 2′-position it may also be possible to alter the lipophilicity and, thereby, the biophysical and biochemical properties of antisense oligonucleotides for specific needs.

While new backbone chemistries continue to be devised in order to address specific drawbacks or to improve the properties of current oligonucleotide modifications, it is important to understand further several aspects of antisense oligonucleotides, including:

- the mechanisms of cellular uptake, transport, and retention of oligonucleotides in various types of cells or tissues including the gastrointestinal tract;
- the impact of pharmacokinetics of intact and metabolized oligonucleotides on *in vivo* therapeutic effectiveness and side effects; and
- the pathways of oligonucleotide metabolism at the cellular and molecular levels.

Development of methods for rapid identification of optimal target sites on mRNAs is also required for continued development and validation of antisense therapeutics.

References

1. Zamecnik, P. and Stephenson, M. (1978) *Proc. Natl Acad. Sci. USA*, **75**, 280.
2. Stephenson, M. and Zamecnik, P. (1978) *Proc. Natl Acad. Sci. USA*, **75**, 285.
3. Zamecnik, P. C. (1996) In Agrawal, S. (Ed.), *Antisense Therapeutics*, pp. 1–11. Humana Press, Totowa, NJ.
4. Agrawal, S. (1996) *Trends Biotechnol.*, **14**, 376.
5. Akhtar, S. and Agrawal, S. (1997) *Trends Pharmacol. Sci.*, **18**, 12.
6. Agrawal, S. (Ed.) (1996) *Antisense Therapeutics.* Humana Press, Totowa,, NJ.
7. Crooke, S. T. (Ed.) (1998) *Antisense Research and Applications.* Springer, New York.
8. Wickstorm, E. (Ed.) (1998). *Clinical Trials of Genetic Therapy with Antisense DNA and DNA Vectors.* Marcel Dekker, New York.
9. Ciba Foundation Symposium 209. (1997) *Oligonucleotides as Therapeutic Agents.* John Wiley & Sons, New York.
10. Stein, C. A. and Krieg, A. M. (Eds) (1998). *Applied Antisense Oligonucleotide Technology.* Wiley–Liss, New York.
11. Bennett, C. F. (1998). *Biochem. Pharmacol.*, **55**, 9.
12. Agrawal, S., Temsamani, H., Galbraith, W. and Tang, J.-Y. (1995). *Clin. Pharmacokinet.*, **28**, 7.
13. Agrawal, S. and Iyer, R. P. (1995). *Curr. Opin. Biotechnol.*, **6**, 12.
14. Seeberger, P. H. and Caruthers, M. H. (1998). In Stein, C. A. and Krieg, A. M. (Eds), *Applied Antisense Oligonucleotide Technology*, pp. 51–71. Wiley-Liss, New York.
15. Agrawal, S. and Tang, J. -Y. (1990). *Tetrahedron Lett.*, **31**, 7541.
16. Iribarren, A. M., Sproat, B. S., Neuner, P., Sulston, I., Ryder, U. and Lamond, A. I. (1990) *Proc. Natl Acad. Sci. USA*, **87**, 7747.

17. Metelev, V., Lisziewicz, J. and Agrawal, S. (1994). *Bioorg. Med. Chem. Lett.*, **4**, 2929.
18. Cummins, L. L., Owens, S. R., Risen, L. M., Lesnik, E. A., Freier, S. M., McGee, D., Guinosso, C. J. and Cook, P. D. (1995). *Nucleic Acids Res.*, **23**, 2019.
19. Kandimalla, E. R., Temsamani, J. and Agrawal, S. (1995). *Nucleosides and Nucleotides*, **14**, 1031.
20. Kean, J. M., Kipp, S. A., Miller, P. S., Kulka, M. and Aurelian, L. (1995). *Biochemistry*, **34**, 14617.
21. Good, L. and Nielsen, P. E. (1997). *Antisense Nucleic Acid Drug Dev.*, **7**, 431.
22. Freier, S. M. and Altmann, K. H. (1997). *Nucleic Acids Res.*, **25**, 4429.
23. Froehler, B. C. and Ricca, D. J. (1992). *J. Amer. Chem. Soc.*, **114**, 8320.
24. Wagner, R. W., Matteucci, M. D., Lewis, J. L. G., Moulds, C. and Froehler, B. C. (1993) *Science*, **260**, 1510.
25. Wagner, R. W. (1997). In *Oligonucleotides as therapeutic agents*, pp. 142–157. Ciba Foundation Symposium 209. John Wiley & Sons, New York.
26. Padmapriya, A. A., Tang, J.-Y. and Agrawal, S. (1994). *Antisense Res. Dev.*, **4**, 185.
27. Agrawal, S. (1993). *Protocols for Oligonucleotides and Analogs: Synthesis and Properties*. Humana Press, Totowa, NJ.
28. Eckstein, F. (Ed.) (1991). *Oligonucleotides and Analogues: A Practical Approach*. IRL Press, Oxford.
29. Iyer, R. P., Egan, W., Regan, J. B. and Beaucage, S. L. (1990). *J. Amer. Chem. Soc.*, **112**, 1253.
30. Eckstein, F., Krieg, A. M., Stein, C. A., Agrawal, S., Beaucage, S., Cook, P. D., Crooke, S., Gait, M. J., Gewirtz, A., Helene, C., Miller, P., Narayanan, R., Nicolin, A., Nielsen, P., Ohtsuka, E., Seliger, H., Stec, W., Tidd, D., Wagner, R. and Zon, J. (1996). *Antisense Nucleic Acid Drug Dev.*, **6**, 149.
31. Agrawal, S. and Temsamani, J. (1997). In Schlingensiepen, R., Brysch, W. and Schlingensiepen, K.-H. (Eds), *Antisense Technology to Therapy*, pp. 224–250. Blackwell Sciences, Vienna.
32. Schweitzer, M. and Engels, J. W. (1997). In Schlingensiepen, R, Brysch, W. and Schlingensiepen, K.-H. (Eds), *Antisense Technology to Therapy*, pp. 78–103. Blackwell Sciences, Vienna.
33. Agrawal, S., Tan, W., Jiang, Z., Yu, D. and Iyer, R. P. (1997). In Schlingensiepen, R, Brysch, W. and Schlingensiepen, K.-H. (Eds), *Antisense Technology to Therapy*, pp. 57–77. Blackwell Sciences, Vienna.
34. Kandimalla, E. R., Venkataraman, G., Sasisekharan, V. and Agrawal, S. (1997). *J. Biomol. Struct. Dyn.*, **14**, 715.
35. Li, Y. and Agrawal, S. (1995). *Biochemistry*, **34**, 10056.
36. Kandimalla E. R. and Agrawal, S. (1995). *Nucleic Acids Res.*, **23**, 1068.
37. Guschlbauer, W., Chantot, J. F. and Thiele, D. (1990). *J. Biomol. Struct. Dyn.*, **8**, 491.
38. Williamson, J. R. (1993). *Curr. Opin. Struct. Biol.*, **3**, 357.
39. Agrawal, S., Iadarola, P. L., Temsamani, J., Zhao, Q. and Shaw, D. R. (1996). *Bioorg. Med. Chem. Lett.*, **6**, 2219.
40. Agrawal, S., Tan, W., Cai, Q., Xie, X. and Zhang, R. (1997). *Antisense Nucleic Acid Drug Dev.*, **7**, 245.
41. Wallace, T. L., Bazemore, S. A., Kornbrust, D. J. and Cossum, P. A. (1996). *J. Pharmacol. Exp. Ther.*, **278**, 1306.

42. Rando, R. F., Ojwang, J., Elbaggari, A., Reyes, G. R., Tinder, R., McGrath, M. S. and Hogan, M. E. (1995). *J. Biol. Chem.*, **270**, 1754.
43. Broaddus, W. C., Chen, Z. J., Prabhu, S. S., Loudon, W. G., Gillies, G. T., Phillips, L. L. and Fillmore, H. (1997). *Neurosurgery*, **41**, 908.
44. Burgess, T. L., Fisher, E. F., Ross, S. L., Bready, J. V., Qian, Y. X., Bayewitch, L. A., Cohen, A. M., Herrera, C. J., Hu, S. S. and Kramer, T. B. (1995). *Proc. Natl Acad. Sci. USA*, **92**, 4051.
45. Maltese, J. Y., Sharma, H., Vassilev, L. and Narayanan, R. (1995). *Nucleic Acids Res.*, **23**, 1146.
46. Bock, L. C., Griffin, L. C., Latham, J. A., Vermaas, E. H. and Toole, J. J. (1992). *Nature*, **355**, 564.
47. Kimura, Y., Sonehara, K., Kuramoto, E., Makino, T., Yamamoto, S., Yamamoto, T., Kataoka, T. and Tokunaga, T. (1994). *J. Biol. Chem.*, **116**, 991.
48. Halpern, H. D. and Pisetsky, D. S. (1995). *Immunopharmacology*, **29**, 47.
49. Krieg, A. M. (1998). In Stein, C. A. and Krieg, A. M. (Eds), *Applied Antisense Oligonucleotide Technology*, pp. 431–448. Wiley–Liss, New York.
50. Agrawal, S. and Zhao, Q. (1998). *Antisense Nucleic Acid Drug Dev.*, **8**, 135.
51. Pisetsky, D. S. and Reich, C. F. (1993). *Life Sci.*, **54**, 101.
52. Zhao, Q., Temsamani, J., Iadarola, P. I., Jiang, Z. and Agrawal, S. (1996). *Biochem. Pharmacol.*, **51**, 173.
53. Krieg, A. M., Yi, A. K., Matson, S., Waldschmidt, T. J., Bishop, G. A., Teasdale, R., Koretzky, G. A. and Klinman, D. M. (1995). *Nature*, **374**, 546.
54. Kline, J. N., Waldschmidt, T. J., Businga, T. R., Lemish, J. E., Weinstock, J. V., Thorne, P. S. and Krieg, A. M. (1998). *J. Immunol.*, **160**, 2555.
55. Dunford, P. J., Mulqueen, M. J. and Agrawal, S. (1997). In: *Antisense 97: Targeting the Molecular Basis of Disease*, Abstract book, p. 40.
56. Wang, Z., Karras, J. G., Colarusso, T. P., Foote, L. C. and Rothstein, T. L. (1997). *Cell. Immunol.*, **180**, 162.
57. Porter, K. R., Kochel, T. J., Wu, S. J., Raviprakash, K., Phillips, I., Hayes, C. G. (1998). *Arch. Virol.*, **143**, 997.
58. Yamamoto, T., Yamamoto, S., Kataska, T. and Tokunaga, T. (1994). *Antisense Res. Dev.*, **4**, 119.
59. Kuramoto, E., Yano, O., Kimura, Y., Baba, M., Makino, T., Yamamoto, S., Yamamoto, T., Kataoka, T. and Tokunaga, T. (1992). *Jpn J. Cancer Res.*, **83**, 1128.
60. Lisziewicz, J., Sun, D., Weichold, F. F., Thierry, A. R., Lusso, P., Tang, J.-Y., Gallo, R. C. and Agrawal, S. (1994). *Proc. Natl Acad. Sci. USA*, **91**, 7942.
61. Felgner, P. L. (1996). *Human Gene Ther.*, **7**, 1791.
62. Yeoman, L. C., Danels, Y. J. and Lynch, M. J. (1992) *Antisense Res. Dev.*, **2**, 51.
63. Bennett, C. F., Mirejovsky, D., Crooke, R. M., Tsai, Y. J., Felgner, J., Sridhar, C. N., Wheeler, C. J. and Felgner, P. L. (1998). *J. Drug Target.*, **5**, 149.
64. Agrawal, S. and Zhang, R. (1997). In Weiss, B. (Ed.), *Antisense Oligodeoxynucleotides and Antisense RNA*, pp. 57–78. CRC Press, Boca Raton, FL.
65. Agrawal, S. (1998). In Stein, C. A. and Krieg, A. M. (Eds), *Applied Antisense Oligonucleotide Technology*, pp. 365–385. Wiley–Liss, New York.
66. Agrawal, S. and Zhang, R. (1998). In Crooke, S. T. (Ed.), *Antisense Research and Applications*, pp. 525–541. Springer, New York.
67. Nicklin, P. L., Craig, S. J., Philips, J. A. (1998). In Crooke, S. T. (Ed.), *Antisense Research and Applications*, pp. 141–168. Springer, New York.

68 . Agrawal, S., Temsamani, J. and Tang, J.-Y. (1991). *Proc. Natl Acad. Sci. USA*, **88**, 7595.
69. Zhang, R., Diasio, R. B., Lu, Z., Liu., T., Jiang, Z., Galbraith, W. and Agrawal, S. (1995). *Biochem. Pharmacol.*, **49**, 929.
70. Sands, H., Gorey-Feret, L. J., Cocuzza, A. J., Hobbs, F. W., Chidester, D. and Trainor, G. L. (1994). *Mol. Pharmacol.*, **45**, 932.
71. Cossum, P.A., Sasmor, H., Dillinger, D., Truong, L., Cummins, L. and Owens, S. R. (1993). *J. Pharmacol. Exp. Ther.*, **267**, 1181.
72. Cossum, P. A., Troung, L., Owens, S. R., Markham, P. M., Shea, J. P. and Crooke, S. T. (1994). *J. Pharmacol. Exp. Ther.*, **269**, 89.
73. Iverson, P. L. (1993). In Crooke, S. T. and Lebleu, B. (Eds), *Antisense Research and Applications*, p. 461. CRC Press, Boca Raton, FL.
74. Agrawal, S. and Iyer, R. P. (1997). *Pharmacol. Ther.*, **76**, 151.
75. Philips, J. A., Craig, S. J., Bayley, D., Christial, R. A., Geary, R. and Nicklin, P. L. (1997). *Biochem. Pharmacol.*, **54**, 657.
76. Grindel, J. M., Musick, T. J., Jiang, Z., Roskey, A. and Agrawal, S. (1998). *Antisense Nucleic Acid Drug Dev.*, **8**, 43.
77. Martin, R. R. (1998). In Stein, C. A. and Krieg, A. M. (Eds), *Applied Antisense Oligonucleotide Technology*, pp. 387–393. Wiley–Liss, New York.
78 . Glover, J. M., Leeds, J. M., Mant, T. G. K., Amin, D., Kisner, D. L., Zuckerman, J. E., Geary, R. S., Levin, A. A. and Shanahan, W. R. (1997). *J. Pharmacol. Exp. Ther.*, **282**, 1173.
79. Zhao, Q., Zhou, R., Temsamani, J., Zhang, Z., Roskey, A. and Agrawal, S. (1998) *Antisense Nucleic Acid Drug Dev.*, **8**, 451.
80. Carome, M. A., Kang, Y. H., Bohen, E. M., Nicholson, D. E., Carr, F. E., Kiandoli, L. C., Brummel, S. E. and Yuan, C. M. (1997). *Nephron*, **75**, 82.
81. Bijsterbosch, M. K., Manogaran, M., Rump, E. T., DeVrueh, R. L., van Veghel, R., Tivel, K. L., Biessen, E. A., Bennett, C. F., Cook, P. D. and van Berkel, T. J. (1997). *Nucleic Acids Res.*, **25**, 3290.
82. Temsamani, J., Tang, J. Y. and Agrawal, S. (1992). *Ann. N.Y. Acad. Sci.*, **660**, 318.
83. Temsamani, J., Tang, J. Y., Padmapriya, A., Kubert, M. and Agrawal, S. (1993). *Antisense Res. Dev.*, **3**, 277.
84. Temsamani, J., Roskey, A., Chaix, C. and Agrawal, S. (1997). *Antisense Nucleic Acid Drug Dev.*, **7**, 159.
85. Cummins, L. L., Winniman, M. and Gaus, H. J. (1997). *Bioorg. Med. Chem. Lett.*, **7**, 1225.
86. Broaddus, W. C., Prabhu, S. S., Fillies, G, T., Neal, J., Conrad, W. S., Chen, Z.-J., Fillmore, H. and Young, H. F. (1998). *J. Neurosurg.*, **88**, 734.
87. Nissbrandt, H., Ekman, A., Erksson, E. and Heilig, M. (1995). *Neuroreport*, **6**, 573.
88. Whitesell, L., Geselowitz, D., Chavany, C., Fahmy, B., Walbridge, S., Alger, J. R. and Neckers, L. M. (1993). *Proc. Natl Acad. Sci. USA,* **90**, 4665.
89. Agrawal, S., Zhao, Q., Jiang, Z., Oliver, C., Giles, H., Heath, J. and Serota, D. (1997). *Antisense Nucleic Acid Drug Dev.*, **7**, 575.
90. Henry, S. P., Monteith, D. and Levin, A. A. (1997). *Anticancer Drug Design*, **12**, 395.
91. Levin, A. A., Monteith, D. K., Leeds, J. M., Nicklin, P. L., Geary, R. S., Butler, M., Templin, M. V. and Henry, S. P. (1998). In Crooke, S. T. (Ed.), *Antisense Research and Applications*, pp. 169–215. Springer, New York.

92. Galbraith, W. M., Hobson, W. C., Giclas, P. C., Schechter, P. J. and Agrawal, S. (1994). *Antisense Res. Dev.*, **3**, 201.
93. Bagasra, O., Whittle, P., Heins, B. and Pomerantz, R. J. (1991). *J. Infect. Dis.*, **164**, 1082.
94. Agrawal, S., Rustagi, P. K. and Shaw, D. R. (1995). *Toxicol. Lett.*, **82/83**, 431.
95. Shaw, D. R., Rustagi, P. K., Kandimalla, E. R., Manning, A. N., Jiang, Z. and Agrawal, S. (1997). *Biochem. Pharmacol.*, **53**, 1123.
96. Schechter, P. J. and Martin, R. R. (1998). In Crooke, S. T. (Ed.), *Antisense Research and Applications*, pp. 233–241. Springer, New York.
97. Sikic, B. I., Yuen, A. R., Advani, R., Halsey, J., Fisher, G. A., Holmlund, J., Dorr, A. (1998). *Proc. American Society of Clinical Oncology*, **17**, 429a.
98. Ellington, A. D. and Szostak, J. W. (1992). *Nature*, **355**, 850.
99. Benimetskaya, L., Tonkinson, J. L., Koziolkiewiez, M., Karwowski, B., Guga, P., Zeltser, R., Stec, W. and Stein, C. A. (1995). *Nucleic Acids Res.*, **23**, 4239.
100. Stein, C. A. (1996). *Trends Biotechnol.*, **14**, 147.
101. Srinivasan, S. K., Tewary, H. K. and Iversen, P. L. (1995). *Antisense Res. Dev.*, **5**, 131.
102. Agrawal, S., Zhang, X., Cai, Q., Kandimalla, E. R., Manning, A., Jiang, Z., Marcel, T. and Zhang, R. (1998). *J. Drug Target.*, **5**, 303.
103. Henry, S. P., Giclas, P. C., Leeds, J., Pangburn, M., Auletta, C., Levin, A. A. and Kornbrust, D. J. (1997) *J. Pharmacol. Exp. Ther.*, **281**, 810.
104. Henry, S. P., Novotny, W., Leeds, J., Auletta, C. and Kornbrust, D. J. (1997). *Antisense Nucleic Acid Drug Dev.*, **7**, 503.
105. Kandimalla, E. R., Shaw, D. R. and Agrawal, S. (1998). *Bioorg. Med. Chem. Lett.*, **18**, 2103.
106. Sands, H., Gorey-Feret, L. J., Ho, S. P., Bao, Y., Cocuzza, A. J., Chidester, D. and Hobbs, F. W. (1995). *Mol. Pharmacol.*, **47**, 636.
107. Sierakowska, H., Sambade, M. J., Agrawal, S. and Kole, R. (1996). *Proc. Natl Acad. Sci. USA*, **93**, 12840.
108. Baker, B. F., Lot, S. S., Condon, T. P., Cheng-Flournoy, S., Lesnik, E. A., Sasmor, H. M. and Bennett, C. F. (1997). *J. Biol. Chem.*, **272**, 11994.
109. Agrawal, S. and Goodchild, J. (1987). *Tetrahedron Lett.*, **28**, 3539.
110. Agrawal, S., Mayrand, S. H., Zamecnik, P. C., Pederson, T. (1990). *Proc. Natl Acad. Sci. USA*, **87**, 1401.
111. Shen, L. X., Kandimalla, E. R. and Agrawal, S. (1998). *Bioorg. Med. Chem.*, **6**, 1695.
112. Altmann, K.-H., Dean, N. M., Fabbro, D., Freier, S. M., Geiger, T., Haner, R., Husken, D., Martin, P., Monia, B. P., Muller, M., Natt, F., Nicklin, P., Phillips, J., Pieles, U., Sasmor, H. and Moser, H. E. (1996). *Chimia*, **50**, 168.
113. Yu, D., Iyer, R. P., Shaw, D. R., Lisziewicz, J., Li, Y., Jiang, Z., Roskey, A. and Agrawal, S. (1996). *Bioorg. Chem.*, **4**, 1685.
114. Agrawal, S., Jiang, Z., Zhao, Q., Shaw, D., Cai, Q., Roskey, A., Channavajjala, L., Saxinger, C. and Zhang, R. (1997). *Proc. Natl Acad. Sci. USA*, **94**, 2620.
115. Crooke, S. T., Graham, M. J., Zuckerman, J. E., Brooke, D., Conklin, B. S., Cummins, L. L., Greig, M. J., Guinosso, C. J., Kornbrust, D., Manoharan, M., Sasmor, H. M., Schleich, T., Tivel, K. L. and Griffey, R. H. (1996). *J. Pharmacol. Exp. Ther.*, **277**, 923.
116. Monia, B. P., Lesnik, E. A., Gonzalez, C., Lima, W.F., McGee, D., Guinosso, C.

J., Kawasaki, A. M., Cook, P. D. and Freier, S. M. (1993). *J. Biol. Chem.*, **268**, 14514.
117. Lesnik, E. A., Guinosso, C. J., Kawasaki, A. M., Sasmor, H., Zounes, M., Cummins, L. L., Ecker, D. J., Cook, P. D. and Freier, S. M. (1993). *Biochemistry*, **32**, 7832.
118. Zhang, R., Lu, Z., Zhang, H., Diasio, R. B., Habus, I., Jiang, Z., Iyer, R. P., Yu, D. and Agrawal, S. (1995). *Biochem. Pharmacol.*, **50**, 545.
119. Kandimalla, E. R., Manning, A., Zhao, Q., Shaw, D. R., Byrn, R. A., Sasisekharan, V. and Agrawal, S. (1997). *Nucleic Acids Res.*, **25**, 370.
120. Agrawal, S., Jiang, Z., Zhao, Q., Shaw, R., Sun, D. and Saxinger, C. (1997). *Nucleosides and Nucleotides*, **16**, 927.
121. Zhang, R., Iyer, R. P., Yu, D., Tan, W., Zhang, X., Lu, Z., Zhao, H. and Agrawal, S. (1996) *J. Pharmacol. Exp. Ther.*, **278**, 971.
122. Agrawal, S. and Zhao, Q. (1998). *Curr. Opin. Chem. Biol.*, **2**, 519.
123. Agrawal, S., Zhang, X., Lu, Z., Hui, Z., Tamburin, M. J., Yan, J., Cai, H., Diasio, R. B., Habus, I., Iyer, R. P., Yu, D. and Zhang, R. (1995). *Biochem. Pharmacol.*, **50**, 571.
124. Zhang, R. and Agrawal, S. (1997). In *Antisense 97: Targeting the Molecular Basis of Disease*, Abstract book, p. 58.
125. Tang, J.-Y., Temsamani, J. and Agrawal, S. (1993). *Nucleic Acids Res.*, **21**, 2729.
126. Zhang, R., Lu, Z., Zhang, X., diasio, R., Liu, T., Jiang, Z. and Agrawal, S. (1995). *Clin. Chem.*, **41**, 836.
127. Chaix, C., Iyer, R. P. and Agrawal, S. (1996). *Bioorg. Med. Chem. Lett.*, **6**, 827.
128. Iyer, R. P., Yu, D. and Agrawal, S. (1994) *Bioorg. Med. Chem. Lett.*, **4**, 2471
129. Iyer, R. P., Yu, D., Devlin, T., Ho, N.-H. and Agrawal, S. (1996) *Bioorg. Med. Chem. Lett.*, **6**, 1917.
130. Iyer, R. P., Ho, N.-H., Yu, D. and Agrawal, S. (1997) *Bioorg. Chem. Lett.*, **7**, 871.
131. Tosquellas, G., Alvarez, K., Dell'Aquila, C., Morvan, F., Vasseur, J. J., Imbach, J.-L. and Rayner, B. (1998). *Nucleic Acids Res.*, **26**, 2069.
132. Tang, J.-Y., Roskey, A., Li, Y. and Agrawal, S. (1995). *Nucleosides and Nucleotides*, **14**, 985.
133. Koziolkiewicz, M., Wojcik, M., Kobylanska, A., Karwowski, B., Rebowska, B., Guga, P. and Stec, W. J. (1997). *Antisense Nucleic Acid Drug Dev.*, **7**, 43.
134. Koziolkiewicz, M., Krakowiak, A., Kwinkowski, M., Boczkowska, M. and Stec, W. J. (1995). *Nucleic Acids Res.*, **23**, 5000.
135. Eckstein, F. (1985). *Annu. Rev. Biochem.*, **54**, 367.
136. Iyer, R. P., Guo, M.-J., Yu, D. and Agrawal, S. (1998). *Tetrahedron Lett.*, **39**, 2491.

9

Retinal neuronal development in *trk*$_B$ antisense 'knockdowns'

DENNIS W. RICKMAN

1. Introduction

Brain-derived neurotrophic factor (BDNF) and neurotrophin-4 (NT-4) are members of a family of trophic molecules, the neurotrophins—potent survival, differentiation and maintenance factors in the developing nervous system (1,2). Neurotrophins also have been shown to influence the elaboration of dendritic morphology (3), the expression of neurochemical phenotype (4–6) and the formation and maintenance of synaptic connections (7,8) of developing neurons. In the development of the mammalian retina, these molecules have emerged as important players. For example, the initial survival of retinal ganglion cells is dependent upon BDNF from central mesencephalic retinal targets (9,10). Furthermore, in the adult retina, intraocular treatment with BDNF appears to prolong the survival of ganglion cells following optic nerve trauma (11,12). NT-4 has been shown to support the survival of adult retinal ganglion cells *in vitro* (13), although no endogenous source of this ligand has been demonstrated in the visual system. Recently, BNDF has been localized to some retinal neurons as well (14), and its expression is up-regulated in response to injury (15).

The specificity of neurotrophin action is mediated through distinct high-affinity receptors which are isoforms of Trk, a receptor tyrosine kinase encoded by the *trk* proto-oncogene (16). BDNF and NT-4 are both preferentially bound by a common isoform denoted Trk$_B$. In the developing rat retina, Trk$_B$ is expressed by most cells of the neuroblastic retina and, later, by most cells in the ganglion cell layer (GCL) and many cells in the inner nuclear layer (INL) (17) (*Figure 1*).

The distribution and temporal patterns of expression of BDNF and Trk$_B$ suggest that BDNF (and/or, perhaps, NT-4) influence the survival and differentiation of both ganglion cells and retinal interneurons (amacrine and bipolar cells) (4, 14, 17, 18).

Recently, gene targeting has allowed the generation of homologous recombinant mice deficient in one or more neurotrophins or their receptors (19).

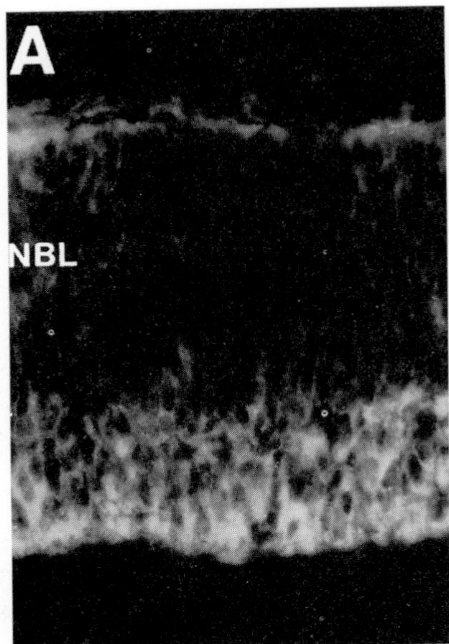

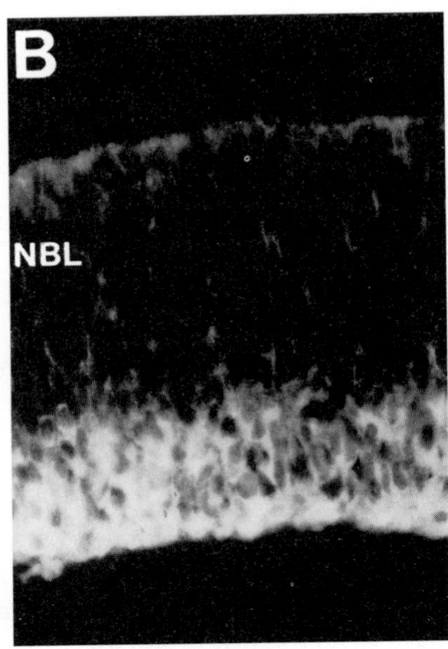

Figure 1. Fluorescence photomicrographs showing localization of Trk$_B$ immunoreactivity in the postnatal rat retina. (A) At postnatal day (PND) 0, Trk$_B$ immunoreactivity was present in numerous well-stained somata throughout the ganglion cell layer (GCL) and in bundles of fibers in the nerve fiber layer (bottom of photomicrograph). In addition, many lightly and moderately stained cells were present in the inner nuclear layer (INL). (B) At PND-10, many heavily stained cells were present in the GCL. Numerous lightly stained cells were seen in the INL at the border of the inner plexiform layer (IPL). Also, a few lightly stained cells were seen in the outer retina (ONL) (scale bar represents 50 μm). Reproduced from Rickman, D. W. and Brecha, N. C. (1995) *Visual Neurosci.*, **12**, 215, with permission of Cambridge University Press.

These models allow the study of neuronal development in animals totally lacking a specific neurotrophin or neurotrophin receptor. In BDNF-deficient mice, there is a substantial reduction in the numbers of motor neurons, resulting in a variety of motor dysfunctions (20). In addition, an analysis of cortical neuronal phenotypes in these animals has shown a decrease in the number of neuropeptide Y (NPY)-containing cells, as well as cells expressing the calcium-binding proteins, parvalbumin and calbindin (20). These molecules are believed to modulate GABA neurotransmission and regulate calcium stores, respectively. These animals generally fail to thrive, and they typically die by the end of the second postnatal week. Mice homozygous for the *trk*$_B$ deletion display an even more deleterious phenotype: they do not feed and die within the first 24–48 h after birth. Therefore a neuronal system in which there is considerable postnatal differentiation or remodeling cannot be thoroughly analyzed with these knockout models. This includes the rodent retina, which undergoes substantial phenotypic differentiation during the first two postnatal weeks and establishes functional intrinsic circuitry, as well as a mature pattern of central connections, during this time (21,22). Consequently, we were challenged to develop an intraocular antisense technique to target trk_B mRNA in the postnatal retina. This approach has allowed us to target both a particular region of the central nervous system and a discrete developmental window.

2. Neuronal differentiation in the rodent retina

In our laboratory, we are interested in the development of a specific functional neuronal circuit in the mammalian retina, namely the rod pathway. This pathway is activated during scotopic (low light level) conditions and utilizes a well-defined modular circuit composed of rod photoreceptors, rod bipolar cells, a characteristic, narrow-field amacrine cell (the AII) and ganglion cells, the retinal efferent neurons. At birth, only the ganglion cell layer has formed, separated from the thick overlying neuroblastic layer by a thin layer of neuropil, the inner plexiform layer (IPL). Initially, in the rat, ganglion cells are produced at three times the number found in the adult retina (21), and axons from these neurons reach their primary central target in the contralateral superior colliculus embryonically (22). Concomitant with development of retinotectal innervation is the maturation of ganglion cell dendritic arborizations within the IPL. During the first two postnatal weeks, these neurons undergo considerable morphological differentiation, establishing both a definitive pattern of target innervation and a characteristic dendritic morphology in the IPL.

During this early postnatal period, there is also the emergence of populations of interneurons, including bipolar and amacrine cells. In the mammalian retina, rod bipolar cells comprise a homogeneous neuronal population that is a convergent element from rod photoreceptors to ganglion cells. Within the IPL of the rat retina, the signal from rod bipolar to ganglion cell is transferred via ribbon synapses through AII amacrine cells (23,24). Thus, the rod pathway in the rat is similar to that in other mammalian species (25).

The AII amacrine cell is a well-characterized, obligatory element of the rod pathway. It is a narrow-field, bistratified neuron that is interposed between rod bipolar cells and ganglion cells (25,26). The AII amacrine cell body is located near the INL/IPL border and gives rise to a single stout primary dendrite that descends into the IPL. In the distal IPL short side branches ('lobular appendages') end in characteristic swellings, while in the proximal IPL the dendrites arborize, forming a dense plexus. The AII makes glycinergic synapses with OFF-cone bipolar cells and OFF-ganglion cells and contacts ON-cone bipolar cells by gap junctions (23,24,27,28). In the rat retina, the AII has been identified by intracellular injection of Lucifer Yellow and by antibodies to parvalbumin (23,29–31). In the rat, parvalbumin immunoreactivity labels two populations of amacrine cells. The predominant population is the AII, while a smaller population of wide-field amacrine cells is also labeled (24,30). Furthermore, in the rat, as in several other mammalian species, the AII amacrine cell body is surrounded by dopaminergic fibers which form characteristic 'rings' at the INL/IPL border (32). In the rat, parvalbumin-immunoreactive neurons are first detected in the INL at about postnatal day (PND) 5, but the final distribution of parvalbumin-immunoreactive cells is not achieved for several weeks (33).

The observation that parvalbumin immunoreactivity is down-regulated in certain brain regions of BDNF-deficient mice, suggested that BDNF might be a regulator of parvalbumin expression in the retina and, perhaps, a regulator of AII amacrine cell differentiation. Indeed, in the early postnatal wild-type mouse retina, antibodies to parvalbumin label numerous cells in the INL and GCL plus a dense plexus of processes in the IPL, whereas in BDNF-knockout animals, parvalbumin immunostaining is very much reduced. However, by PND-10, parvalbumin fails to label any cells in the mouse retina. Thus we were again challenged to devise an alternative strategy for analyzing the development of this neuronal phenotype in the mammalian rod pathway.

3. Antisense oligonucleotides in suppression of retinal proteins

The recent development of a method for targeting specific mRNA species provided us with the opportunity to study the role of neurotrophic factors and their receptors in the postnatal differentiation of specific neuronal populations in the rat retina. For our studies this was important for three reasons:

(1) Neurotrophin- and *trk*-deficient mice did not survive through the temporal window of retinal differentiation.
(2) The specific phenotypic marker (parvalbumin) that we were interested in was not expressed in the mouse retina (as in many other mammalian species).
(3) The rat retina is a well-understood functional model in terms of anatomy and physiology.

Thus we were not confined to an analysis of the BDNF- or *trk*$_B$-knockout mouse retina. Although much is known about the development of the mouse retina, particularly in terms of photoreceptor development and synaptogenesis in the outer retina, less is known about the morphology of retinal ganglion cell types and discrete populations of immunohistochemically identifed phenotypes of retinal interneurons.

Previous studies in other laboratories have used antisense oligodeoxynucleotides (ODNs) to suppress expression of specific retinal proteins by introducing into the eye an ODN whose sequence is complementary to a targeted mRNA (34,35). In theory, this antisense strand of DNA hybridizes to the targeted mRNA and prevents its translation and/or destablilizes the mRNA such that it is rapidly degraded. Both processes prevent expression of the protein encoded by the targeted mRNA.

In developing chick retina, intraocular treatment with an antisense ODN to a neuronal-specific protein (synaptosome-associated protein, SNAP-25) on two consecutive days suppressed expression of SNAP-25 by 75% for 4 days *in vivo* (36). In the adult rabbit, introcular injection of an antisense ODN to kinesin, an axoplasmic transport-related ATPase, reduced kinesin expression by 87% in 16 h (37). In order to selectively target the expression of trk_B, the high-affinity receptor for BDNF, in the rat retina, we have used intraocular injections of antisense ODN directed to a specific region of the trk_B mRNA.

4. Design of a specific antisense oligonucleotide targeted to the trk_B mRNA

Generally, ODNs oriented in the antisense direction are designed to bind to single-stranded RNA and are assumed to act by preventing translation of a specific mRNA. In order to achieve this goal, we strove to meet several criteria:

(1) The ODN must be designed to optimize its entry into the cell, presumably by receptor-mediated endocytosis. It should be of sufficient length to recognize a unique mammalian RNA sequence, yet small enough to be readily taken up (18- to 20-mer).

(2) The ODN must be able to resist degradation by nucleases; this can be accomplished by modifying the nucleic acid phosphate group. We chose to use thiolated ODNs in which one non-bridging internucleotide oxygen was replaced with a sulfur resiue. This alteration preserves the poly-anionic character and aqueous solubility of the molecule, but also increases the resistance of the molecule to nuclease metabolism.

(3) To avoid toxicity, we used sterile ODNs that had been purified by high performance liquid chromatography (HPLC).

The nucleotide sequence of rat full-length trk_B was obtained from the GenBank database. ODNs, in the sense and antisense orientations, were designed as follows: We first identified the initiator methionine (AUG) (nucleotide 665). From that point, we counted 15 nucleotides in both the 3′ and 5′ directions. Within that span we searched for an 18- to 20-mer that had:

- an equal number of purines and pyrimidines;
- a terminal purine at each end; and
- a minimum number of single nucleotide repeats.

For full-length trk_B, such an ODN spanned the nucleotides 651–670. A trk_B sense nucleotide was identified as 5′-ACTGGCAGCTCGGGATGTCG-3′.

The antisense nucleotide, complementary to that sequence, was 5′-CGACATCCCGAGCTGCCAGT-3′. As an additional control, we used the same criteria to identify a sequence from the non-coding region. The determined ODNs were then synthesized by a commercial supplier (National Biosciences, Plymouth, MN, USA).

4.1 Delivery of oligonucleotides to the eye

Oligonucleotides oriented in either the sense or antisense direction were injected into the vitreal chamber of neonatal and early postnatal rats following a defined regimen (PND-0; PND-0, PND-3 and PND-7; or PND-5 and PND-10). Rat pups were lightly anesthetized by inhalation of Metafane. With the aid of a dissecting microscope, the palpebral fissure was visualized and opened with a scalpel. Using a lateral approach, the ODN solution was delivered with a Hamilton syringe equipped with a sterile 30 gauge needle. Care was taken not to pierce the lens capsule, and 2 μl of a 10 μM solution was slowly injected into the vitreal cavity. The eye was then coated with antibiotic ointment and the animal was returned to the litter. When multiple injections were performed over several days, we attempted to use the same scleral injection site in order to minimize trauma to the eye. Eyes that demonstrated evidence of infection were not analyzed.

On various days following injection (PND-10 or PND-15), animals were killed and their retinas were fixed in 4% paraformaldehyde and processed for immunohistochemistry using polyclonal antibodies specific to the Trk isoforms (Santa Cruz Biotechnology, Santa Cruz, CA, USA). Alternatively, retinas were dissected and RNA was extracted for Northern blot analysis and probed using a ^{32}P-labeled PCR-derived fragment of *trk*$_B$ cDNA (nucleotides 1362–1558 of full-length *trk*$_B$).

4.2 Suppression of Trk$_B$ expression in the retina

Immunostaining revealed that in retinas treated with a *trk*$_B$ sense ODN, both Trk$_A$ and Trk$_B$ were present at normal levels. As in the normal, untreated retina, staining was present in numerous neurons in the GCL and INL and in fibers in the IPL and nerve fiber layer. In retinas treated with a specific *trk*$_B$ antisense ODN, 5′-CGACATCCCGAGCTGCCAGT-3′, Trk$_A$-immunoreactivity was present at normal levels while Trk$_B$ was greatly reduced in all retinal regions (*Figure 2*). This homogeneity of Trk$_B$ suppression was a surprising finding, but indicated that intravitreal delivery of an ODN was an effective route to target the retina. We examined retinas on sequential days and determined that our treatment regimens created temporal windows of Trk$_B$ suppression. The effect was noted as soon as 48 h following a single antisense ODN treatment and persisted for at least 72 h. In retinas examined after 96 h, however, immunostaining appeared no different from that in sense-treated or untreated controls.

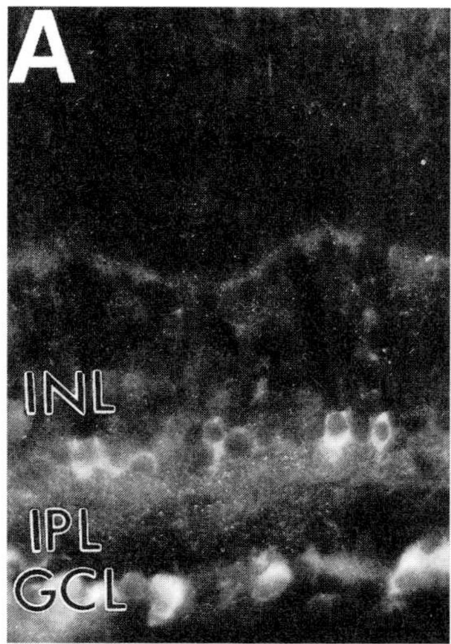

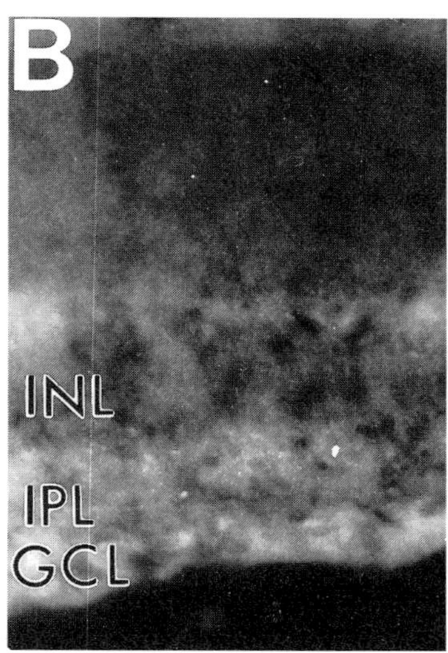

Figure 2. Fluorescence photomicrograph showing normal and antisense-suppressed Trk_B immunoreactivity in the postnatal day (PND) 10 rat retina. (A) Trk_B immnoreactivity in a retina that received intraocular injection of a trk_B sense strand of DNA on PND-0, -3 and -7. Immunostaining is localized to cells in both the ganglion cell layer (GCL) and inner nuclear layer (INL). (B) Trk_B immunoreactivity in the contralateral retina that received intraocular injection (10 μM) of a trk_B antisense strand of DNA on PND-0, -3 and -7. No specific immunostaining was observed. Reproduced, with permission, from Rickman, D.W. and Bowes Rickman, C. (1996) *Proc. Natl Acad. Sci. USA*, **93**, 12564. Copyright 1996 National Academy of Sciences, USA.

To determine if Trk_B protein suppression was a result of an effect on trk_B gene transcription, we also analyzed the levels of trk_B mRNA by Northern blot at 24 h intervals following antisense treatment (*Figure 3*). At all time points examined (PND-1, PND-2 and PND-10) no differences were detected between sense- and antisense-treated retinas. This suggested that the observed suppression of Trk_B expression was a result of an effect on protein translation and not gene transcription.

4.3 Effects on a retinal neuronal phenotype

Intraocular treatment with either trk_B sense or antisense ODNs did not result in any obvious morphological alterations of the retina. As described earlier, our primary interest is in the development of a specific functional circuit in the mammalian retina—the rod pathway. Studies of BDNF-knockout mice had revealed that certain immunohistochemically identified neuronal phenotypes were altered in selected brain regions. Specifically, the calcium-binding proteins, parvalbumin and calbindin, were down-regulated in widespread, but different, neuronal populations (20). In the rat retina, both of these calcium-

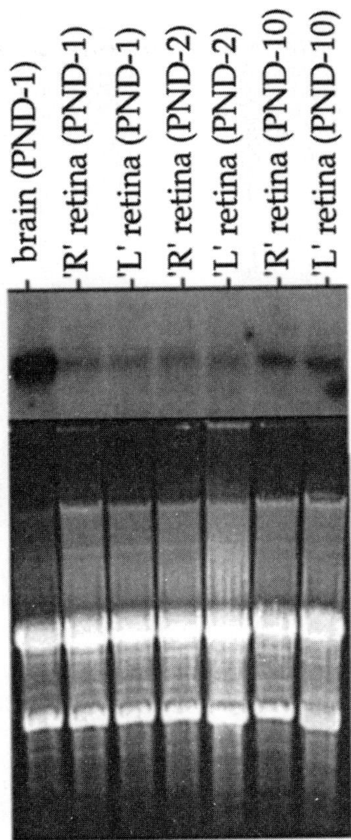

Figure 3. Northern blot (above) and denaturing agarose gel (below) of rat total RNA (10 μg/lane). The rat tissue from which total RNA was isolated and the age at time of isolation are indicated above each lane. In each case, the right eye ('R') received *trk*$_B$ antisense ODN injection and the left eye ('L') received no injection on postnatal day (PND)-0. Retinas were then isolated on PND-1 or -2. The last two lanes show RNA from retinas that received subsequent injections on PND-3 and -7. These retinas were isolated on PND-10. The Northern blot was probed with a PCR-derived, ^{32}P-labeled fragment of *trk*$_B$ cDNA (nucleotides 1362–1558 of full-length *trk*$_B$). There was no difference in size or relative abundance of *trk*$_B$ mRNA 24 or 48 h following antisense treatment, nor following multiple antisense injections. Reproduced, with permission, from Rickman, D.W. and Bowes Rickman, C. (1996) *Proc. Natl Acad. Sci. USA*, **93**, 12564. Copyright 1996 National Academy of Sciences, USA.

binding proteins label populations of retinal interneurons. Parvalbumin immunoreactivity reveals, primarily, a dense population of narrow-field, bistratified amacrine cells, the AIIs (29).

In normal, untreated retinas and in retinas treated with the sense ODN, numerous heavily stained cells in the GCL (presumed ganglion cells), as well

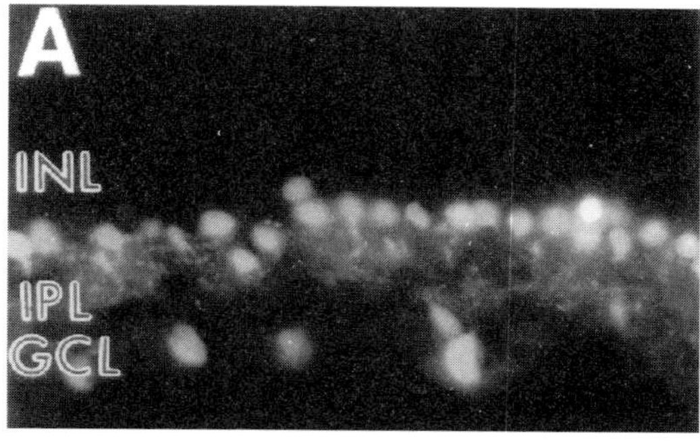

Figure 4. Fluorescence photomicrographs showing the localization of parvalbumin immunoreactivity in the rat retina. (A) The pattern of parvalbumin immunoreactivity in the postnatal day (PND)-10 rat retina that received intraocular injection of *trk*$_B$ sense ODN on PND-0, -3 and -7. Parvalbumin immunoreactivity is localized primarily to numerous cells at the border of the inner nuclear layer (INL) and inner plexiform layer (IPL) (presumed AII amacrine cells), and to some cells in the ganglion cell layer (GCL). (B) The pattern of parvalbumin immunoreactivity in the PND-10 rat retina that received intraocular injection of *trk*$_B$ antisense ODN on PND-0, -3 and -7. The number of parvalbumin-immunoreactive cells in the INL is greatly reduced. In addition, most labeled cells are only faintly stained. Reproduced, with permission, from Rickman, D.W. and Bowes Rickman, C. (1996) *Proc. Natl Acad. Sci. USA*, **93**, 12564. Copyright 1996 National Academy of Sciences, USA.

as some smaller, lightly stained cells (small ganglion cells or displaced amacrine cells) were present. In retinas treated with the *trk*$_B$ antisense ODN, however, parvalbumin immunoreactivity was greatly reduced (*Figure 4*). This was evidenced by both a reduced number of immunostained cells and by a decreased intensity of immunostaining. Studies using an antibody to calbindin yielded identical patterns of immunostaining in both sense- and antisense-treated retinas. Together, these studies suggest that the ligands for Trk$_B$, BDNF and, perhaps, NT-4 have very selective effects on phenotypic expression in specific populations of retinal neurons. These subtle alterations in retinal neuronal phenotypic expression could not have been appreciated with other currently available techniques. The selectivity of this downstream effect on parvalbumin expression provides further evidence of the specificity of our antisense treatment.

5. Summary of results

5.1 Knockdowns versus knockouts

The development of an antisense ODN approach for targeting specific mRNAs has provided us with a unique experimental opportunity that was not available with other conventional technologies. In many instances, knockout animals with null mutation of a specific gene are suitable models to answer a developmental question. However, this technique can be problematic. In the case of trk_B knockouts, for example, animals fail to survive, hence resulting in a lethal mutation.

Furthermore, one must be conservative in the interpretation of effects on a particular cellular phenotype in systemic knockouts. In our own studies of neurotrophins, we are confronted with a system in which there are numerous, confounding, redundancies. Retinal ganglion cells, for example, appear to express both the Trk_A and Trk_B isoforms of the high-affinity neurotrophin receptor (17). In BDNF-deficient animals the number of retinal ganglion cells is not reduced, suggesting that multiple trophic factors contribute to their survival.

Finally, it is difficult to determine the cascade of genetic regulatory events triggered by deletion of a single gene during the developmental period. Thus a single deletion may result in the up- or down-regulation of numerous other mRNAs and encoded proteins.

5.2 Targeting to the retina

In our system, an advantage of the antisense technique over conventional knockout methods is the relative ease of targeting to a discrete tissue. In studies of the central nervous system, the retina is a particularly accessible target, requiring minimal surgical intervention. Furthermore, the retina, and other ocular structures, present a minimal barrier to uptake from the vitreous fluid. This may be particularly attractive in areas of the anterior chamber and retinal pigmented epithelium which are involved in fluid flow.

Our initial studies used 'naked' ODNs, but recently developed methods allow one to incorporate antisense ODNs into viral vectors for prolonged delivery to a target tissue (38). Presumably, long-term suppression of a specific gene product could be achieved using this technique. Such an approach holds not only experimental, but also therapeutic, promise. Another advantage of the antisense strategy is the ability to target a specific temporal window. For our studies of the AII amacrine cell, we relied upon prior knowledge of the ontogeny of parvalbumin immunoreactivity in the retina and designed our experiments to target trk_B mRNA during that developmental window.

5.3 Interpretation of results

A key consideration in the interpretation of antisense experiments is the design of appropriate control studies. These might include the corresponding sense strand or a random, missense ODN of similar characteristics (length, purine:pyrimidine ratio, etc.) to the particular experimental antisense ODN. The interpretation of results also requires determination of the time-course and degree of the suppressive effect. This can be accomplished by immunohistochemical or Western blot analysis. In addition, Northern blot analysis can provide an indication of the intracellular action of antisense ODNs. The ODN may act solely at the level of protein translation or it may, in turn, have a suppressive effect upon mRNA transcription. In our own studies, presented here, we concluded that application of antisense ODNs targeted to the trk_B mRNA resulted in suppression of Trk_B protein, but had no effect upon trk_B gene transcription. Hence, levels of Trk_B protein returned to normal in a short period of time.

Another important control is the demonstration of a specific downstream effect of antisense treatment. In our studies, we observed a specific suppressive effect upon the calcium-binding protein, parvalbumin. On the other hand, another retinal calcium-binding protein, calbindin, was unaffected by antisense treatment. This is a convincing observation, and may serve well when other analyses are not feasible.

Acknowledgements

This work was supported by NIH grant EY11389 and Regeneron Pharmaceuticals Inc.

References

1. Maisonpierre, P.C., Belluscio, L., Friedman, B., Alderson, F.R., Wiegand, S.J., Furth, M.E., Lindsay, R.M. and Yancoupoulos, G.D. (1990). *Neuron*, **5**, 501.
2. Eide, F.F., Lowenstein, D.H. and Reichardt, L.F. (1993). *Exp. Neurol.*, **121**, 200.
3. Snider, W.D. (1988). *J. Neurosci.*, **8**, 2628.
4. Rickman, D.W. and Bowes Rickman, C. (1996). *Proc. Natl Acad. Sci. USA*, **93**, 12564.
5. Lindsay, R.M. and Harmar, A.J. (1989). *Nature*, **341**, 149.
6. Vedder, H., Affolter, H.-U. and Otten, U. (1993). *Neuropeptides*, **24**, 351.
7. Garofalo, L., Ribeiro-da-Silva, A. and Cuello, A.C. (1992). *Proc. Natl Acad. Sci. USA*, **89**, 2639.
8. Lohof, A.M., Ip, N.Y. and Poo, M.-M. (1993). *Nature*, **363**, 350
9. Cohen-Cory, S. and Fraser, S.E. (1994). *Neuron*, **12**, 747.

10. Rickman, D.W., Lauterbor, J., Brecha, N.C. and Gall, C.M. (1992). *Soc. Neurosci. Abstr.*, **18**, 225.
11. Mey, J. and Thanos, S. (1993). *Brain Res.*, **602**, 302.
12. Mansour-Robaey, S., Clarke, D.B., Wang, Y.-C., Bray, G.M. and Aguayo, A.J. (1994). *Proc. Natl Acad. Sci. USA*, **91**, 1632.
13. Cohen, A., Bray, G.M. and Aguayo, A.J. (1994). *J. Neurobiol.*, **25**, 953.
14. Perez, M.-T.R. and Caminos, E. (1995) *Neurosci. Lett.*, **183**, 96.
15. Gao, H., Qiao, X., Hefti, F., Hollyfield, J.G. and Knusel, B. (1997). *Investig. Ophthalmol. Vision Sci.*, **38**, 1840.
16. Barbacid, M. (1994). *J. Neurobiol.*, **25**, 1386.
17. Rickman, D.W. and Brecha, N.C. (1995). *Visual Neurosci.*, **12**, 215.
18. Cellerino, A. and Kohler, K. (1997). *J. Comp. Neurol.*, **385**, 1.
19. Snider, W.D. (1994). *Cell*, **77**, 627.
20. Jones, R.J., Farinas, I., Backus, C. and Reichardt, L.F. (1994). *Cell*, **76**, 989.
21. Perry, V.H., Henderson, Z. and Linden, R. (1983). *J. Comp. Neurol.*, **219**, 356.
22. Yhip, J.P.A. and Kirby, M.A. (1990). *Vision Neurosci.*, **4**, 313.
23. Chun, M.H., Han, S.H., Chung, J.W. and Wassle, H. (1993). *J. Comp. Neurol.*, **332**, 421.
24. Stretoi, E., Raviola, E. and Dacheux, R.F. (1992). *J. Comp. Neurol.*, **325**, 152.
25. Wässle, H. and Boycott, B.B. (1991). *Physiol. Rev.*, **71**, 447.
26. Boos, R., Schneider, H. and Wässle, H. (1993). *J. Neurosci.*, **13**, 2874.
27. Famiglietti, E.V. and Kolb, H. (1975). *Brain Res.*, **84**, 293.
28. Sterling, P. (1983). *Annu. Rev. Neurosci.*, **6**, 149.
29. Wässle, H., Grünert, U. and Rohrenbeck, J. (1993). *J. Comp. Neurol.*, **332**, 407.
30. Sanna, P.P., Keyser, K.T., Celio, M.R., Karten, H.J. and Bloom, F.E. (1993). *Brain Res.*, **600**, 141.
31. Endo, T., Kobaysahi, M., Kobayshi, S. and Onaya, T. (1986) *Cell Tiss. Res.*, **243**, 213.
32. Voigt, T. and Wässle, H. (1987). *J. Neurosci.*, **7**, 4115.
33. Guo, Q.X., Yu, M.C., Garey, L.J. and Jen, L.S. (1992). *Exp. Brain Res.*, **90**, 359.
34. Eng, L.F. (1993). In Waxman, S.G. (Ed.), *Molecular and Cellular Approaches to the Treatment of Neurological Diseases*, pp. 293–310. Raven, New York.
35. Wahlestedt, C. (1994). *Trends Pharmacol. Sci.*, **15**, 42.
36. Osen-Sand, A., Catsicas, M., Staple, J.K., Jones, K.A., Ayala, G., Knowles, J., Grenningloh, G. and Catsicas, S. (1993). *Nature,* **364**, 445.
37. Amaratana, A., Morin, P. J., Kosik, K. S. and Fine, R. E. (1993). *J. Biol. Chem.*, **268**, 17427.
38. Phillips, M.I. (1997). *Hypertension,* **29**, 177.

10

Pluronic gel as a means of antisense delivery

DAVID L. BECKER, JUN SHENG LIN and COLIN R. GREEN

1. Introduction

Antisense oligodeoxynucleotides (ODNs) have considerable potential as agents for the manipulation of specific gene expression (1,2). There are, however, still some difficulties in the technique which need to be overcome, such as the short half-life of ODNs and how to deliver the ODNs consistently and reliably to target tissues. Unmodified phosphodiester oligomers (POs) typically have an intracellular half-life of only 20 min owing to intracellular nuclease degradation (2) and phosphorothioate and methylphosphonate ODNs are often used, being readily available and nuclease resistant. In general, though, these have a weaker affinity than PO ODNs, can be less efficient at entering the cells and can cause non-specific inhibition by binding to essential proteins (2,3). Because the probes are rapidly broken down within the cells, they need to be constantly replenished. This is linked to a second problem: the probes need to be delivered accurately and consistently to the target tissues over a period of time if the treatment is going to be effective.

We have developed a novel method using Pluronic gel to deliver antisense ODNs to a variety of tissues which goes some way to overcoming these problems (4). Pluronic F-127 gel (BASF Corp.) has the advantage that it is liquid at low temperatures, but rapidly sets at physiological temperatures. It therefore provides a delivery vehicle that is simple to use and applicable to a number of systems, including the developing chick embryo (*in ovo*), tissues *in vivo*, tissue culture and organ culture. Our approach overcomes the effect of intracellular nuclease activity by providing, for a period, a constant source of unmodified ODNs from the gel, thereby reducing artefacts which can occur at higher dose levels including non-specific imperfectly matched mRNA binding (5,6) and accumulation of nucleotide and nucleoside breakdown products which can affect cell proliferation and differentiation (2). The gel can be accurately placed on to the target tissue, thereby providing accurate spatio-temporal control of gene expression. In a modification of the technique, plugs of ODN-containing gel can be delivered directly into tissues. The Pluronic gel–antisense oligonucleotide approach may have a wide variety of applications provided that sufficient attention is paid to the antisense ODN design and that appropriate control experiments are carried out (2).

We have used antisense to modify the expression of an electrical synapse or gap junction protein (connexin 43) in a variety of nervous system applications, including the early nervous system of the developing chick embryo (*in ovo*), (Fig. 1) the rat brain *in vivo*, brain slices in organ culture and dissociated neurons in tissue culture. Our start point was to characterize the time course of the expression pattern of this connexin in these systems using immunocytochemistry combined with confocal microscopy (4). Once the expression pattern has been determined, antisense applications are targeted, spatially and temporally, to take effect prior to peak expression of the connexin during a particular developmental or wound healing event. In the developing chick embryo these events include the fusion of the spinal cord, the migration of neural crest and the development of the early eye cup and the otocyst, during all of which high levels of connexin 43 are expressed. FITC tagging of the ODNs demonstrated their entry into the treated tissues. Immunostaining and confocal microscopy are used to reveal the time course of knockdown and recovery of the connexin in the target tissue (Fig. 2). By blocking translation, rather than transcription, we thus appear to have eliminated compensation by other homologous proteins. Reduction in connexin 43 expression in the developing chick embryos results in developmental defects in the tissues in which it is normally expressed. These defects include failure of neural tube fusion, neural crest associated defects, reductions in cell proliferation within the developing eye cup and problems with the invagination of the otocyst, indicating a role for this connexin during these developmental events (4, 12).

2. Methods

Protocol 1. Pluronic gel and antisense preparation

Equipment and reagents

- Pluronic F-127 gel (BASF corp)
- PBS (made up with molecular grade water)
- Oligodeoxynucleotides (ODN's) Antisense, sense and random controls
- Ice
- 0.5–10 μl Eppendorf pipette
- Sterile crystal tips

Method

1. Prepare a 25–50%[a] solution of Pluronic F-127 gel (BASF Corp.) in phosphate-buffered saline (molecular grade water).[b]
2. Add ODNs, antisense, sense or random controls, at desired concentration,[c] and thoroughly vortex several times.[d]

3. Aliquot gel into 1500 μl molecular grade Eppendorf tubes and store at –80°C until ready for use.

[a] The percentage concentration of gel determines the softness and persistence of the gel. Higher concentrations of gel set more quickly and remain in place longer before dissolving. Different concentrations should be tested for your system but for most purposes a 30% solution is best.
[b] The gel can take 24–48 h to dissolve owing to the properties of the gel, which is only liquid between 0°C and 4°C. It is best made up on a shaker in a cold room.
[c] We have found that ODN concentrations of 0.5–1.0 μM are most effective. With concentrations above 10 μM we have observed non-specific toxic effects but this may vary with the ODN sequence. Preliminary screening for the characterization of ODN efficacy is essential and should be carried out at concentrations between 0.05 and 50 μM.
[d] For some ODNs addition of 1% DMSO to the gel increases the efficacy of the antisense, presumably by increasing the amount that enters the tissue.

Protocol 2. Pluronic gel application to chick embryos *in ovo*

Equipment and reagents

- Fertilized white leghorn chicken eggs
- Egg incubator
- 70% Alcohol
- Fine forceps
- Fine scissors
- Sellotape
- 10 ml and 1 ml Syringe
- 27G and 27W grade needles
- 30% India ink in PBS (Sterile)
- Ice
- ODNs in Pluronic gel
- 0.5–10 μl Eppendorf pipette
- Sterile crystal tips

Method

1. Incubate fertilized White Leghorn eggs at 38°C and stage them according to Hamburger and Hamilton stages (7). On removal from the incubator, rotate eggs ten times to ensure that the embryo is floating free at the top of the egg.
2. Clean eggs with 70% alcohol and then, using fine sterile forceps, make a small hole in the blunt end of the egg, where the air sac is found. Insert a 27 ga hypodermic needle vertically through the hole to the bottom of the egg and withdraw a small amount (<1 ml) of albumin.
3. Place cellophane tape over the top of the egg and make a small hole through the tape and shell using forceps. Now, using small fine scissors, cut a larger hole or window from this start point in the top of the shell[a] (8).
4. Using fine forceps, gently open the vitelline and amniotic membranes over the area to be treated. Take care not to damage the embryo or associated blood vessels.[b]
5. Apply 5–10 μl of Pluronic gel to the target site using a chilled 0.5–10 μl Eppendorf with a crystal tip.[c] Because the gel sets rapidly at temperatures above 4°C it is essential to work swiftly during the

Protocol 2. *Continued*

application process. Drops of gel, between 5–10 μl, can be placed with high accuracy on parts of an embryo, tissue or organ culture. Drops will mould around the site of application and set in place as they do so (*Figure 1*). The volume of the drops can be varied as required for the experiment and applications can be repeated at later time points if required.

6. Seal eggs with cellophane tape and replace them in the incubator until ready for analysis. In most cases embryos can be analyzed after 48 h.[d]

[a] Take care not to point the scissors downwards or you will cut through all of the membranes and reduce the chances of the embryo surviving.
[b] At very early stages of development, a 30% India ink/PBS solution can be injected under the amniotic sac using a 27 ga needle to reveal the outline and therefore the stage of the embryo.
[c] Keep the Eppendorf tips on ice during the experiment. Use a fresh tip for every application.
[d] An exception is for the time-course analysis of connexin protein knockdown and recovery when embryos are examined at 2, 4, 8, 18, 24, 36 and 48 h.

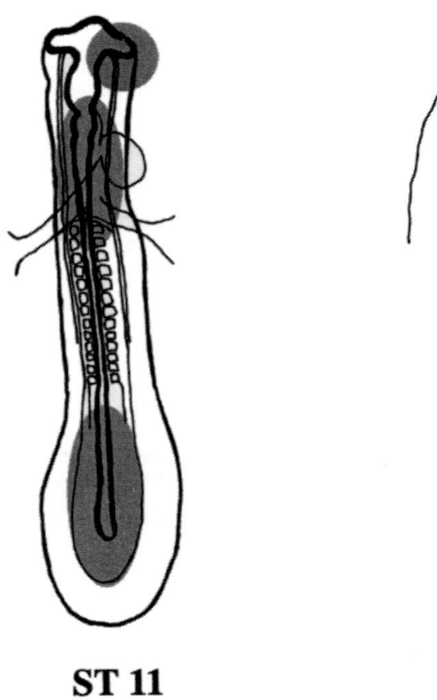

Figure 1. Line diagrams of stage 11 (ST 11) and stage 13 (ST 13) chick embryos indicating sites and extent of placement of Pluronic gel. Gel positioning is indicated with shading. Five-microliter drops can cover half of the face or one end of the neural tube whereas 10 μl would be required to cover the whole of the whole of the early neural tube adequately.

Protocol 3. Application of Pluronic gel plugs into rat brain lesions

Equipment and reagents

- Appropriate anaesthetics and operating instruments
- Stereotaxic frame
- Dental Drill
- Micromanipulator
- 27G 1/2 gauge needle with flattened (cut off) tip
- 1 ml syringe
- Cut down yellow tip to couple Eppendorf to syringe
- Ice
- ODNs in Pluronic gel
- 0.5–10 μl Eppendorf pipette
- Sterile crystal tips
- PBS (sterile)
- Hydrogen peroxide

Method

1. Anesthetize the animal and hold its head in a stereotaxic clamping device. Shave the region around the lesion site, slit the skin with a scalpel and pull it back to leave the skull plates clear. Drill a 0.5 mm diameter hole through the skull plate using a hand drill or dentist's drill. Make a lesion using a 27G 1/2 gauge syringe needle attached to a micrometer stage.[a]
2. File the tip from a 27G 1/2 gauge syringe needle so that it is flat (*Figure 3*). Cool the needle on ice. Attach the syringe needle to an Eppendorf pipette via a cut-down yellow pipette tip. Use this device to suck 10 μl ice-cold Pluronic gel containing the ODN of interest (or a control ODN) into the precooled needle. Allow the gel to set as the needle warms to room temperature.
3. Transfer the needle with the gel plug at its tip to a 1 ml syringe containing sterile PBS. Place a sleeve over the needle shaft so that it can be lowered into the lesion with the sleeve (coming up against the skull) preventing over-penetration. Gentle pressure on the syringe plunger will eject the gel plug out of the needle into the lesion.[b]
4. Treat the wound with hydrogen peroxide to stop any bleeding and suture the skin back into place. Monitor animals carefully and leave until ready to be killed.[c]

[a] In our experiments lesions were made 2 mm into the cortex. The micrometer allows accurate directional control and the precise stereotaxic penetration depth in creating the lesion.
[b] This can be felt, though not seen, by the operator. The gel cannot be expelled using the volumetric pipette.
[c] For our experiments, where we expected to knock down connexin 43 expression for up to 48 h after lesioning, animals were killed at 24 and 48 h and at 12 days.

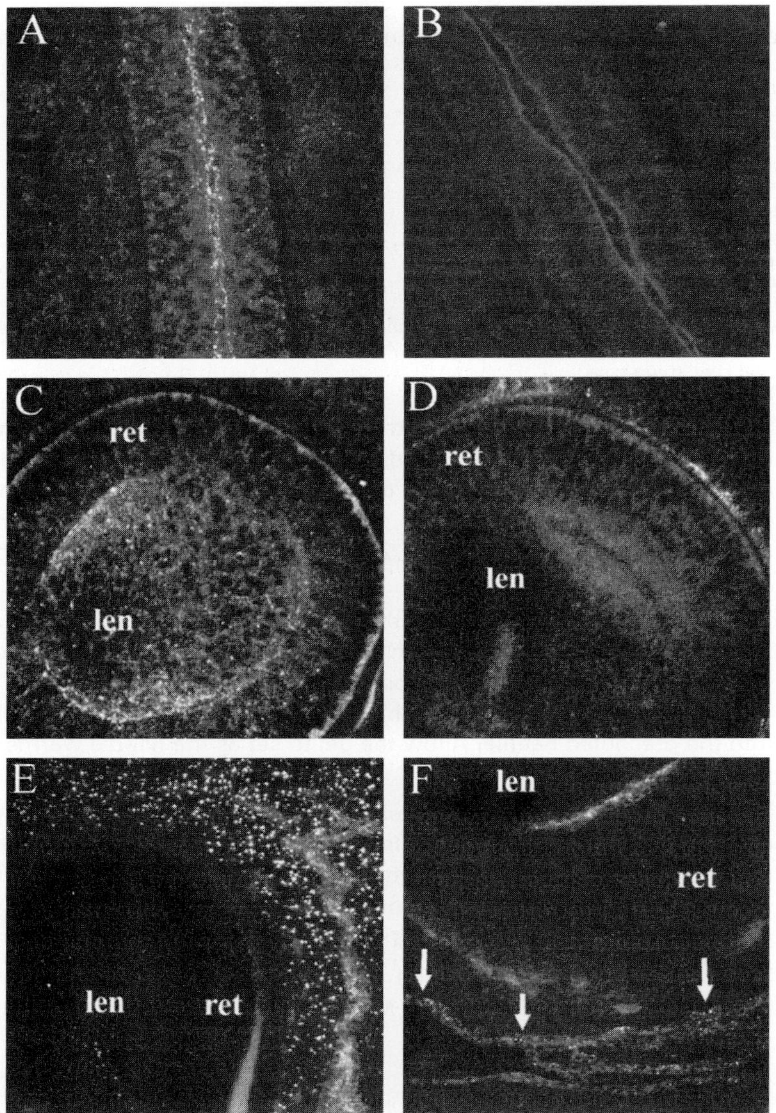

3. Tips for a successful experiment

1. Several control experiments should always be carried out in parallel, including the use of Pluronic gel alone, Pluronic gel with sense, and Pluronic gel with random ODNs. Ideally the application and analysis of the experiment should be carried out blind.

Figure 2. Immunohistochemical localization of gap junction proteins in the chick embryo eye and spinal cord after connexin 43-specific antisense oligonucleotide or control oligonucleotide applications. Confocal laser scanning microscopy images of the neural tube of the chick show that it has high ectodermal connexin 43 expression around the point of fusion in normal embryos and embryos treated with sense control (A); the level of expression is dramatically reduced following treatment with antisense oligonucleotides 18 h prior to antibody labeling (B) (note the poor fusion of the cord). Reduction in connexin 43 expression is very specific, as shown by immunohistochemical labeling of developing eyes in stage 18–19 chick embryos treated with antisense ODN over the head region at stage 11–12. Connexin 43 labeling is high in the retina ('ret') and newly invaginated lens ('len') of control-treated embryos (C). Embryos treated with connexin 43-specific antisense ODN show a major reduction in connexin 43 protein labeling in the retina and lens (D) but levels of connexin 32 (E) and connexin 26 (F, arrows) are the same as in controls (expressed in the mesenchyme and epithelium, respectively, at this stage). Reproduced in a modified form from (4) Dev. Genetics 24, 33–42 (1999) with permission.

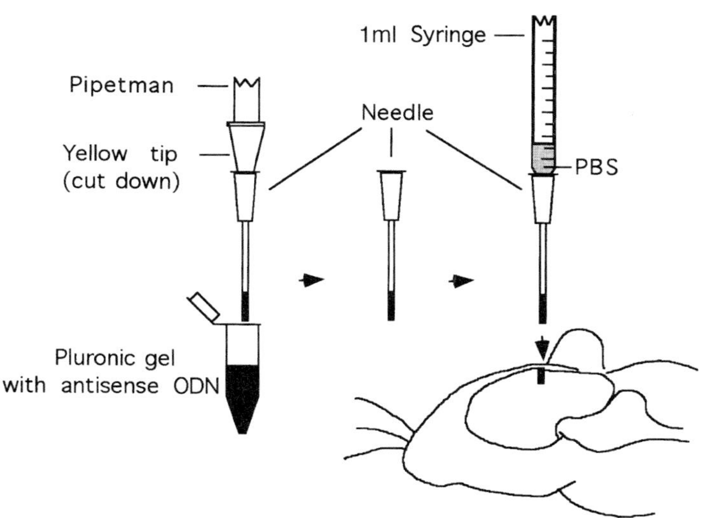

Figure 3. A method for loading a Pluronic gel plug containing antisense ODN into an organ, in this case the rat brain. A precise volume of gel containing the ODN is sucked up into a precooled 27G 1/2 syringe needle which has been filed down so as to have a flattened tip. The modified needle is attached to an Eppendorf pipette via a cut-down yellow tip, allowing precise volumes to be sucked into the needle. The gel is allowed to set as the needle warms up, and the needle is transferred to a 1 ml syringe containing PBS. The needle is then inserted into a pre-prepared lesion in the organ and gentle pressure applied to the syringe plunger until the gel plugs 'pop' out. The volumetric pipette itself cannot apply sufficient pressure to displace the gel plug, but carefully applied hydraulic pressure from the syringe will inject the gel plug into the lesioned organ.

Protocol 4. Application to brain slices or dissociated neurons in culture

Equipment and reagents

- Dissection kit
- Vibratome or wire brain slicer
- Chilled oxygenated Ringer's solution
- Tissue culture facilities
- Opti-MEM low serum medium (Gibco, UK)
- Ice
- ODNs in Pluronic gel
- 0.5–10 µl Eppendorf pipette
- Sterile crystal tips

Method

1. Kill the animal humanely by cervical dislocation or decapitation, then dissect the brain free as quickly as possible and place it in chilled oxygenated Ringer's solution.
2. Take slices rapidly using either a Vibratome or wire slice and transfer them to appropriate tissue culture medium. Incubate as appropriate for the tissue. Allowed to acclimatize in an incubator at 37°C for 1 h. Alternatively, dissociate the tissue, plate it out at appropriate cell densities required for tissue culture and allow cells to adhere to the dish or attain desired confluence.
3. Remove the standard medium and rinse the slices or cells with Opti-MEM low serum medium[a] (Gibco, UK). Remove the Opti-MEM and quickly apply Pluronic gel to the desired part of the slice or area of the cultured cells using the application conditions described in *Protocol 2*. Replace the Opti-MEM and return the preparation to the incubator for 24–48 h before analysis.

[a] Serum-free medium is preferable as this reduces the effects of nuclease activity in the medium and thereby extends the lifespan of the ODNs.

2. Use immunocytochemistry to determine where and when the target protein is expressed; if possible, quantify the levels at which the protein is normally expressed.
3. By adding ink to the gel in order to make it more visible, one can determine how long the gel remains in place in a particular system. If the gel is placed on a tissue undergoing a lot of movement, it will of course dissipate more rapidly.
4. We find that antisense sequences between 18 and 30 bases long work best. Sequences should be analyzed for their specificity and the probability of forming stem–loop structures or stable secondary structures; they should not homodimerise. It has been reported that some sense oligonucleotides can form stable DNA triplets (9) inhibiting transcription.
5. Use FITC-tagged ODNs to demonstrate the entry of the ODNs into the

target tissue. Confocal microscopy can be used in order to determine the time course of entry and the depth of penetration of the tagged probes.

6. Use immunocytochemistry to determine both the specificity and time course of knockdown and recovery of the target protein. Direct immunocytochemistry using confocal microscopy is more rapid and has distinct advantages over Western blotting: (i) information can be gained regarding the spatial distribution of the protein knockdown in relation to the target site and (ii) protein expression can be quantified rapidly from the confocal microscope image (10,11). If possible, check that the expression of other related proteins is not affected by the antisense or whether other proteins are undergoing compensatory up-regulation for the knocked down protein.
7. Northern blots and RNase protection assays are of little use in determining the efficacy of all ODNs as the mRNA is not always destroyed by their action. Measurement of target protein levels is the best assay for antisense efficacy.
8. In developmental experiments the efficacy of the ODNs is improved if they are applied to tissues just prior to the expression of the target protein. For tissues with a low turnover rate of the target protein, antisense can prove ineffective unless this strategy is adopted.

Acknowledgments

Dr D. L. Becker is a Royal Society University Research Fellow and thanks the Royal Society for its support. Dr C. R. Green thanks the New Zealand Marsden fund for their support.

References

1. Stein, C.A. (1992) *Leukemia*, **6**, 967.
2. Wagner, R.W. (1994) *Nature*, **372**, 333.
3. Milligan, J.F., Matteucci, M.D., and Martin, J.C. (1993) *J. Med. Chem.*, **36**, 1923.
4. Becker, D.L., McGonnel, I., Makarenkova, H., Patel, K., Tickle, C., Lorimer, J., and Green, C.R. (1999) *Dev. Genet.* **24**, 33.
5. Boiziau, C., Moreau, S., and Toulme, J.-J. (1994) *FEBS Lett.*, **340**, 236.
6. Woolf, T.M., Melton, D.A., and Jennings, C.G.B. (1992) *Proc. Natl Acad. Sci. USA*, **89**, 7305.
7. Hamburger, V. and Hamilton, H. (1951) *J. Morphol.*, **88**, 49.
8. Tickle, C.T. (1993) In Stern, C.D. and Holland, P.W.H. (Eds), *Essential Developmental Biology. A Practical Approach*, pp. 119–126. Oxford University Press.
9. Neckers, L. and Whitesell, L. (1993) *Amer. J. Physiol.*, **265**, L1.
10. Becker, D.L., Evans, W.H., Green, C.R., and Warner, A. (1995) *J. Cell Sci.*, **108**, 1455.
11. Green, C.R., Bowles, L., Crawley, A., and Tickle, C. (1994) *Dev. Biol.*, **161**, 12.
12. Becker, D. L. and Mobbs, P. (1999) *Exp. Neurol.*, **156**, 326.

11

Delivery of antisense by viral vectors for prolonged antisense effects *in vivo*

M. IAN PHILLIPS, XIAOPING TANG and DAGMARA MOHUCZY

1. Introduction

Gene therapy for hypertension is being studied with antisense inhibition aimed at components of the renin–angiotensin system in the brain and periphery (1–4). Hypertension is a polygenic disease with genes overexpressing or underexpressing steroids, peptides and lipids. In the expression of genes encoding components of the renin–angiotensin system, at least two mutations have been linked to hypertension. These include the angiotensin converting enzyme genes, D (deletion) mutation, and the angiotensinogen T235 variant (5). Inserting genes, such as the renin gene or the angiotensinogen gene, into transgenic animals results in their developing hypertension (6).

The opposite of gene insertion is gene knockout. Knocking out genes for angiotensinogen production results in hypotension in mice (7). However, the limitation of the transgenic knockout approach is that, in order to survive embryonic and fetal development, the animals compensate for the lost gene by modulation of expression of other genes. Antisense inhibition offers a different approach from knockout because it can be used in adult animals, whereas knockout must be done in embryos and therefore the adult knockout animal undergoes its entire development without a specific gene ever being expressed. The effect of antisense inhibition has been called 'knockdown' because there is rarely a complete inhibition of specific protein.

A new development has been the production of a hybrid of these techniques with transgenic rats bearing an antisense gene to angiotensinogen (8). In the spontaneously hypertensive rat (SHR), angiotensin II expression is increased in the brain but normal in the periphery (9). In addition, angiotensin II type 1 receptors (AT_1 receptors) are expressed more abundantly in the brain of the SHR than in the brains of normotensive rats (10). The apparently increased activity of angiotensin in brain tissue of SHR gave us a starting point for testing the effectiveness of antisense inhibition in lowering blood pressure in hypertensive animals. Earlier experiments (11) had shown that a single injection into the brain of a nonspecific angiotensin antagonist, Sar1-Ile8 angiotensin II, produced a brief but significant decrease in blood pressure at a dose which was ineffective when given peripherally. Normotensive rats did not respond to central injections of angiotensin II antagonists. Therefore, it was hypothesized that in the SHR hypertension is associated with an overactive brain renin–angiotensin system. We designed antisense oligodeoxynucleotides (ODNs) to specifically inhibit AT_1 receptors or angiotensinogen to produce longer-lasting effects than a single injection of the pharmacological antagonist.

Antisense inhibition has been developed, particularly in cell culture applications, to the point where it is being tested in clinical trials for HIV and cancer (12,13). The pros and cons of its use have been reviewed elsewhere (14). Before 1992, however, antisense knockdown approaches had not been applied *in vivo* with any success. There was much concern about the efficiency of cellular uptake of ODNs. In 1992–3, three or four laboratories simultaneously and independently made and tested antisense ODNs in the brain (15,16,17,18). Cellular uptake proved not to be a limiting factor in the central nervous system. The first demonstration of an antisense approach for hypertension was the use of antisense ODNs designed to inhibit angiotensinogen mRNA and angiotensin to AT_1 receptor mRNA in the brain (19).

Antisense ODNs have many potential attractive features as a new class of therapeutic agents. To prolong the effect of antisense inhibition for weeks or months, DNA (partial or full-length) can be inserted in the antisense direction in viral vectors. This chapter discusses both the use of antisense oligonucleotides and the use of viral vectors with details of the production of plasmid and recombinant adeno-associated virus (AAV) vectors.

2. Antisense oligonucleotides

2.1 Designing antisense molecules

The following characteristics of antisense ODNs need to be incorporated into their design:

- the DNA sequence should be specific and unique
- uptake into cells should be efficient
- the effect in cells should be stable
- there should be no non-specific binding to proteins
- hybridization of the ODN should be specific for the target mRNA
- the targeted protein and/or mRNA level should be reduced
- the ODN should be not toxic
- no inflammatory or immune response should be induced

- the ODN should be more effective than appropriate sense and mismatch ODN controls

The concept of antisense inhibition assumes that a short DNA sequence in the antisense direction binds to the specific mRNA of the target protein in the cytoplasm, and prevents either ribosomal assembly or read-through of the message (20). These antisense ODNs are therefore targeted to the gene initiation codon (AUG) or to part of the coding region downstream from it. Other approaches involved the formation of triple-helical structures with antisense molecules constructed to the promoter region of a specified DNA.

Antisense ODNs are 15–20 bases long, but longer or full-length DNA in the antisense direction is used in viral vectors. When designing antisense molecules, one has to consider two antagonistic factors: the affinity of ODN for its target sequence (which is dependent on the number and composition of complementary bases) and the availability of the target sequence (which is dependent on the folding of the mRNA molecule) (21).

Several reports suggested that antisense ODNs targeted to different regions of the RNA have different efficiencies (22,23). These differences may be related to the predicted secondary structure of the target mRNA (24–26). The folding of the mRNA influences target sequence availability. The RNA double helices that are responsible for the secondary structure of the mRNA incorporate a weaker G–U base pairing next to A–U and G–C, and are generally short and rarely perfect. Therefore the design should avoid G-repeats. Burgess *et al.* (27) showed that the effects of repeated G-sequences in ODNs may be due to non-antisense mechanisms.

Proper testing of antisense requires a sense ODN and a mismatch ODN control for every antisense ODN. An ODN that has strong (Watson–Crick) base pairing with 100% complementarity will form the more thermodynamically favorable structure with its target RNA (28).

Antisense ODNs have several potential sites of action:

(1) They could inhibit translation by hybridizing to the specific mRNA for which they are designed, and then hybridization would prevent either ribosomal assembly or ribosomal sliding along the mRNA. In this case the antisense ODNs would be acting in the cytosol and would not affect measurable mRNA levels. Indeed, there are several articles reporting antisense effects without detectable change in target mRNA levels (17).

(2) They could act by reducing mRNA levels. This can occur by RNase H digestion of the RNA portion of the mRNA–antisense DNA hybrid. RNase H is found in the cytoplasm as well as in the nucleus, and is normally involved in DNA duplication, where it cleaves RNA that has bound to DNA. Activation of RNase H is advantageous, because the enzyme leaves the antisense ODN intact, so it is free to hybridize with another mRNA, making the reaction catalytic rather than stoichiometric.

(3) Studies of cellular uptake of labeled ODNs have shown that most antisense ODNs quickly migrate to the cell nucleus, suggesting an intranuclear site of action (29). Antisense DNA may hybridize to its target mRNA or pre-mRNA in the nucleus, forming a partially double-stranded structure which would inhibit its transport out of the nucleus into the cytoplasm, thus preventing translation.

(4) Antisense ODNs targeted to intron–exon junction sites prevent the splicing process and, consequently, the maturation of the transcript. Therefore, antisense molecules might inhibit pre-RNA splicing or the transport of mRNA from the nucleus to the cytoplasm.

An alternative anti-gene strategy is to target the DNA with triplex-forming ODNs to block DNA transcription. Effective antisense ODNs have been designed targeting exon–intron splicing sites (30) or the major groove of the DNA (31) but triplex formation can be corrected by DNA repair mechanisms.

Currently, the three regions that are considered to be the best targets for designing effective antisense ODNs are the 5′ cap region, the AUG translation initiation codon and the 3′ untranslated region of the mRNA (32–34). Since most mRNAs have an AUG initiator codon site, targeting 12–15 of the neighboring bases should produce inhibitory ODNs. Routinely, all designed ODNs must be checked against the GenBank and other databases for existing sequences to avoid any homology with other mRNAs. Essentially, antisense design usually boils down to trial-and-error testing in a model first (but see Chapter 2). A general rule suggested by our own experience is that for a 15-mer ODN, three different sites should be tested to find at least one that will work. Obviously, it is desirable to have a rapid screening test *in vitro* or *in vivo* for the specific protein that the antisense ODN has been designed to inhibit. Controls are a sense ODN and a mismatch ODN (with one or more nucleotides different from the antisense ODN), or a scrambled ODN where the entire sequence is random.

2.2 Stability of oligonucleotides

ODNs in their natural form as phosphodiesters are subject to rapid degradation in the blood, intracellular fluid or cerebrospinal fluid by exonucleases and endonucleases. Phosphodiester ODNs have a half-life of only minutes in blood and tissue culture media. The half-life of ODNs is somewhat longer in cerebrospinal fluid, and intact ODNs can be detected 24 h after injection into the cerebral ventricles (34).

Several chemical modifications have been proposed to prolong the half-life of ODNs in biological fluids and enhance uptake while retaining their activity and specificity. The most widely used modified ODNs are phosphorothioates, in which one of the oxygen atoms in the phosphodiester bond between nucleotides is replaced with a sulfur atom. These phosphorothioate ODNs are more stable in biological fluids than normal ODNs. The half-life of a 15-mer phosphorothioate ODN is 9 h in human serum, 4 days in tissue culture medium (35) and 19 h in cerebrospinal fluid (36). Phosphorothioate ODNs can be synthesized with automated DNA synthesizers but the product may contain impurities unless purified on an affinity gel. ODNs should be checked to ensure that they are pure.

One or more of the oxygen atoms in the phosphodiester bond can be replaced with a variety of other compounds, such as methyl groups (methylophosphoriate), alkyl phosphotriester, phosphoramidate or boranophosphate, all of which expand the half-life of ODNs in *in vivo* experiments. Some clever new designs are being tried in which the ODN has a dumb-bell shape produced by a hairpin extension at the 3′ end (37). It is hoped that these third- or fourth-generation ODNs will be more stable and have enhanced uptake kinetics and better affinity for the target (38; see Chapter 8).

2.3 Cellular uptake of oligonucletoides

In order to hybridize with the target mRNA, antisense ODNs have to cross the cell membrane. Saturable uptake of ODNs reaches a plateau within 50 h, occurs rapidly and, depending on the cells, can be efficient (39). Uptake is faster for shorter ODNs than for longer ones (39). Decreasing the temperature prevents ODN uptake, indicating that there is an active uptake mechanism. An 80 kDa ODN-binding protein has been proposed to be the receptor molecule for ODN uptake (39). An efflux mechanism has also been described indicating temperature-dependent secretion of the ODNs from the cells to the extracellular space (35).

2.4 Pharmacology of antisense ODNS

In pharmacological terms, antisense inhibition can be considered to be a drug–receptor interaction, where the ODN is the drug and the target sequence is the receptor. For binding to occur between the two, a minimum level of affinity is required which is provided by hydrogen bonding between the Watson–Crick base pairs and base stacking in the double helix that is formed. In order to achieve pharmacological activity, a minimum number of 12–15 bases can provide the minimum level of affinity (40). Longer sequences are more specific but above 20 bases problems of cell uptake begin to reduce the effectiveness of ODNs.

One of the main advantages of antisense inhibition is the specificity of the antisense ODN target sequence interaction provided by the Watson–Crick base pairing. An ODN of 12–15 nucleotides length is specific enough statistically to be complementary to a single sequence (13). Increasing the length of the ODN should result in higher level of specificity, but it also decreases its uptake into cells (39). With viral vectors, however, the uptake problem is overcome because the virus freely enters cells by binding to viral receptors on cell membranes. Therefore, in a viral vector a full-length DNA-antisense sequence can be used. The mechanism of action of antisense DNA differs from that of the antisense ODN. The antisense DNA produces an antisense mRNA which competes negatively with mRNA in the cytoplasm.

2.5 Toxicity

Antisense ODNs can inhibit protein synthesis in cultured cells in nmol/L doses. The therapeutic window for antisense ODNs is rather narrow (40). When testing for the optimal dose, small increments in the high nmol/L range should be tested (34). High concentrations may produce non-specific binding to cytosolic proteins and give misleading results.

Phosphodiester ODNs are degraded to their naturally occurring nucleotide building blocks relatively quickly, therefore no toxic reaction is expected from even high doses of phosphodiester. Studies on phosphorothioated ODNs in rats show that following intravenous injection, phosphorothioated ODNs are taken up from the plasma mainly by the liver, fat and muscle tissues. Phosphorothioate ODNs are excreted through the urine in 3 days, mainly in their original form. An apparently mild increase in plasma lactate dehydrogenase (LDH) and, to a lesser extent, indicators of a possible transient liver toxicity with very high doses of phosphorotioated ODNs were observed (41). Whole new classes of ODN backbone modification are being developed to avoid the possible liver toxicity in humans with phosphorothioates (38,40; see Chapter 8).

2.6 Delivery of antisense

2.6.1 Naked DNA

Direct injection of the antisense DNA has been used in the experiments described below (41–45). For injections into the brain, naked DNA appears to be very successful. In a number of studies, using different antisense ODNs, there has been efficient uptake and effective reduction in protein as well as inhibition of the physiological parameters studied. Uptake is so efficient that one difficulty with intracerebroventricular injections is that the DNA tends to be taken up close to the site of injection and not to spread to other parts of the brain. While this has little impact for hypertension therapy, it is an important consideration in antisense strategies for the treatment of brain diseases, such as Parkinson's disease, thalamic pain, Alzheimer's disease and gliomas.

Chao and colleagues (45) have reported success with direct gene delivery of DNA plasmid for human tissue kallikrein in reducing blood pressure of SHR. They used naked DNA constructs, one with a metallothionine metal response element, the other with a Rous sarcoma virus 3′ long terminal repeat (LTR) promoter. They injected the DNA intravenously. Expression of human kallikrein was identified in several tissues. Blood pressure was significantly reduced for 6 weeks and reached a maximum of –46 mmHg reduction (45). These authors have also shown that intravenous injection of the atrial natriuretic peptide (ANP) gene as naked DNA reduces hypertension in young SHR (but not in adult SHR) (4).

2.6.2 Liposomes

Liposomes, which are self-assembling particles of bilipid layers, have been used for encapsulating antisense ODN for delivery in blood. Antisense directed to angiotensinogen mRNA in liposomes has proved to be a successful approach. Tomita *et al.* (46) used liposome encapsulation of angiotensinogen antisense and a Sendai virus injected into the portal vein. Blood pressure decreased for several days. However, they did not compare their results with the effects of naked DNA. Wielbo *et al.* (2) compared liposome-encapsulated antisense and naked DNA given intra-arterially. They found that liposome encapsulation was effective, whereas naked DNA was not, under the same conditions. Twenty-four hours after injection of 50 μg of liposome-encapsulated antisense ODN, blood pressure decreased by 25 mmHg. Neither empty liposomes nor liposome-encapsulated scrambled ODN nor unencapsulated antisense ODN had a significant effect on blood pressure. Confocal microscopy of rat liver tissue 1 h after intra-arterial injection of 50 μg of unencapsulated fluorescein isothiocyanate (FITC) antisense, or liposome-encapsulated FITC-conjugated antisense, showed intense fluorescence in liver tissue sinusoids with the liposome-encapsulated ODN. Levels of protein (angiotensinogen and angiotensin II in the plasma) were significantly reduced in the liposome-encapsulated ODN group. Antisense alone, lipids alone, and scrambled ODN in liposomes had no effect on protein levels.

Liposome development with cationic lipids allow high transfection efficiency of plasmid DNA. The short, single-stranded antisense ODNs are not in fact encapsulated but complexed with bilamellar vesicles by electrostatic interactions. This simplifies the production of the antisense delivery system and allows for a variety of routes of delivery including aerosol nasal sprays and parenteral injections.

3. Viral vectors for antisense DNA delivery

Several viruses have been tested for gene delivery; although each has its advantages, none of them is ideal. The perfect viral vector should fulfil all of the following criteria:

- it should be safe, so if it is known to cause disease it must be re-engineered to be harmless
- it should not elicit an immune or inflammatory response
- it should not integrate into the genome randomly, as this would risk disrupting other cellular genes and mutagenesis
- it must be replication-deficient so that it will not spread to other tissues or infect other individuals

- ideally it would deliver a defined gene copy number into each infected cell
- it must be efficiently taken up in target tissue, so it must infect the target cells with high frequency
- it should be easy to manipulate and produce in pure form
- it should to be able to accommodate the gene of interest, along with its regulatory sequences
- the recombinant DNA has to be packaged with high efficiency into the viral capsid proteins.

3.1 Retroviruses

Retroviruses have been used primarily because of their high efficiency in delivering genes to dividing cells (47); they permit insertion and stable integration of single-copy genes. Although effective in cell culture systems, retroviruses integrate randomly into the genome, which raises concerns about their safety for practical use *in vivo*. Retroviruses can only act in dividing cells, making them ideal for tumor therapy but less desirable where other cells are dividing that need to be protected.

In hypertension research retroviruses are being investigated in developing SHR. Our colleagues at the University of Florida delivered retrovirus vector (LNSV) containing an antisense DNA to AT_{1b} receptor mRNA (48). Injections in the heart of 6 week old SHR resulted in effective long-term inhibition of AT_1 receptor mRNA and significant inhibition of the development of hypertension. Several measures indicated that the AT_1 receptors in vessels were reduced in responsiveness by the treatment (48).

3.2 Adenoviruses

Adenovirus vectors have been tested successfully in their natural host cells, respiratory endothelia, as well as in other tissues such as vascular smooth and striated muscle, and brain (49–51). Adenovirus is a double-stranded DNA with 2700 distinct adenoviral gene products. It infects most mammalian cell types because most cells have membrane receptors. The viruses enter the cell by receptor-induced endocytosis and translocate to the nucleus. Most adenovirus vectors in their current form are episomal, that is, they do not integrate into the host DNA. They provide high levels of expression, but the episomal DNA will invariably become inactive after some time. In some species, e.g. mice, this time may be long relative to their life span, but in humans it is a limitation of the virus as a vector. Repeated infections result in an inflammatory response with consequent tissue damage. This is because the adenovirus expresses genes that lead to immune cell attacks. This further limitation makes current recombinant adenovirus unsuitable for long-term treatment and several gene therapy trials using adenovirus vectors have failed to produce acceptable results. Preliminary studies with adenovirus vectors for delivery of AT_1 receptors in mRNA antisense have been tested in rats and reduce developing hypertension in SHR (52). The adenovirus is easy to produce and therefore useful for animal studies of mechanisms. However, the adenovirus as a vector has too many limitations at present to be successful in human gene therapy. Further engineering of the adenovirus may eventually avoid these limitations.

3.3 Adeno-associated virus

AAV has been gaining attention because of its safety and efficiency (53). It has been successfully used for delivering antisense RNA against alpha-globin (54) and HIV LTR (55), and is our vector of choice for delivering antisense targeted to the AT_1 receptor in hypertensive rat models.

AAV is a parvovirus, discovered as a contamination of adenoviral stocks. It is widespread (it is estimated that antibodies are present in 85% of people in the USA) and has not been linked to any disease. Its replication is dependent on the presence of a helper virus, such as adenovirus or herpes virus. Five serotypes have been isolated, of which AAV-2 is the best characterized. AAV has a single-stranded linear DNA which is encapsidated into capsid proteins VP1, VP2 and VP3 to form an icosahedral virion of 20–24 nm in diameter (53).

The AAV DNA is approximately 4.7 kb long. It contains two open reading frames and is flanked by two inverted terminal repeats (ITRs). There are two major genes in the AAV genome: *rep* and *cap*. *rep* codes for proteins responsible for viral replication, whereas *cap* codes for capsid proteins VP1–3. Each ITR forms a T-shaped hairpin structure. These terminal repeats are the only essential *cis*-components of the AAV for chromosomal integration. Therefore, the AAV can be used as a vector with all viral coding sequences removed and replaced by the cassette of genes for delivery. Three viral promoters have been identified and named p5, p19 and p40, according to their map position. Transcription from p5 and p19 results in production of Rep proteins, while transcription from p40 produces the capsid proteins (53). For more powerful expression we have inserted a cytomegalovirus (CMV) promoter. Other promoters are being tested which are specific to certain cells including arginine vasopressin (AVP) promoter for cells synthesizing AVP, neuron specific enolase and glial fibrillary acid protein.

Upon infection of a human cell, the wild-type AAV integrates into the q arm of chromosome 19 (56,57). Although chromosomal integration requires the terminal repeats, the viral components responsible for site-specific integration have been recently targeted to the Rep proteins (58). With no helper virus present, AAV infection remains latent indefinitely. Upon superinfection of the cell with helper virus, the AAV genome is excised, replicated, packaged into virions and released to the extracellular fluid. This fact is the basis of recombinant AAV production for research.

Several factors prompted researchers to study the possibility of using recombinant AAV as an expression vector:

(1) *Its simplicity*: all that is necessary for gene delivery is the presence of the 145 bp ITRs, which represent only 6% of the AAV genome. This leaves room in the vector for a DNA insertion of up to 4.4 kb. While this carrying capacity may limit the size of gene that the AAV can deliver, it is amply suited to delivering small genes and antisense cDNA. It is sufficient to ensure a specific response, a potent promoter and a selective marker such as a neomycin resistance gene.

(2) *Its safety*: there is a relatively complicated rescue mechanism. Not only adenovirus (wild type) but also AAV genes are required to mobilize the recombinant AAV. The spread of recombinant AAV vectors to non-target areas can be limited to certain tissues. AAV is not pathogenic and not associated with disease. The elimination of viral coding sequences in producing a +AAV minimizes immune reactions to viral gene expression, and therefore recombinant AAV does not evoke an inflammatory response (in contrast to the recombinant adenovirus).

(3) *Its very broad host range*: AAV apparently infects all mammalian tissues tested, except vascular endothelial cells (59). It remains intact for long periods of time.

A limitation of AAV is its production. Although it can be purified and concentrated (which are advantages) it also has to be rendered free of adenovirus, and therefore its production is more complicated than that of other vectors.

The advantages, particularly its safety, make AAV appear to be one of the best candidates for delivery of genes for long-term therapy. Recently, Flotte and colleagues (60) have established gene therapy Phase I trials for cystic fibrosis using AAV gene delivery in patients.

4. Methods for antisense delivery by AAV

The general concept for antisense gene delivery in the AAV vector and the steps involved are shown in *Figure 1*. To illustrate these steps, a brief description is given that is applicable to hypertension. Further details are presented in reference 60.

4.1 Construction of plasmids

After subcloning the target gene into an AAV-based vector, highly purified plasmid is needed for virus packaging. To achieve this, we recommend the method described in *Protocol 1*.

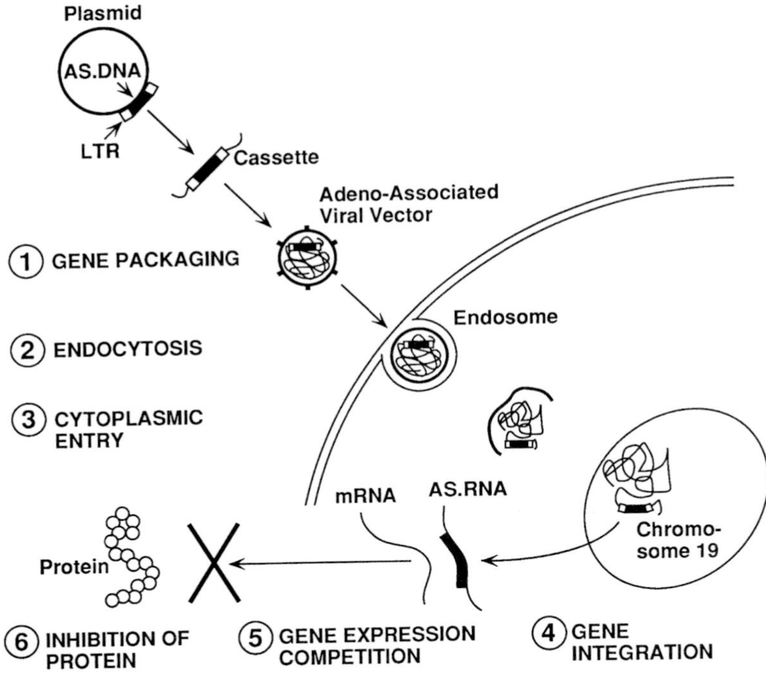

Figure 1. Gene delivery of antisense DNA (AS.DNA) with adeno-associated viral vector (AAV). (1) Gene packaging: plasmid containing the long terminal repeats (LTR) characteristic of AAV with cDNA subcloned in the antisense direction. The final cassette also contains promoters, such as the CMV or TK promoter. The packaging cell line is transfected with AAV-based plasmid and helper plasmid with *rep* and *cap* genes, and transduced with adenovirus as a helper virus. (2) Endocytosis: the viral vector fuses with the cell membrane by binding to adhesion molecules and becomes an endosome within the bilipid layer. (3) Cytoplasmic entry: the vesicle 'opens' in the cytoplasm, releasing the vector which is transported to, and enters the nucleus. (4) Gene integration: AAV integrates with chromosome 19. It is not known if the addition of foreign DNA interferes with this integration. (5) Gene expression competition: genomic DNA in chromosome 19 produces an antisense RNA (AS.RNA). This competes with the natural mRNA and prevents it from producing its product. (6) Inhibition of protein: binding of antisense RNA to the mRNA prevents sliding through ribosomal assembly to produce protein. This gene delivery system should be result in reduction in the amount of the protein, specifically targeted by the antisense DNA.

Protocol 1. Large-scale plasmid preparation

Equipment and reagents

- LB (Luria–Bertani) medium with 100 μg/ml ampicillin
- Lysozyme buffer (25 mM Tris pH 7.5, 10 mM EDTA, 15% sucrose or glucose)
- Lysozyme (12 mg/ml in lysozyme buffer)
- 0.2 N NaOH–1% SDS
- 3 M sodium acetate, pH 4.8–5.2
- Chloroform

- 40% PEG 8000
- 5.5 M LiCl
- Isopropanol
- TE pH 7.4 (10 mM Tris–Cl with 1 mM EDTA)
- Cesium chloride
- Ethidium bromide (10 mg/ml)
- 4.9 ml Optiseal centrifuge tube (Beckman, cat. no. 326185)
- 3 ml syringe with a 18 gauge needle
- Isoamyl alcohol
- Ethanol, 100% and 75%
- Phenol:chloroform (25:24, v/v)
- J2-HS centrifuge with JA-20.1 and JA-14 rotors (Beckman) or equivalent
- Ultracentrifuge with NVT90 rotor (Beckman) or equivalent
- 250 ml polypropylene centrifuge bottles
- 50 ml polypropylene centrifuge bottles

Method

1. Grow bacteria containing the appropriate plasmid in 1 liter of LB medium with 100 μg/ml ampicillin.
2. Pellet bacteria at 3000***g*** at 4°C for 15 min.
3. Resuspend bacteria in 20 ml of lysozyme buffer.
4. Add 4 ml of lysozyme (12 mg/ml in lysozyme buffer) and mix.
5. Place on ice for 5 min until the mixture becomes viscous.
6. Add 48 ml of 0.2 N NaOH–1% SDS. Mix using a glass pipette as a stirring rod.
7. Place on ice for 5–10 min.
8. Add 36 ml of 3 M sodium acetate, pH 4.8–5.2; mix with the same pipette.
9. Add 0.2 ml of chloroform; mix.
10. Place on ice for 20 min.
11. Spin at 3000***g*** at 4°C for 20 min.
12. Transfer supernatant into a fresh bottle.
13. Add 33 ml of 40% PEG 8000, mix, and incubate on ice for 10 min.
14. Spin at 14 000***g*** at 4°C for 10 min.
15. Discard supernatant, dissolve pellet in 10 ml of sterile water, then add 10 ml of 5.5 M LiCl.
16. Place on ice for 10 min.
17. Spin at 14 000 g at 4°C for 10 min.
18. Save supernatant, transfer equal amounts (each 10 ml) into two 30 ml Corex (or plastic) tubes, add 6 ml of isopropanol to each tube; mix.
19. Incubate at room temperature for 10 min.
20. Spin at 10 000***g*** at room temperature for 10 min.
21. Dissolve each pellet in 3.7 ml of TE pH 7.4.
22. Add 4.2 g of cesium chloride to each tube, mix and dissolve, add 0.24 ml of ethidium bromide (10 mg/ml), mix.
23. Transfer the solution in each tube into a 4.9 ml Optiseal centrifuge tube.
24. Spin in NVT90 rotor (Beckman) at 78 000 r.p.m., 15°C for 4 h.

Protocol 1. *Continued*

25. After centrifugation, you will see three bands: the upper one contains protein, the middle one is nicked and linear DNA, and the lowest one is closed circular plasmid DNA. Carefully remove the plasmid band using a 3 ml syringe with a 18 gauge needle and transfer it into Eppendorf tubes (two tubes, each about 0.5 ml).
26. Extract three or four times with an equal volume of isoamyl alcohol, discarding the organic phase (top layer) every time until all pink color is removed.
27. Transfer into one 30 ml Corex (or plastic) tube, add 2.5 vols (2.5 ml) of water, mix and add two combined volumes of ethanol (7 ml).
28. Place on ice for 30 min.
29. Pellet plasmid DNA at 12 000***g*** for 15 min at 4°C.
30. Discard supernatant and dissolve pellet in 500 μl of TE (pH 7.4).
31. Transfer into Eppendorf tube, add 500 μl of phenol:chloroform (25:24, v/v), vortex and spin for 2 min at top speed in a microcentrifuge.
32. Save the top aqueous layer and transfer into a fresh Eppendorf tube.
33. Add 50 μl of 3 M sodium acetate buffer, pH 4.8–5.2 and mix; add 1 ml ethanol and mix.
34. Pellet the plasmid DNA at top speed in a microcentrifuge for 5 min at 4°C.
35. Discard the supernatant, wash the pellet with 75% ethanol and vacuum dry.
36. Dissolve the pellet in 1 ml of TE.

We constructed plasmids for both AT_1 receptor antisense (paAT_1) and angiotensinogen antisense (paAo) in the AAV-derived expression vector. Initially we used a plasmid containing a 750 bp cDNA inserted into the AAV genome in the antisense direction downstream from the AAV promoter. NG108-15 (neuroblastoma–glioma) cells or H4 hepatoma cells were transfected with paAT_1 or paAo, respectively, using lipofectamine (61,62). In both cases, there were significant reductions in the appropriate proteins, namely AT_1 receptor and angiotensinogen. To test that the cells expressed AAV, we used the *rep* gene product as a marker. Immunocytochemical staining with a Rep protein antibody showed that the majority of cells in culture fully expressed the vector. A further development of the AAV vector was the insertion of more powerful and specific promoters than the p40 promoter. AAV with a CMV promoter and neomycin resistance (neo^r) gene as a selectable marker is being used in our current experiments. The AAV cassette contains either 750 bp of rat AT_1 cDNA in the antisense direction (*Figure 2*), or a marker, either the *gfp* gene, which encodes green fluorescent protein (63)

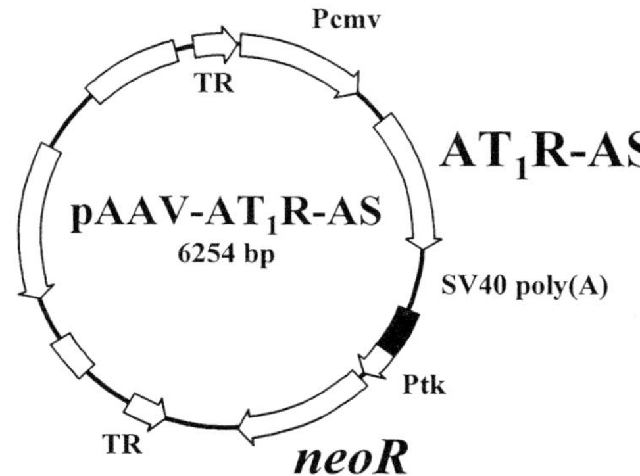

Figure 2. Plasmid vector pAAV-AT_1R-AS contains a 750 bp fragment of the AT_{1A} receptor cDNA in the antisense orientation. Abbreviations: TR, AAV terminal repeat; Pcmv, human cytomegalovirus early promoter; SV40 poly(A), polyadenylation signal from simian virus 40; Ptk, thymidine kinase promoter; *neo*^{r}, neomycin phosphotransferase gene from Tn*5*. Other promoters have been substituted for CMV, including the arginine vasopressin (AVP), neuron specific enolase (NSE) and glial fibrillary acid protein (GFAP) promoters.

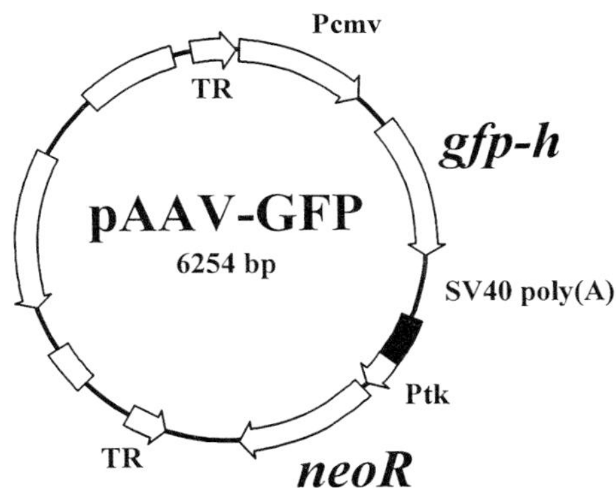

Figure 3. Schematic diagrams of recombinant AAV vector containing the *gfp* gene. In the recombinant AAV–*gfp* vector almost all of the parental wild-type AAV genome (except the terminal repeats) has been deleted and replaced with *gfp*, the gene encoding *Aequorea victoria* green fluorescent protein, driven by a CMV promoter (Pcmv). Also, a thymidine kinase promoter (Ptk) has been inserted into the neomycin resistance gene (*neo*^{r}). *gfp* serves as a reporter gene *in vitro* or *in vivo*, while *neo*^{r} serves for selection *in vitro*.

(*Figure 3*) or the *lac*Z gene (64). NG108-15 cells transfected with AAV plasmid containing the *gfp* and *neo*^{r} genes were selected by antibiotic, G418 (600 μg/ml), and the selected clones viewed for GFP expression. Very few cells died during selection. Two weeks after transfection all of the cells were expressing GFP. The transfection efficiency of this pAAV-*gfp* construct in different cell lines, including ATt20 (mouse pituitary cells), L929 (mouse fibroblasts), HEK 293 (human embryonic kidney cells) and NG108-15, is over 50% (65).

4.2 Preparation of pAAV-AT_1R-AS

The 749 bp fragment of the angiotensin receptor cDNA (–183 to 566) was amplified using polymerase chain reaction (PCR) and ligated to an AAV-derived vector in the antisense orientation, in place of *gfp*. The resulting plasmid vector (pAAV-AT_1R-AS) contained AAV terminal repeats, a CMV promoter (Pcmv), the DNA encoding AT_1 receptor mRNA in the antisense direction and a *neo*^{r} gene. The plasmid DNA was purified on CsCl gradient.

pAAV-AT_1R-AS was tested for AT_1 receptor inhibition *in vitro*, using NG108-15 (66) and vascular smooth muscle cells (67). The cells had significantly ($P < 0.01$) fewer angiotensin II AT_1 receptors than the control cells. No effect was seen on AT_2 receptors.

AAV-based plasmids are used to prepare recombinant virus, by the method described in *Protocol 2*. In this method, human embryonic kidney (HEK293) cells are transfected with plasmid vector containing the gene of interest in the antisense orientation and AAV terminal repeats (pAAV-AS), together with helper plasmid delivering the *rep* and *cap* genes, which are necessary for AAV replication, *in trans* using the calcium phosphate method (see *Protocol 2A*). Eight hours after transfection, adenovirus is added at a multiplicity of infection (MOI) of 5.

Protocol 2. Preparation of recombinant adeno-associated virus

Equipment and reagents

- 15 cm cell culture plates
- Sonicator
- Ultracentrifuge with SW41 rotor
- Syringe (6 ml)
- Dot-blot apparatus and vacuum pump
- Nylon membrane pre-soaked in distilled water and then 20 × SSC
- Whatman 3MM filter paper
- Microwave oven
- Centricon-30 tubes (Amicon)
- HEK293 cells grown in DMEM with 10% heat inactivated FBS and penicillin/streptomycin
- Plasmid to be transfected
- Helper plasmid
- 0.1 × TE (1 mM Tris-Cl, 0.1 mM EDTA pH 8.0)
- HBS, pH 7.4
- 2 × HBS
- 2 M $CaCl_2$
- Tris–Cl (50 mM, pH 8.4) with 150 mM NaCl
- Ammonium sulfate pH 7.0, saturated at 4°C
- Cesium chloride, solid and solutions of density 1.5 and 1.39 g/ml
- 20 × SSC (3 M NaCl, 0.3 M sodium citrate pH 7.0)
- 10% SDS
- 0.5 M NaOH with 1.5 M NaCl
- 0.5 M Tris–HCl pH 7.2 with 1.5 M NaCl
- [^{32}P]dCTP-labeled AAV probe, labeled by random priming using a kit
- Phosphate-buffered saline (PBS)
- Cell culture incubator with the temperature 37 °C and 5% CO_2
- Cell culture hood
- Inverted microscope
- 2 × HBS pH 7.05 (280 mM NaCl, 10 mM KCl, 1.5 mM $Na_2HPO_4{\cdot}2H_2O$, 12 mM dextrose and 50 mM HEPES)
- 0.05 % porcine trypsin with 0.02% EDTA
- kit for ^{32}P random-primed labeling of linear double-stranded DNA
- 50 × Denhardt's reagent (5 g Ficoll 400, 5 g polyvinylpyrrolidone, 5 g bovine serum albumin fraction V in 500 ml water)
- Prehybridization buffer (5 × Denhardt's solution diluted from 50 × concentrate in 6 × SSC, 0.5% SDS, 100 μg/ml denatured, fragmented salmon sperm DNA)
- Hybridization buffer (6 × SSC, 0.5% SDS, 100 μg/ml denatured, fragmented salmon sperm DNA)
- Washing buffer (2 × SSC with 0.1% SDS)

A. *Transfection of HEK293 cells*

1. Split low passage number HEK293 cells grown in DMEM with 10% heat inactivated FBS and 100 U/ml penicillin or 100 μg/ml streptomycin, onto 15 cm cell culture plates, so they are about 70% confluent the following day.
2. For each plate, mix 20 μg of plasmid, and 20 μg of helper plasmid (containing *rep* and *cap* genes) in a final volume 876 μl of 0.1 × TE.
3. Add 1 ml of 2 × HBS and mix.
4. Dropwise, and with mixing, add 124 μl of 2 M $CaCl_2$.
5. Incubate for 15–20 min at room temperature so that a precipitate forms; mix once by pipetting.
6. Add 2 ml of the mixture to the plate of cells, swirl gently and return cells to the incubator.
7. Eight hours after transfection, replace medium with fresh medium and add adenovirus at an MOI of 5.
8. When cytopathic effects are observed (usually after 2–3 days), harvest cells in medium and purify recombinant AAV as described in *Protocol 2B*.

B. *Purification of recombinant AAV*

1. Harvest cells using a rubber policeman and place in centrifuge bottles.
2. Centrifuge cell suspension at 900***g*** at 4°C for 15 min.
3. Resuspend the cell pellet in 1 ml of 50 mM Tris–Cl pH 8.4 with 150 mM NaCl and freeze–thaw three times.
4. Sonicate the cell suspension for 30 sec three times on ice
5. Spin down cell debris by centrifugation at 2000***g*** at 4°C for 10 min. Transfer the supernatant to a new tube.
6. Repeat freeze–thawing, sonicating and spinning down the pellet once. Combine supernatants.
7. Calculate 33% of the volume of supernatant; slowly, and with continuous mixing, add this volume of ammonium sulfate pH 7.0, saturated at 4°C, and incubate slurry at 4°C for 15 min.
8. Spin the sample at 8000***g***, 4°C for 15 min. Transfer the supernatant to a new tube.
9. Dropwise and with mixing, add 67% of the initial volume of supernatant of ammonium sulfate pH 7.0, saturated at 4°C.
10. Incubate on ice for 20 min. Centrifuge the solution at 17,500***g*** at 4°C for 20 min. Discard supernatant and turn the tube upside down on a paper towel to make sure that all fluid is removed.
11. Dissolve the pellet from 10 plates in 8.5 ml of HBS, pH 7.4.

Protocol 2. *Continued*

12. Mix with 5.5 g of solid CsCl and transfer to centrifuge tubes (density should be 1.39 g/ml).
13. Underlay with 1 ml of CsCl solution of 1.5 g/ml density; use a marker pen to mark the level of the cushion on the outside of the tube.
14. Spin the sample in an SW41 rotor at 40 000 r.p.m. at 18°C for 40 h. You will see a white diffuse band of proteins at the top and a sharp white band of adenovirus below.
15. Using a 6 ml syringe, withdraw the fluid that lies from about one-third of the way up the tube to about 2 mm below the adenovirus band.
16. Mix the sample with 1.39 g/ml CsCl and spin in an SW41 rotor at 40 000 r.p.m. at 18°C for 40 h.
17. Gently, without disturbing the CsCl gradient, place a needle in the upper part of the tube, tape it (so you can control the speed of fluid dripping later on), puncture the bottom of the tube with a needle and start to collect fluid. Collect five 1 ml fractions, then ten 0.5 ml fractions.
18. Check these fractions for AAV using hybridization with a [^{32}P]dCTP-labeled random primed AAV probe (see *Protocol 2C*) using dot-blot apparatus.

C. *Dot blotting to identify fractions containing AAV*

1. Assemble dot-blot apparatus with Whatman 3MM filter paper under a nylon filter pre-soaked in distilled water and then 20 × SSC.
2. Add 200 μl of 20 × SSC per well and apply slow vacuum to remove the fluid.
3. Add 5 μl aliquots of each fraction from the CsCl gradient and apply a slow vacuum to remove the fluid.
4. Remove the nylon filter from the manifold, place on Whatman 3MM filter paper soaked as follows: 10% SDS for 3 min, 0.5 M NaOH with 1.5 M NaCl for 5 min, 0.5 M Tris–HCl pH 7.2 with 1.5 M NaCl for 5 min. Air dry filter for 10 min., briefly wash in 4 × SSC for 10 sec and air dry for 10 min. Microwave the filter for 4 min with 0.5 L of water in a beaker placed near by.
5. Radiolabel the probe using random-primed labeling kit to specific radioactivity 10^9 cpm/μg or greater.
6. Incubate the wet filter in prehybridization buffer for 1 h at 65°C.
7. Remove prehybridization buffer and replace with hybridization buffer.

8. Denature radiolabeled probe (1–2 ng/ml) by heating for 5 min at 100°C and rapidly cooling in ice water.
9. Add probe to the hybridization buffer and incubate overnight at 65°C.
10. Wash filter in a washing buffer 2–3 times, 10 min each time at room temperature.
11. Expose the filter to autoradiography film at –80°C. The packaged AAV virions should be present near the middle of the gradient.
12. Combine positive fractions and concentrate virus using Centricon-30 (Amicon) at 4350***g*** for 30 min at 4°C.
13. Overlay the filter with concentrated virus with 0.5 ml of PBS and spin again for 2 min at 500***g***. Collect the virus.

Protocol 3. Virus titer assay

The titer of the virus is calculated using HEK293 cells or PC12w, wild type AAV and adenovirus.

Equipment and reagents

- HEK293 or PC12w cells
- 24-well plate
- Adenovirus
- Wild-type and recombinant AAV
- Trypsin–EDTA
- PBS
- Nylon filter presoaked in PBS
- Vacuum pump
- Whatman 2MM paper soaked in 0.5 N NaOH with 1.5 M NaCl
- Whatman paper soaked in 1 M Tris–HCl pH 7.0 with 2 × SSC
- ^{32}P-labeled probe specific for the gene of interest (labeled by random priming using a kit)
- Cell culture incubator with the temperature 37°C and 5% CO_2
- Cell culture hood
- Inverted microscope
- 0.05 % porcine trypsin with 0.02% EDTA
- Kit for ^{32}P random-primed labeling of linear double-stranded DNA
- 50 × Denhardt's reagent (5 g Ficoll 400, 5 g polyvinylpyrrolidone, 5 g bovine serum albumin fraction V in 500 ml water)
- Prehybridization buffer (5 × Denhardt's solution diluted from 50 × concentrate in 6 × SSC, 0.5% SDS, 100 μg/ml denatured, fragmented salmon sperm DNA)
- Hybridization buffer (6 × SSC, 0.5%, 100 μg/ml denatured, fragmented salmon sperm DNA)
- Washing buffer (2 × SSC with 0.1% SDS)

Method

1. Seed 5 × 10^4 cells in each well of a 24-well plate and incubate for 24 h.
2. Infect all but one well with adenovirus at an MOI of 20.
3. Infect all but one well (a different one from that in step **2**) with wild-type AAV at an MOI of 4.
4. Make serial 5-fold dilutions of recombinant AAV in PBS and infect 8–10 wells, which contain already adenovirus and wild-type AAV.

Protocol 3. *Continued*

Infect some cells with undiluted recombinant AAV but without adenovirus or without wild-type AAV. Incubate cells for 24 h.

5. Spin down the medium, discard supernatant, combine pellet with pre-washed and trypsinized cells from the plate (100 μl trypsin–EDTA per well), add 10 ml of PBS and disperse into single cell suspension.
6. Transfer cell suspension on to nylon filter presoaked in PBS and apply low vaccum.
7. Place filter on Whatman 2MM paper soaked in 0.5 N NaOH with 1.5 M NaCl for 5 min at room temperature.
8. Transfer filter to the top of Whatman paper soaked in 1 M Tris–HCl pH 7.0 with 2 × SSC for 5 min at room temperature.
9. Air-dry the filter.
10. Hybridize the filter with ^{32}P-labeled probe specific for your gene of interest (random primed according to the kit instruction) (see Protocol 2C).
11. Expose the filter to autoradiography film at –80°C. Count the spots and multiply by the dilution factor for each well.

In our studies, recombinant AAV-AT_1R-AS was tested for AT_1 receptor inhibition *in vitro* using vascular smooth muscle cells (67). Transduced cells, without G418 selection, expressed the transgene for at least 8 weeks, had a decreased number of AT_1 receptors and reduced calcium response to angiotensin II stimulation.

Expression *in vivo* was tested by direct injection into the brain. An AAV vector with a *lac*Z gene driven by an AVP promoter was constructed. The vector expressed β-galactosidase in neurons of the paraventricular nucleus and supraoptic nucleus. The expression was in magnocellular cells which normally express AVP (64). The expression was observed at 1 day, 1 week and after 1 month with no diminution of signal. This is an example of how AAV can be developed for specific tissue and/or cell gene expression and shows that AAV vectors can deliver foreign genes into adult brain for long periods of time.

To test for effectiveness *in vivo*, recombinant AAV-AT_1R-AS was microinfused into the lateral ventricles of adult male SHR. Control rats received AAV with the *gfp* reporter gene but without the antisense gene ('mock' vector) in vehicle (artificial cerebrospinal fluid). Blood pressure was measured by the tailcuff method. There was a significant decrease in systolic blood pressure in one group of rats which received the recombinant antisense AAV vector. No effect was observed in the controls. Systolic blood pressure decreased by 23 ± 2 mmHg in the first week after administration. This drop in blood pressure was prolonged in four rats for 9 weeks, whereas controls had no reduction in blood pressure. This was considerably longer than the longest effect observed with antisense ODN. Recombinant AAV–*gfp* expression in the hypothalami of the control rat group was detectable by reverse transcription–nested PCR 11 months after injection. Further, intracardiac injection of recombinant antisense AAV in SHR significantly reduced blood pressure and slowed the development of hypertension for several weeks (68,69). This result demonstrates that recombinant antisense AAV, in a single application, is effective in chronically reducing hypertension. Further such studies will undoubtedly provide interesting and important insights into gene regulation associated with hypertension as well as many other pathological processes.

Acknowledgments

This work has been supported by NIH (MERIT) grant HL23774 and grants from the American Heart Association, Florida Affiliate. The authors thank Ed Meyer, Allyson Peele, Birgitta Kimura, Leping Shen and Sara Galli for help in developing these methods and Gayle Butters for word processing.

References

1. Phillips, M.I. (1997) *Hypertension* **29**, 177.
2. Wielbo, D., Simon, A., Phillips, M.I. and Toffolo, S. (1996) *Hypertension* **28**, 147.
3. Morishita, R., Gibbons, G.H., Kaneda, Y., Ogihara, T. and Dzau, V.J. (1994) *Gene* **149**, 13.
4. Lin, K.-F., Chao, J. and Chao, L. (1995) *Hypertension*, **26**, 847.
5. Junemaitre, X., Soubrier, F., Kotelvtsev, Y.V., Lifton, R.P., Williams, C.S., Charru, A., Hunt, S.C., Hopkins, P.N., William, R.R., Lalouel, J.M. and Corvol, P. (1992) *Cell*, **71**, 169.
6. Kim, H.S., Krege, J.H., Kluckman, K.D., Hagaman, J.R., Hodgin, J.B., Best, C.F., Jennette, J.C., Coffman, T.M., Maeda, N. and Smithies, O. (1995) *Proc. Natl Acad. Sci. USA*, **92**, 2735.
7. Tanimoto, K., Sugiyama, F., Goto, Y., Ishida, J., Takimoto, E., Yagami, K., Fukamizu, A. and Murakami, K. (1994) *J. Biol. Chem.*, **269**, 31334.
8. Schinke, M., Bohm, M., Bricca, G., Ganten, D. and Bader, M. (1996) *Hypertension*, **27**, 508.
9. Phillips, M.I. and Kimura, B. (1988) *J. Hypertension*, **6**, 607.
10. Nazarali, A.J., Gutkind, J.S., Correa, F.M. and Saavedra, J.M. (1990) *Amer. J. Hypertension*, **3**, 59.
11. Phillips, M.I., Mann, J.F.E., Haebara, H., Hoffman, W.E., Dietz, R., Schelling, P. and Ganten, D. (1977) *Nature*, **270**, 445.
12. Wagner, R.W. (1994) *Nature*, 372, 333.
13. Crooke, S.T. (1992) *Annu. Rev. Pharmacol. Toxicol.*, **32**, 329.
14. Stein, C.A. and Cheng, Y.-C. (1993) *Science*, **261**, 1004.
15. Chiasson, B.J., Hooper, M.L., Murphy, P.R. and Robertson, H.A. (1992) *Eur. J. Pharmacol.*, **277**, 451.
16. Wahlestedt, C., Pich, E.M., Koob, G.F., Yee, F. and Heilig, M. (1993) *Science*, **259**, 528.

17. Wahlestedt, C., Golanov, E., Yamamoto, S., Yee, F., Ericson, H., Yoo, H., Inturrisi, C.E. and Reis, D.J. (1993) *Nature*, **363**, 260.
18. McCarthy, M.M., Masters, D.B., Rimvall, K., Schwartz-Giblin, S. and Pfaff, D.W. (1994) *Brain Res.*, **636**, 209.
19. Gyurko, R., Wielbo, D. and Phillips, M.I. (1993) *Regul. Peptides*, **49**, 167.
20. Simons, R.W. (1988) *Gene*, **72**, 35.
21. Stull, R.A., Taylor, L.A. and Szoka, F.C. (1992) *Nucleic Acids Res.*, **20**, 3501.
22. Cowsert, L.M., Fox, M.C., Zon, G. and Mirabelli, C.K. (1993) *Antimicrob. Agents Chemother.*, **37**, 171.
23. Wakita, T. and Wands, J.R. (1994) *J.Biol.Chem.*, **269**, 14205.
24. Lima, W.F., Monia, B.P., Ecker, D.J. and Freier, S.M. (1992) *Biochemistry*, **31**, 12055.
25. Rittner, K. and Sczakiel, G. (1991) *Nucleic Acids Res.*, **19**, 1421.
26. Jaroszevski, J.W., Syi, J.L., Ghosh, M., Ghosh, K. and Cohen, J.S. (1993) *Antisense Res. Dev.*, **3**, 339.
27. Burgess, T. and Farrell, C. (1995) *Proc. Natl Acad. Sci. USA*, **92**, 4051.
28. Singer, M. and Berg, P. (1992) In *Genes and Genomes*, pp. 54–59. University Science Books, Mill Valley, CA.
29. Iversen, P.L., Zhu, S., Meyer, A. and Zon, G. (1992) *Antisense Res. Dev.*, **2**, 211.
30. Colige, A., Sokolov, B.P., Nugent, P., Baserge, R. and Prockop, D.J. (1993) *Biochemistry*, **32**, 7–11.
31. Helene, C. (1991) *Anticancer Drug Res.*, **6**, 569.
32. Bennett, C.F., Condon, T.P., Grimm, S., Chan, H. and Chiang, M. Y. (1994) *J. Immunol.*, **152**, 3530.
33. Bacon, T.A. and Wickstrom, E. (1991) *Oncogene Res.*, **6**, 13.
34. Wahlestedt, C. (1994) *Trends Pharmacol. Sci.*, **15**, 42.
35. Li, B., Hughes, J.A. and Phillips, M.I. (1996) *Neurochem. Intl*, **31**, 393.
36. Campbell, J.M., Bacon, T.A. and Wickstrom, E. (1990) *J. Biochem. Biophys. Methods*, **20**, 259.
37. Takaku, H. (1996) *Neurotide*, **15**, 519.
38. Stein, C.A. (1996) *Chem. Biol.*, **3**, 319.
39. Loke, S.L., Stein, C.A., Zhang, X.H., Mori, K., Nakanishi, M., Subasinghe, C., Cohen, J.S. and Neckers, L.M. (1989) *Proc. Natl Acad. Sci. USA*, **86**, 3474.
40. Wagner, R.W., Matteucci, M.D., Lewis, J.G., Gutierrez, A.J., Moulds, C. and Froehler, B.C. (1993) *Science*, **260**, 1510.
41. Iversen, P.L., Mata, J., Tracewell, W.G. and Zon, G. (1994) *Antisense Res. Dev.*, **4**, 43.
42. Phillips, M.I., Wielbo, D. and Gyurko, R. (1994) *Kidney Intl*, **46**, 1554.
43. Ambuhl, P., Gyurko, R. and Phillips, M.I. (1995) *Regul. Peptides*, **59**, 171.
44. Wielbo, D., Sernia, C., Gyurko, R. and Phillips, M.I. (1995) *Hypertension*, **25**, 314.
45. Wang, C., Chao, L. and Chao, J. (1995) *J. Clin. Invest.*, **95**, 1710.
46. Tomita, N., Morishita, R., Higaki, J., Kaneda, Y., Mikami, H. and Ogihara, T. (1994) *Hypertension*, **24**, 397.
47. Mulligan, R.C. (1993) *Science*, **260**, 926.
48. Katovich, M.J., Lu, D., Lyer, S. and Raizada, M.K. (1996) *FASEB J.*, abstract 1588.
49. Brody, S.L., Jaffe, H.A., Eissa, N.T. and Daniel, C. (1994) *Nature Genet.*, **1**, 42.
50. Quantin, B., Perricaudet, L.D., Tajbakhsh, S. and Mandel, J.-L. (1992) *Proc. Natl Acad. Sci USA*, **89**, 2581.

51. Le Gal La Salle, G., Robert, J.J., Berrard, S., Ridoux, V., Stratford-Perricaudet, L.D., Perricaudet, M. and Mallet, J. (1993) *Science*, **259**, 988.
52. Lu, D., Yu, K. and Raizada, M.K. (1995) *Proc. Natl Acad. Sci. USA*, **92**, 1162.
53. Muzyczka, N. and McLaughin, S. (1988) In Gluzman, Y. and Hughes S.H. (Eds), *Current Communications in Molecular Biology: Viral Vectors*, pp. 39–44. Cold Spring Harbor Laboratory Press, Cold Spring Harbor, NY.
54. Ponnazhagan, S., Nallari, M.L. and Srivastava, A. (1994) *J. Exp. Med.*, **179**, 733.
55. Chatterjee, S., Johnson, P.R. and Wong, K.K. (1992) *Science.*, **258**, 1485.
56. Muzyczka, N. (1992) *Curr. Top. Microbiol. Immunol.*, **158**, 97.
57. Samulski, R.J., Zhu, X., Xiao, X., Brook, J.D., Housman, D.E., Epstein, N. and Hunter, LA. (1991) *EMBO J.*, **10**, 3941.
58. Linden, R.M., Winocour, E. and Berns, K.I. (1996) *Proc. Natl Acad. Sci. USA*, **93**, 7966.
59. Lebkowski, J.S., McNally, M.M., Okarma, T.B. and Lerch, B. (1988) *Mol. Cell. Biol..*, **8**, 3988.
60. Flotte, T.R., Carter, B., Conrad, C., Guggino, W., Reynolds, T., Rosenstein, B., Taylor, G., Walden, S. and Wetzel, R. (1996) *Human Gene Ther.*, **7**, 71145.
61. Gyurko, R. and Phillips, M.I. (1995) *FASEB J.*, abstract 1915.
62. Gyurko, R., Wu, P., Sernia, C., Meyer, E. and Phillips, M.I. (1994) Abstract presented at the American Heart Association 48th Annual Council for High Blood Pressure.
63. Zolothukhin, S., Potter, M., Hauswirth, W.W., Guy, J. and Muzyczka, N. (1996) *J. Virol.*, **70**, 4646.
64. Wu, P., Du, B., Phillips, M.I. and Terwilliger, E.F. (1996) *Soc. Neurosci.*, **22**, abstract 133.2.
65. Mohuczy, D. and Phillips, M.I. (1996) *FASEB J.*, **10**, A447.
66. Zelles, T., Mohuczy, D. and Phillips, M.I. (1996) *Soc. Neurosci.*, 83, abstract 41.18.
67. Mohuczy, D., Gelband, C. and Phillips, M. I. (1999) *Hypertension*, **33**, 354.
68. Phillips, M.I., Mohuczy-Dominiak, D., Coffey, M., Wu, P., Galli, S.M. and Zelles, T. (1997) *Hypertension*, **29**, 374.
69. Kimura, B., Mohuczy, D. and Phillips, M.I. (1998) *FASEB J.*, abstract 522.

12

Regulation of gene expression in the CNS by natural antisense RNAs

PAUL R. MURPHY, RAI KNEE and AUDREY W. LI

1. Introduction

Antisense oligodeoxynucleotides (ODNs) hold great promise as research tools and therapeutic agents, but the design of effective antisense ODNs and appropriately inactive control ODNs has been problematic. Sense ODNs have been widely used as negative controls in a variety of applications because they are complementary to the 'non-coding' DNA strand and should be unable to hybridize to the target mRNA. However, sense ODNs may have unanticipated effects alone, or in combination with antisense ODNs (1). One possible mechanism for sense ODN activity which has been largely overlooked is the potential interaction with antisense RNAs transcribed from the target gene. Antisense RNA transcription occurs in a significant number of prokaryotic genes, and may be a significant mechanism of gene regulation of eukaryotes as well. In the course of investigating the regulation of *FGF-2* gene expression in malignant glioma cells, we have isolated an antisense RNA transcribed from the mammalian *FGF-2* gene locus. An understanding of the function of antisense mRNA expression may provide insights into the rational design of antisense ODNs. In this chapter we will review the literature pertaining to gene regulation by naturally occurring antisense RNA transcripts, and describe our investigation of *FGF-2* antisense RNA expression in mammalian tissues.

2. Evolution of antisense RNA expression

The strategy of molecular targeting of RNA with complementary nucleic acid sequences has probably been in use since protein-based life evolved. Transfer RNA is essentially an antisense RNA which base-pairs with mRNA to initiate and propagate translation (2). More complex interactions of sense and antisense RNAs have since evolved, and are now generally accepted to be a common mechanism of gene regulation in prokaryotes (reviewed in ref. 3). Interaction of the complementary RNA molecules regulates gene expression through steric hindrance of transcription or translation, or by rapid degradation by double-stranded RNA-specific RNase III.

Antisense RNA has, until recently, been regarded as a relatively unusual event. However, the frequency of antisense RNA expression is considerably more common than was originally recognized, and is not limited to prokaryotes. Merino *et al.* (4) recently analyzed the sequence databases of several prokaryotic and eukaryotic organisms for evidence of overlapping antisense open reading frames (ORFs). The study included only database entries greater than 300 nucleotides in length which coded for proteins; extragenic regions and genes for tRNAs and rRNAs were excluded. It was found that gene coding sequences with in-phase, overlapping antisense ORFs are present at a remarkably high frequency (>5%) in every genome examined, from *Escherichia coli* to human.

The origin of these antisense genes is not yet clear. However, it has been suggested that new, phylogenetically restricted genes with more specialized function have arisen by a process of 'overprinting' existing ancient housekeeping genes, whose development predates the divergence of prokaryotes and eukaryotes (5). Analysis of the phylogenetic relationship of a variety of overlapping coding sequences supports this hypothesis; for each pair of overlapping sequences, one is restricted to a single lineage, while the other is more diverse (5). This overprinting hypothesis is supported by recent examples of overlapping sense–antisense gene pairs discussed below, which contain overlapping antisense ORFs for phylogenetically ancient enzymes involved in nucleotide metabolism, DNA repair or transcriptional regulation, coupled with more recently evolved genes involved in growth factor signalling. Whatever their evolutionary origin, it is clear that an understanding of the function of naturally occuring antisense RNAs may provide insight into the rational design of effective antisense therapeutics.

3. Mechanisms of natural antisense action

The list of eukaryotic genes which contain an overlapping antisense-transcribed partner is considerable, and is likely to grow as the repository of sequenced genes becomes more complete. As recent reviews on the subject indicate, the biological significance of eukaryotic antisense RNAs is poorly understood. However, it is becoming clear that the antisense RNAs may be tentatively assigned to one of three classes based on function:

- Class I antisense RNAs are believed to form stable heteroduplexes with their cognate sense RNAs and, by a process of steric hindrance, regulate post-transcriptional processing or translation.

- Class II antisense RNAs may regulate mRNA stability of their complementary partner by targeted digestion with double-strand-specific RNase, or by extensive RNA editing by double-stranded RNA-specific adenosine deaminase (DRADA) activity.
- Class III antisense RNAs are those which encode translated gene products. Several members of both Class I and Class II antisense RNAs must also be included in this group, demonstrating that antisense RNAs can serve both regulatory and protein-coding functions.

We will briefly review examples of both Class I and Class II RNAs, and then describe our own work on FGF-2 and its antisense partner, which appears to function as both a Class II and Class III RNA.

3.1 Class I antisense RNAs: regulation of mRNA processing and translation

3.1.1 c-*erbA*/*Rev-erbA*

The thyroid hormone receptor/*c-erbA* gene locus is the best characterized example of gene regulation by a Class I antisense RNA. Rat and human thyroid hormone receptors (TRs) are encoded by two genetic loci, c-*erbA*α and c-*erbA*β (6–9). The c-*erbA*β gene transcribes two mRNAs encoding two thyroid hormone β-receptor forms which have a tissue-specific, developmentally regulated pattern of expression. The c-*erbA*α locus generates two different mRNAs in the 'sense' orientation, of which the first, α1, encodes the authentic TR and the second, α2, encodes a TR which lacks thyroid hormone binding ability. The first eight exons of the c-*erbA*α gene are common to both RNA forms, but exon 9 is unique to TRα1 and exon 10 is unique to TRα2. The ligand-binding domain in the COOH terminus of TRα1 is replaced by an unrelated sequence in TRα2, which cannot bind ligand, but acts as a dominant-negative regulator of TRα1 and TR-β expression. *In vitro*, α2 splicing is extremely efficient, raising the possibility that formation of α2 mRNA is favored over α1 in the absence of specific regulation. An antisense mRNA, *rev-erbA*α, transcribed from the complementary strand of the c-*erbA*α gene, is believed to regulate the differential splicing of TR-α1 and -α2 isoforms. The 3′-terminal exon of the *rev-erbA*α antisense mRNA is complementary to 263 of 360 nucleotides of the α2-specific exon 10. *Rev-erbA*α RNA inhibits α2 pre-mRNA splicing in HeLa cell nuclear extracts (10). This inhibition of splicing was also observed with a shorter antisense RNA complementary only to the 3′ exon of α2 mRNA, indicating that splicing is sensitive to relatively limited RNA duplex formations. *Rev-erbA*α mRNA is widely expressed in the brain (specifically in the neocortex), and may be involved in the repression of the α2 mRNA in this tissue (11).

In addition to its regulatory role at the RNA level, the *rev-erbA*α transcript encodes an orphan member of the steroid/thyroid hormone nuclear receptor family with sequence-specific DNA-binding and transcriptional repressor activity (12,13). It has been proposed that the *erbA/rev-erbA* locus was generated by translocation of one of the genes into the other, in the process creating the alternative exon 10 (14). In support of this hypothesis, phylogenetic analysis of the ligand-binding domains of these receptors indicates that TRα1 and *rev-erbA*α are the original genes and that exon 10 (specifying TRα2) arose more recently (5). The recent discovery of *rev-erbA*α-related genes encoding other members of the nuclear receptor superfamily (15,16) further supports this hypothesis.

3.1.2 N-*myc*

The N-*myc* proto-oncogene, a homolog of c-*myc*, is amplified in human neuroblastomas (17). The N-*myc* antisense gene, termed N-*cym*, originates within intron 1 and extends back through exon 1 of the N-*myc* gene, with extensive overlap between the 5′ ends of the transcriptional units (18). Balanced transcription in both orientations appears to be co-regulated from a bidirectional promoter in the vicinity of exon 1 (19). Bidirectional promoters have been reported for other eukaryotic genes (20,21). Antisense gene transcription produces distinct 1.0 and 1.8 kb polyadenylated RNA transcripts, and also smaller, more abundant non-adenylated species by initiation at multiple sites predominantly within intron 1. The antisense RNA transcripts form stable heteroduplexes with the N-*myc* transcript, and it has been suggested that the antisense transcript may inhibit N-*myc* pre-mRNA splicing (18).

Only N-*myc* sense transcripts which retain intron 1 selectively form RNA duplexes with N-*cym* antisense transcript over the region extending from the 5′ end of N-*myc* to the 5′ end of N-*cym*. These longer N-*myc* transcripts contain an in-frame AUG translation-initiation codon which is preferentially used *in vitro* to generate an N-terminally extended N-*myc* protein *in vitro* (22). However, this longer N-Myc protein is not detected *in vivo*, suggesting that the N-*cym* antisense transcript may also prevent translation from the intronic AUG.

3.1.3 GnRH (Gonadotropin releasing hormone)

Antisense RNA transcripts derived from the opposite strand of the GnRH gene (designated SH) were first detected in rat heart (23), and subsequently in the preoptic area of the hypothalamus (24). Regulation of GnRH pre-mRNA processing or translation in the hypothalamus by interaction with SH transcripts does not seem likely because of the very low levels of antisense transcripts compared with that of the proGnRH RNA species (25). However, GnRH and its antisense transcript are also co-expressed in peripheral tissues where the level of antisense expression is comparable to or greater than that of the sense RNA (26,27). The apparent localization of GnRH antisense RNA in the nucleus raises the possibility that it may play a role in the regulation of GnRH mRNA processing in some tissues. In the rat Nb2 lymphoma cell line, which co-expresses GnRH and SH transcripts, the half-life of the GnRH RNA is very short, suggesting that the antisense RNA may also regulate GnRH mRNA stability.

3.1.4 The Wilms' tumor suppressor gene

The Wilms' tumor suppressor gene (*WT1*) encodes a 52–54 kDa nuclear protein with transcriptional regulatory function and presumptive tumor repressor activity (28,29). The expression of *WT1* is tightly regulated developmentally during nephrogenesis, and loss of *WT1* is associated with malignancy. Large (7–10 kb) antisense RNA transcripts complementary to a portion of intron 1 and all of exon 1 of the *WT1* gene are expressed in the fetal kidney and in some Wilms' tumor samples (30). Since the antisense RNAs do not contain significant ORFs it has been suggested that they may regulate WT1 protein synthesis by the formation of inhibitory double-stranded RNA complexes with *WT1* transcripts. The antisense promoter is located in the first intron of the *WT1* gene, and has features consistent with other developmentally regulated promoters (29). Furthermore, the presence of high-affinity WT1-binding sites suggests that the activity of the antisense promoter may be regulated by *WT1* itself. This is supported by the demonstration that elevated levels of *WT1* gene expression induce antisense transcription. Transfection and expression of the *WT1* exon 1 antisense RNA in *WT1*-expressing cell lines down-regulate WT1 protein levels, consistent with a role of the antisense RNA in regulating WT1 protein accumulation.

3.1.5 Insulin-like growth factor II

Transcription of insulin-like growth factor II (IGF-II) antisense RNAs has been identified in a broad distribution of species from chickens to humans (31,32), suggesting an evolutionary conservation of the antisense gene. The antisense RNA is transcribed most abundantly at day 18 of mouse embryonic development, then declines progressively during postnatal development to undetectable levels after day 10. The chicken IGF-II antisense RNA shows a similar developmental pattern of expression, with RNA levels being highest in the late stages of embryonic development. IGF-II antisense RNA transcripts have been suggested to play a role during fetal development in the attentuation of IGF-II translation (33).

3.2 Class II antisense RNAs: regulation of mRNA stability

It has been suggested that Class II antisense RNAs form cytoplasmic heteroduplexes with their complementary partners, and regulate transcript stability or half-life. This may result by direct targeting of the RNA heteroduplex by a double-stranded RNA-specific RNase activity as suggested for *Dictyostelium* EB4 RNA (see below). Alternatively, the duplex may be targeted by extensive RNA editing by the unwindase/deaminase activity of DRADA (34,35). The latter mechanism results in the conversion of a number of adenosine residues to inosine, which is thought to hasten the degradation process.

3.2.1 EB4-PSV

The 2.2 kb EB4-PSV mRNA of *Dictyostelium discoideum* is constitutively transcribed during growth and development, but the mRNA does not accumulate due to the instability of the transcript (36). However, when the cells form aggregates and begin to establish a prestalk pattern, the mRNA becomes more stable and begins to accumulate. Disruption of the pattern by mechanical disaggregation causes rapid loss of EB4 RNA, although transcription remains unchanged. A 1.8 kb antisense RNA is transcribed from the same gene locus as EB4, and its abundance is reciprocally related to the abundance of the EB4 transcript during development; as the EB4 mRNA accumulates during aggregation and prestalk formation, the antisense RNA decreases to undetectable levels. Mechanical disaggregation results in rapid accumulation of the antisense RNA accompanied by rapid disappearance of the EB4 transcript. Loss of EB4 RNA following disaggregation is prevented by inhibition of RNA transcription, supporting the notion that the antisense RNA is involved in the regulation of EB4 transcript stability. The rate of transcription of the antisense RNA is lower than the rate of sense transcription in aggregated cells and prestalk formations, but in disaggregated cells antisense transcription exceeds sense transcription by a factor of 5-fold, sufficient to drive the efficient formation of sense:antisense hybrids. There is no significant modification of adenosine residues in the region of the antisense RNA complementary to EB4, indicating that DRADA activity is not involved in the destabilization process. A cytoplasmic double-strand-specific RNase activity has been identified in *Dictyostelium* that could mediate the rapid degradation of EB4 sense:antisense hybrids.

3.2.2 Proliferating cell nuclear antigen

Proliferating cell nuclear antigen (PCNA) is an auxiliary protein of DNA polymerase-γ, which is required for DNA processivity in eukaryotic cells. The long 3′ untranslated region (UTR) of PCNA mRNA shares a 521 nt region of overlap at its 3′ end with a noncoding antisense RNA termed yellow cresent (YC) (37). The antisense YC RNA has been suggested to function in limiting the localization of maternal PCNA to cellular regions during ascidian development. The temporal up-regulation of YC RNA coincides with PCNA mRNA attenuation in the myoplasm following fertilization. Since this occurs at a time when double-strand-specific RNases are activated, YC RNA may play a role in the control of mRNA stability to facilitate PCNA localization during embryogenesis.

3.2.3 Hoxa-11

The *Abdominal-B (Abd-B)* type Hox genes of the *Antennapedia*-like homeobox class play an important role in specifying regional identity during limb development (38,39). The antisense strand of the murine *Hoxa-11* gene gives rise to elaborately spliced mRNAs, which are more abundant than *Hoxa-11* sense transcripts in mouse embryos, suggesting a possible regulatory role for the antisense transcript during development (40). The reciprocal pattern of sense and antisense expression in developing limbs is consistent with the proposed role of the antisense RNA in regulating *Hoxa-11* transcript stability.

3.2.4 FGF-2

The *FGF-2* gene is perhaps the best-documented example of antisense regulation of RNA stability by RNA editing. The *Xenopus* oocyte contains two maternal *FGF-2* mRNA transcripts (4.2 and 2.3 kb in length) and a 1.5 kb antisense RNA (41,42). The antisense gene consists of at least four exons separated by large introns (43). The sense and antisense transcripts share a 900 bp region of overlap such that a portion of the 3′ UTR of each transcript overlaps with coding sequence at the 3′ end of the transcript from the opposite DNA strand.

The antisense transcript is present in 20-fold excess over the sense transcript in the amphibian oocyte, and the two mRNAs form a stable double-stranded RNA duplex at their 3′ ends (42). Duplex formation does not prevent translation of *FGF-2*, but does appear to target the *FGF-2* mRNA (and presumably the antisense mRNA (35)) for modification by a double-stranded RNA-specific unwindase activity (42). This enzyme, which is ubiquitously expressed in eukaryotes (44), specifically binds double-stranded RNA molecules and unwinds them (34,35). During the unwinding process about 50% of the available adenosine residues are covalently converted to inosines, a process which prevents subsequent re-annealing of the duplex (45). Interestingly, unwindase activity is restricted to the nucleus of *Xenopus* oocytes until germinal vesicle breakdown which occurs at oocyte maturation. The appearance of modified *FGF-2* mRNA sequences (adenosine → inosine) in the oocyte occurs only after maturation, and immediately before the abrupt degradation of *FGF-2* sense mRNA transcripts, raising the possibility that antisense-directed unwindase activity targets *FGF-2* mRNA for rapid degradation (42).

Antisense *FGF-2* transcripts complementary to exon 3 of the *FGF-2* gene are also expressed during chicken embryogenesis (46). The sense and antisense transcripts co-localize in some tissues and both transcripts are expressed in a developmentally regulated manner. In the adult, levels of *FGF-2* sense and antisense transcripts are inversely proportional. Furthermore, tissue levels of FGF-2 protein are inversely related, supporting the possibility that the antisense RNA regulates *FGF-2* mRNA and protein levels. Interestingly,

Savage *et al.* (47) have reported that cellular FGF-2 protein levels in developing chick mesoderm were lowest during the G_1 phase of the cell cycle, and suggest that the antisense message may direct the degradation of *FGF-2* mRNA at the end of each cell cycle (48).

4. Does antisense RNA regulate FGF-2 expression in mammalian tissue?

Basic fibroblast growth factor (FGF-2) is a potent pleiotropic factor involved in a host of developmental processes including mesoderm induction, neurite outgrowth, and differentiation (reviewed recently by Basilico and Moscatelli (49)). Transcriptional and post-transcriptional mechanisms operate to keep *FGF-2* mRNA at low or undetectable levels in most differentiated tissues postnatally. However, inappropriately elevated expression of FGF-2 is associated with autocrine growth of CNS tumors including malignant gliomas and schwannomas (50). We have previously observed that FGF-2 overexpression in human glioma cells is associated with increased *FGF-2* mRNA stability (51). It is possible that disruption of antisense regulation of *FGF-2* expression might be responsible for the elevated levels of FGF-2 expression in some CNS tumors. We were therefore interested in identifying mammalian equivalents of the *FGF* antisense RNA. An understanding of the mechanisms regulating *FGF-2* mRNA expression and turnover may provide insights into the treatment and management of primary tumors.

4.1 Detection and cloning of the mammalian FGF antisense RNA

FGF gene organization and sequence are highly conserved among vertebrates and the *FGF-2* gene is transcribed into multiple polyadenylated mRNA transcripts in all species so far examined, including human (52), rat (53) and *Xenopus laevis* (42). The two major transcripts in human tissues (7 kb and 3.7 kb) differ from each other only in the length of the 3′ UTR which may be up to 6 kb in length (54,55). Comparison of the full-length 7 kb human *FGF-2* cDNA sequence with the *Xenopus* antisense *FGF-2* gene transcript indicated two regions which share significant complementarity (*Figure 1a*). These two regions of the *FGF-2* gene are separated by 4300 nucleotides which should be spliced out of the putative antisense RNA. Using primers specific for the predicted antisense splice variant, we amplified a 301 bp cDNA fragment of the human *FGF* antisense RNA. The cDNA product was sequenced and shown to have 73% identity with exons 3 and 4 of the *Xenopus laevis* antisense RNA (56).

The 301 bp cDNA was used as a probe to isolate a full-length 1.1 kb cDNA from a neonatal rat liver cDNA library (57). The rat cDNA has >90%

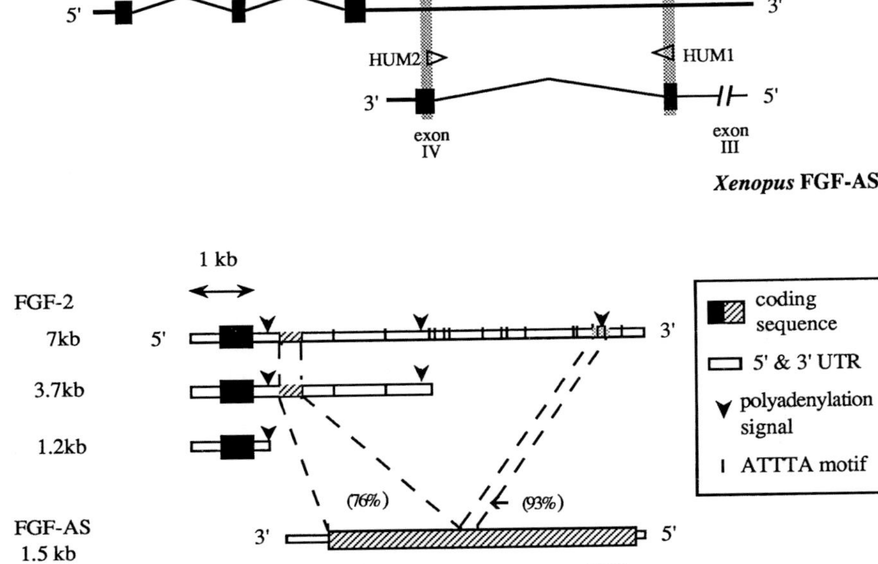

Figure 1. Prediction and identification of the mammalian *FGF-2* antisense RNA. (a) Regions of complementarity of the *Xenopus laevis* antisense RNA with the human *FGF-2* mRNA can be used to predict the location of mammalian antisense exons. The location of primer sequences for RT-PCR amplification of the antisense cDNA are indicated. (b) The full-length rat antisense *FGF* transcript is complementary to discrete regions of the *FGF-2* 3′-UTR.

homology to the human 301 kb cDNA fragment, and 67% overall homology to the *Xenopus FGF* antisense cDNA. However, the extent of overlap (425 nucleotides) is considerably less than the 900 nucleotides reported in *Xenopus*, and the overlapping region does not extend into the *FGF-2* coding region. The antisense RNA is complementary to two widely separated regions of the *FGF-2* mRNA; one 60 nucleotide region includes the most distal polyadenylation signal motif of the 7 kb sense transcript, while the other lies just downstream of the proximal *FGF-2* polyadenylation signal motif (*Figure 1b*). The association of the antisense RNA with potential polyadenylation sites in the *FGF-2* mRNA is intriguing. It is possible that the antisense transcript is involved in regulating post-transcriptional processing of the primary *FGF-2* transcript, possibly by directing alternative polyadenylation signal usage. Remarkably, in two brain-derived *FGF-2* cDNA sequences deposited

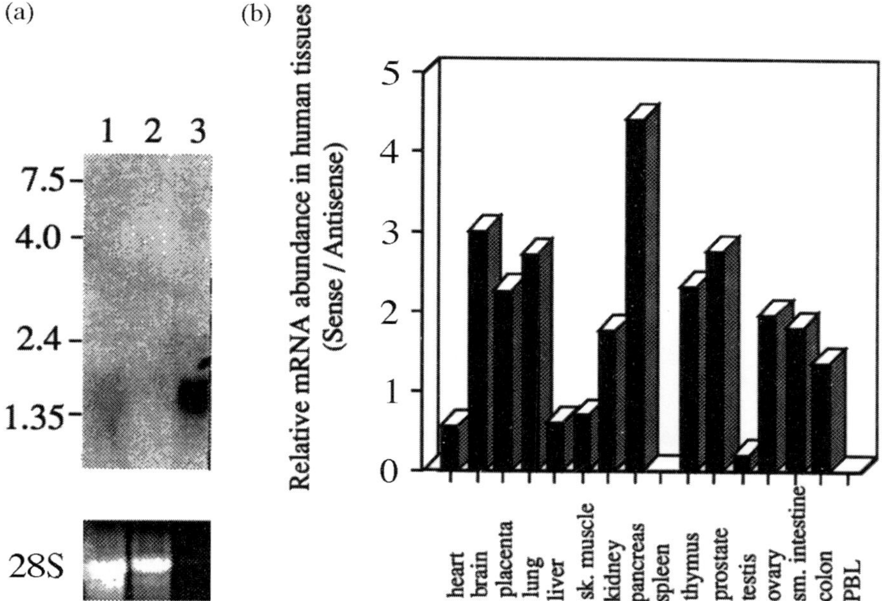

Figure 2. The *FGF* antisense RNA is polyadenylated and expressed in a tissue-specific manner in mammalian tissues. (a) Northern blot containing liver total RNA (lane 1), poly(A)$^-$ RNA (lane 2) and poly(A)$^+$ RNA (lane 3) was hybridized with an antisense-specific cRNA probe. Numbers on the left indicate the size (in kb) of RNA markers. (b) The ratio of sense and antisense mRNA abundance in human tissues was determined by densitometric scanning of multiple-tissue Northern blots.

in GenBank, the proximal polyadenylation signal motif shows signs of editing (AATAA**A** → AATAA**G**) in a position consistent with the 5′ neighbor preference of DRADA (58). Modification of the proximal polyadenylation signal could be responsible for the preferential expression of the longer (3.7 and 7 kb) transcripts in brain and other tissues.

Using RT-PCR, we established that antisense transcripts are present in unfertilized human oocytes at levels which greatly exceed *FGF-2* transcripts (59), consistent with the situation originally reported in *Xenopus* oocytes. Northern hybridization with an antisense-strand specific cRNA established that the 1.5 kb antisense RNA is polyadenylated and expressed in a tissue-specific pattern in mammalian tissues (*Figure 2*).

4.2 Reciprocal expression of FGF-2 sense and antisense expression in brain

The antisense RNA was undetectable in a human malignant glioma cell line (U87-MG) which contains abundant *FGF-2* mRNA (56). *FGF-2* transcripts in

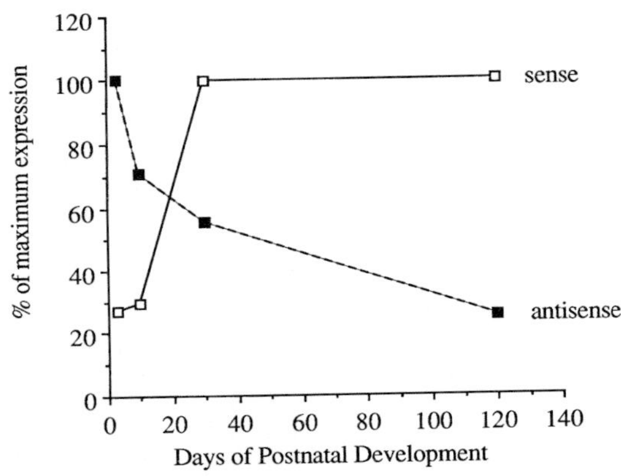

Figure 3. Reciprocal pattern of expression of FGF-2 mRNA (sense) and antisense RNA in the developing rat CNS.

this cell line have a remarkably long half-life, perhaps attributable to lack of the regulatory antisense RNA (51). We were, therefore, interested in determining the expression of FGF and its cognate antisense RNA in normal brain. FGF-2 bioactivity in the developing rat brain is reported to increase more than 10-fold in the first 3 weeks of postnatal development. This is accompanied by an increase in abundance of the longest *FGF-2* transcript (6 kb in rat) and a corresponding decrease in the 1.8 kb transcript (53). Consistent with this, we found that the abundance of the 6 kb *FGF-2* RNA increased dramatically in brain between days 10 and 30 of postnatal development. Remarkably, the increase in sense RNA abundance was accompanied by a reciprocal decline in the level of antisense RNA (*Figure 3*), strongly suggestive of a functional interaction. It is possible that expression of the antisense RNA regulates differential degradation of the various *FGF-2* mRNA species, resulting in enhanced turnover of the 6 kb transcript in the embryonic brain. Alternatively, antisense-mediated control of polyadenylation site usage cannot be ruled out. In either case, the decline in antisense RNA abundance postnatally appears to be associated with differential accumulation of the major 6 kb *FGF-2* transcript in the CNS. Our findings are supported by a recent *in situ* hybridization study which reported an inverse relationship between *FGF-2* sense and antisense RNA in the CNS of the developing rat (60). The pattern of antisense RNA expression in brain is distinct from what we have observed in peripheral tissues, where antisense RNA abundance rises dramatically postnatally (61). This may reflect the fact that *FGF-2* mRNA is abundantly expressed postnatally only in the CNS.

4.3 The antisense RNA encodes a nuclear protein with antimutator activity

The *FGF* antisense RNA is also a Class III RNA, encoding a functional protein which we call GFG. The antisense sequence contains a long ORF which is predicted to encode a 35 kDa translation product. The deduced amino acid sequence contains a conserved MutT domain characteristic of a family of prokaryotic and eukaryotic nucleotide hydrolases. The prototype of this gene family, the *E. coli* MutT protein, plays an important antimutator role by removing mutagenic nucleotides from the DNA precursor pools (62). Insertional inactivation of this protein results in a 1000-fold increase in the rate of spontaneous mutations in *E. coli* (63). GFG has 48–78% identity (within the MutT domain) with a variety of MutT-related proteins (*Figure 4a*), and complete conservation of the invariant amino acids which define the MutT domain (64). Antisera against the MutT domain or against the COOH-terminal region of GFG immunoprecipitate the *in vitro* translated GFG gene product, and detect a 35 kDa immunoreactive band in Western blots of extracts from a variety of rat tissues (57,65,66). Furthermore, the antisense protein is predominantly nuclear, consistent with a possible role in nucleotide metabolism or DNA repair. To test for MutT-related enzymatic activity, we determined the ability of the GFG cDNA to function in MutT-deficient *E. coli*. Expression of recombinant GFG in *mutT*-deficient SBMutT⁻ *E. coli* more than halved the mutation rate in these bacteria compared with vector-transformed cells (*Figure 4b*). Deletion of the MutT domain eliminated the

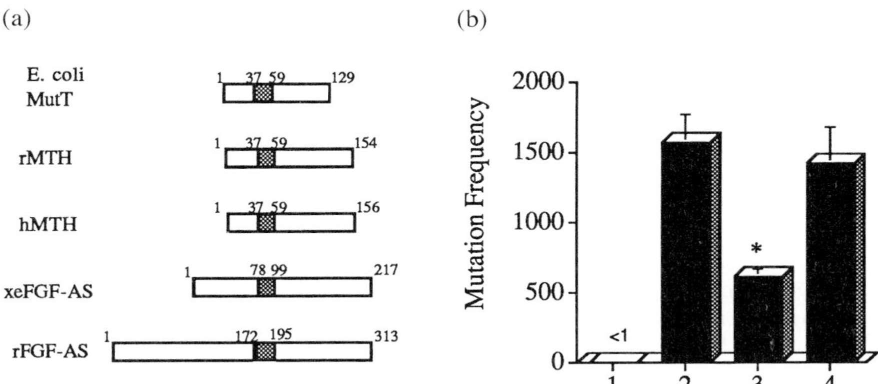

Figure 4. The *FGF* antisense RNA encodes a functional MutT-related protein with antimutator activity. (a) The *E. coli* MutT protein and its mammalian homologs (MTH) contain a conserved enzymatic MutT domain (shaded box) also found in the *Xenopus* and rat *FGF* ORFs. (b) The mutation frequency of MutT-deficient *E. coli* (2) is 1500 times higher than that of wild-type bacteria (1). Recombinant FGF antisense protein (3) significantly reduced the mutation rate, whereas antisense protein without the MutT domain was ineffective (4).

antimutator activity of the construct, confirming that the activity observed is attributable to the catalytic activity of the MutT domain.

It is interesting to note that other DNA repair enzymes, including ERCC-1, RAD10 and MutM, have also been associated with antisense RNA partners. The human MutM RNA is transcribed from the antisense strand of the *camK1* gene. Although intriguing, the significance of this association remains uncertain.

5. Summary

Reports of eukaryotic genes which are bidirectionally transcribed continue to increase as the various sequence databases become more comprehensive. Many of the antisense transcripts are strict Class III RNAs, encoding functional proteins and playing no role in regulation of their sense RNA partners. However, a significant number of sense/antisense RNA partners appear to be involved in either Class I or Class II regulatory interactions. The best examples of Class I (*rev-erbB*) and Class II (*FGF-2*) antisense RNAs both appear to play dual roles as regulatory RNAs and Class III antisense RNAs encoding translated proteins. In both cases, one of the RNAs is evolutionarily more ancient than the other partner, supporting the concept that antisense RNA expression developed by a process of 'overprinting' of existing genes, and that antisense RNA regulation developed secondarily. None the less, regulation of gene expression by natural antisense RNA transcripts appears to be a physiologically meaningful mechanism. This is strongly supported by the recent demonstration that double-stranded RNA ODNs targeted to the coding region potently and specifically inhibit gene expression in *Caenorhabditis elegans* (1). Although the mechanism of this activity is not clear, its effects appear to be amplified by activation of physiological mechanisms. An understanding of the mechanisms of action of antisense RNA may provide valuable insights into the design of antisense therapeutics.

References

1. Fire, A., Xu, S., Montgomery, M.K., Kostas, S.A., Driver, S.E. and Mello, C.C. (1998) *Nature* **391**, 806.
2. Zamecnik, P.C. (1995) In Agrawal, S. (Ed.), *Methods in Molecular Medicine: Antisense Therapeutics*, pp. 1–11. Humana Press, Inc, Totama, NJ.
3. Simons, R.W. and Kleckner, N. (1988) *Annu. Rev. Genet.* **22**, 567.
4. Merino, E., Balbas, P., Puente, J.L. and Bolivar, F. (1994) *Nucleic Acids Res.* **22**, 1903.
5. Keese, P.K. and Gibbs, A. (1992) *Proc. Natl Acad. Sci. USA* **89**, 9489.
6. Weinberger, C., Thompson, C.C., Ong, E.S., Lebo, R., Gruol, D.J. and Evans, R.M. (1986) *Nature* **324**, 641.
7. Nakai, A., Sakurai, A., Bell, G.I. and DeGroot, L.J. (1988) *Mol. Endocrinol.* **2**, 1087.

8. Murray, M.B., Zilz, N.D., McCreary, N.L., MacDonald, M.J. and Towle, H.C. (1988) *J. Biol. Chem.* **263**, 12770.
9. Hodin, R.A., Lazar, M.A., Wintman, B.I., Darling, D.S., Koenig, R.J., Larsen, P.R., Moore, D.D. and Chin, W.W. (1989) *Science* **244**, 76.
10. Munroe, S.H. and Lazar, M.A. (1991) *J. Biol. Chem.* **266**, 22083.
11. Bradley, D.J., Young, W.S.I. and Weinberger, C. (1989) *Proc. Natl Acad. Sci. USA* **86**, 7250.
12. Harding, H.P. and Lazar, M.A. (1995) *Mol. Cell. Biol.* **15**, 4791.
13. Downes, M., Burke, L.J., Bailey, P.J. and Muscat, G.E.O. (1996) *Nucleic Acids Res.* **24**, 4379.
14. Laudet, V., Hanni, C., Coll, J., Catzeflis, F. and Stehelin, D. (1992) *EMBO J.* **11**, 1003.
15. Pena-de-Ortiz, S. and Jamieson, G.A.J. (1997) *J. Neurobiol.* **32**, 341.
16. Bonnelye, E., Vanacker, J.-M., Desbiens, X., Begue, A., Stehelin, D. and Laudet, V. (1994) *Cell Growth Differentiation* **6**, 1357.
17. Kohl, N.E., Kanda, N., Schreck, R., Bruns, G., Latt, S. and Gilbert, F. (1983) *Cell* **35**, 359.
18. Krystal, G.W., Armstrong, B.C. and Battey, J.F. (1990) *Mol. Cell. Biol.* **10**, 4180.
19. Armstrong, B.C. and Krystal, G.W. (1992) *Cell Growth Differentiation* **3**, 385.
20. Burbelo, P.B., Martin, G.R. and Yamada, Y. (1988) *Proc. Natl Acad. Sci. USA* **5**, 9679.
21. Linton, J.P., Yen, J.-Y.J., Selby, E., Chen, Z., Chinsky, J.M., Liu, K., Kellems, R.E. and Crouse, G.F. (1989) *Mol. Cell. Biol.* **9**, 3058.
22. Makela, T.P., Saksela, K. and Alitalo, K. (1989) *Mol. Cell. Biol.* **9**, 1545.
23. Adelman, J.P., Bond, C.T., Douglass, J. and Herbert, E. (1987) *Science* **235**, 1514.
24. Bond, C.T., Hayflick, J.S., Seeburg, P.H. and Adelman, J.P. (1989) *Mol. Endocrinol.* **3**, 1257.
25. Jakubowski, M. and Roberts, J.L. (1994) *J. Biol. Chem.* **269**, 4078.
26. Kelly, A.C., Rodgers, A., Dong, K.W., Barrezueta, N.X., Blum, M. and Roberts, J.L. (1991) *DNA Cell Biol.* **10**, 411.
27. Wilson, T.M., Yu-Lee, L. and Kelley, M.R. (1995) *Mol. Endocrinol.* **9**, 44.
28. Haber, D., Sohn, R., Bucker, A., Pelletier, J., Call, K. and Housman, D. (1991) *Proc. Natl Acad. Sci. USA* **88**, 9618.
29. Malik, K.T.A., Wallace, J.I., Ivins, S.M. and Brown, K.W. (1995) *Oncogene* **11**, 1589.
30. Eccles, M.R., Grubb, G., Ogawa, O., Szeto, J. and Reeve, A.E. (1994) *Oncogene* **9**, 2059.
31. Rivkin, M., Rosen, K.M. and Villa-Komaroff, L. (1993) *Mol. Reprod. Dev.* **35**, 394.
32. Taylor, E.R., Seleiro, E.A.P. and Brickell, P.M. (1991) *J. Mol. Endocrinol.* **7**, 145.
33. Baccarini, P., Fiorentino, M., D'Errico, A., Mancini, A.M. and Grigioni, W.F. (1993) *Amer. J. Pathol.* **143**, 1535.
34. Bass, B.L. and Weintraub, H. (1987) *Cell* **48**, 607.
35. Bass, B. and Weintraub, H. (1988) *Cell* **55**, 1089.
36. Hildebrandt, M. and Nellen, W. (1992) *Cell* **69**, 197.
37. Swalla, B.J. and Jeffery, W.R. (1996) *Dev. Biol.* **178**, 23.
38. Dolle, P., Izpisua-Belmonte, J.-C., Falkenstein, H., Renucci, A. and Duboule, D. (1989) *Nature* **342**, 767.
39. Yokouchi, Y., Sasaki, H. and Kuroiwa, A. (1991) *Nature* **353**, 443.

40. Hsieh-Li, H.M., Witte, D.P., Weinstein, M., Branford, W., Li, H., Small, K. and Potter, S.S. (1995) *Development* **121**, 1373.
41. Kimelman, D., Abraham, J., Haaparanta, T., Palisi, T. and Kirschner, M. (1988) *Science* **242**, 1053.
42. Kimelman, D. and Kirschner, M.W. (1989) *Cell* **59**, 687.
43. Volk, R., Koster, M., Poting, A., Hartmann, L. and Knochel, W. (1989) *EMBO J.* **8**, 2983.
44. Wagner, R.W., Yoo, C., Wrabetz, L., Kamholz, J., Buchhalter, J., Hassan, N.F., Khalili, K., Kim, S.U., Perussia, B., McMorris, F.A. *et al.* (1990) *Mol. Cell. Biol.* **10**, 5586.
45. Polson, A.G., Crain, P.F., Pomerantz, S.C., McCloskey, J.A. and Bass, B.L. (1991) *Biochemistry* **30**, 11507.
46. Borja, A.Z.M., Meijers, C. and Zeller, L. (1993) *Dev. Biol.* **157**, 110.
47. Savage, M.P., Hart, C.E., Riley, B.B., Sasse, J., Olwin, B.B. and Fallon, J.F. (1993) *Dev. Dynam.* **198**, 159.
48. Savage, M.P. and Fallon, J.F. (1995) *Dev. Dynam.* **202**, 343.
49. Basilico, C. and Moscatelli, D. (1992) *Adv. Cancer Res.* **59**, 115.
50. Murphy, P.R., Myal, Y., Sato, Y., Sato, R., West, M. and Friesen, H.G. (1989) *Mol. Endocrinol.* **3**, 225.
51. Murphy, P.R., Guo, J.Z. and Friesen, H.G. (1990) *Mol. Endocrinol.* **4**, 196.
52. Murphy, P.R., Sato, R., Sato, Y. and Friesen, H.G. (1988) *Mol. Endocrinol.* **2**, 591.
53. Powell, P.P., Finklestein, S.P., Dionne, C.A., Jaye, M. and Klagsbrun, M. (1991) *Mol. Brain Res.* **11**, 71.
54. Prats, H., Kaghad, M., Prats, A.C., Klagsbrun, M., Lelias, J.M., Liauzun, P., Chalon, P., Tauber, J.P., Amalric, F., Smith, J.A. and Caput, D. (1989) *Proc. Natl Acad. Sci. USA* **86**, 1836.
55. Kurokawa, T., Sasada, R., Iwane, M. and Igarashi, K. (1987) *FEBS Lett.* **213**, 189.
56. Murphy, P. and Knee, R. (1994) *Mol. Endocrinol.* **8**, 852.
57. Knee, R., Li, A. and Murphy, P. (1997) *Proc. Natl Acad. Sci. USA* **94**, 4943.
58. Polson, A.G. and Bass, B.L. (1994) *EMBO J.* **13**, 5701.
59. Knee, R.S., Pitcher, S.E. and Murphy, P.R. (1994) *Biochem. Biophys. Res. Commun.* **205**, 577.
60. Grothe, C. and Meisinger, C. (1995) *Neurosci. Lett.* **197**, 175.
61. Li, A., Seyoum, G., Shiu, R. and Murphy, P. (1996) *Mol. Cell. Endocrinol.* **118**, 113.
62. Mo, J.-Y., Maki, H. and Sekiguchi, M. (1992) *Proc. Natl Acad. Sci. USA* **89**, 11021.
63. Yanofsky, C., Cox, E.C. and Horn, V. (1966) *Proc. Natl Acad. Sci. USA* **55**, 274.
64. Koonin, E.V. (1993) *Nucleic Acids Res.* **21**, 4847.
65. Li, A.W., Too, C.K.L. and Murphy, P.R. (1996) *Biochem. Biophys. Res. Commun.* **223**, 19.
66. Li, A., Too, C., Knee, R., Wilkinson, M. and Murphy, P. (1997) *Mol. Cell. Endocrinol.* **133**, 177.

13

Aptamers: another use for oligonucleotides

RICHARD C. CONRAD

1. Introduction

Two decades ago, the biological function of nucleic acids was thought to be reserved to base pairing with other nucleic acids or to interactions with proteins that had evolved to bind nucleic acids. The discovery in the early 1980s of 'ribozymes,' RNA molecules capable of performing specific chemical reactions on themselves or other RNA molecules, provided an inkling that perhaps the role of nucleic acids had been underestimated. It is now clear that nucleic acids possess structural as well as functional complexity beyond that envisioned for them in the early days of molecular biology. With the advent of simple means for replication of nucleic acids *in vitro* and the ability to chemically synthesize large amounts of nucleic acids in the 100 nucleotide (nt) range, novel nucleic acids with previously unknown binding functionalities can be created and propagated *in vitro*. Variations of these and other techniques can be used to find these novel binding nucleic acids, using a procedure of cycled amplification and selection steps referred to as SELEX (systematic evolution of ligands by exponential enrichment). The actual nucleic acid ligands are called aptamers.

The number of aptamers is steadily mounting in the literature. The 'targets' of these aptamers range from proteins known to bind nucleic acids, to proteins not thought to associate with nucleic acids *in vivo*, to small molecules. There are many potential uses for aptamers. With nucleic acid-binding targets, a 'perfect' target sequence can be found to investigate the genome for undiscovered interaction sites, or the molecular interactions involved can be characterized by comparing different aptamers with similar binding affinity. At a basic research level, aptamers for small molecules can be used to ask questions about molecular evolution and recognition, by comparing aptamers of similar sequence that have different binding specificities, or similar binding specificities and disparate sequences. Most germane to this volume is the utility of aptamers that bind novel ('non-nucleic acid-binding') proteins. Often these types of aptamers have dissociation constants in the low nanomolar range. These can be labeled radioactively or in some other manner, and used to find their target in a macro- or microscopic physiological milieu. When they are found to inhibit the function of their target protein, as they often do, they serve as easily replaceable reagents for *in vitro* or *in vivo* inhibition studies. In this capacity, they serve a function analogous to antisense oligonucleotides, but inhibiting at the level of protein function rather than gene expression. For *in vivo* studies, their application as inhibitors presents the same problems as antisense oligonucleotides in terms of toxicity and bioavailability, with identical solutions being attempted (chemical modification of bases and backbone). An added bonus is that the initial selection of the aptamer can be performed with many of these modifications in place, creating a more highly tailored aptamer for the purpose at hand.

This chapter is meant to serve as a primer for the selection of aptamers, providing a basic approach to SELEX. For brevity's sake, only the most common methodology, finding RNA aptamers using nitrocellulose filter immobilization, is presented. Further procedures detailing isolation of DNA or modified RNA aptamers and usage of alternative selection modalities, such as affinity resins or immunoprecipitations, can be found in references 1–3. Although the procedures involved are not new, they are somewhat modified to suit the needs at hand. My aim is to try to provide cautionary notes along the way, so as to avoid pitfalls that bring about failure or misleading results.

2. Overview

The procedure as outlined depends on the ability of the researcher to isolate desired nucleic acid molecules from a huge pool of molecules with a randomly distributed assortment of sequences and, hence, structures. The relatively few molecules so isolated are then replicated to create thousands to millions of copies. This new pool of nucleic acids, though enriched in the desired species, needs to be passed through additional cyclical rounds of selection and amplification, until an end point is met. *Figure 1a* presents a cartoon version of this process. The cycle is represented as having an 'informational' side, where the ability of nucleic acids to serve as their own template is paramount, and a 'structural/functional' side, where the ability of the nucleic acids to fold and bind to complementary shapes is important. At the top, at the end of the informational phase, is the pool of molecules. This would be a huge collection of random sequences with only one copy each in the first round, and a collection of selected sequences amplified by replication of the individual molecules in subsequent rounds. By placing this pool in a solution with enough ionic strength to mitigate phosphate–phosphate repulsion in the backbone, heating the sample, and cooling, the individuals in the pool fold into accessible structures (**renaturation**), as indicated on the right side. In the figure, various squiggles represent various three-dimensional shapes that can

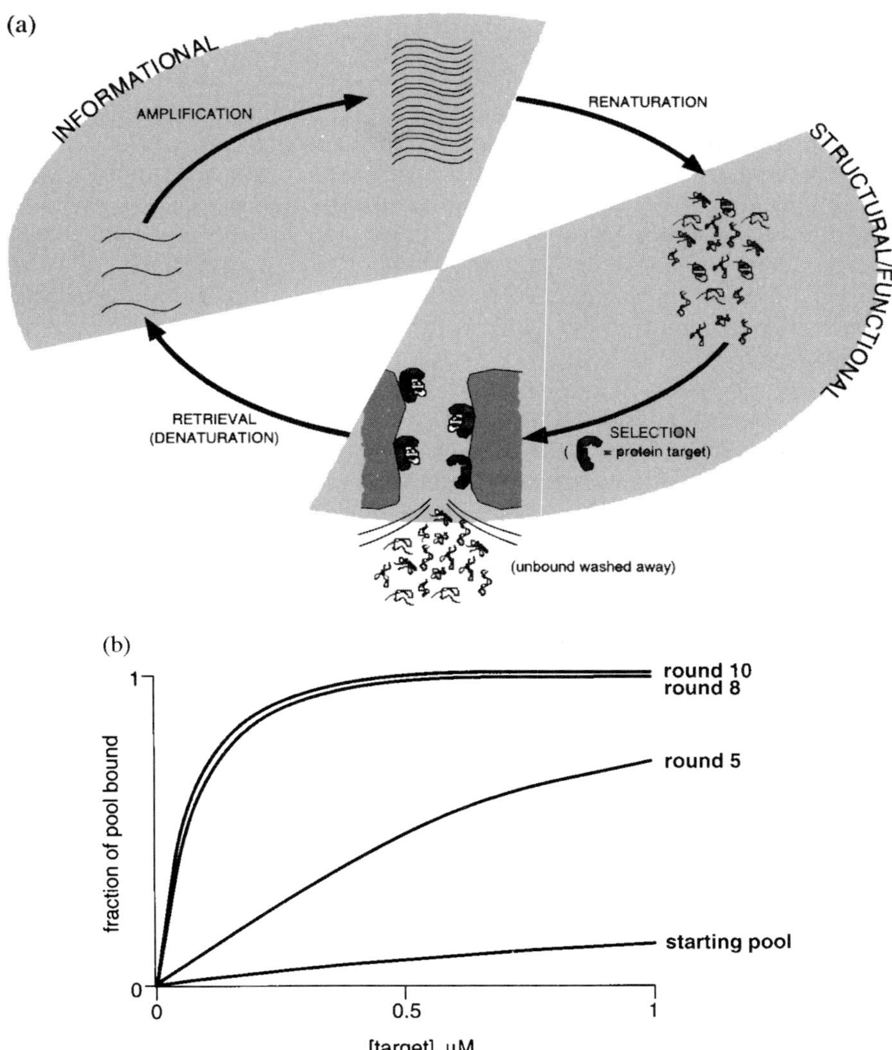

Figure 1. (a) Highly diagrammatic representation of the SELEX process. Consult the text for details. (b) A series of binding curves representing the course of a hypothetical SELEX experiment through many rounds. Such data would be obtained through the procedures outlined in Section 6.1.

be formed by nucleic acids, each dictated by their sequence. These can now be mixed with the protein target and, after sufficient time is allowed for binding, the protein can be collected on a nitrocellulose filter (**selection**). The bottom of the figure indicates a pore in the nitrocellulose, where the protein molecules are adsorbed on the surface, and the bound nucleic acid is immobilized with them. After rinsing away unbound nucleic acids, the filter can be extracted with a denaturant, freeing the bound nucleic acids (**retrieval**) and returning them to the informational part of the cycle, as shown on the left side of *Figure 1a*, where the cycle is completed by replicating these molecules as much as a million-fold (**amplification**) to create a new pool.

Each round of SELEX provides an enrichment of representation of high-affinity binders, rather than an immediate selection of only the best binders. The number of rounds required to reach a frequent enough representation of good binders varies with design used for the original pool (referred to as the 'library') and also with target. Generally, libraries with limited degeneracy require three or four rounds (2,4,5), while for those with contiguous regions of random sequence over 20 nt, 8–12 rounds are the norm, and up to 17 rounds have been reported (6). The need for so many rounds is explained to some extent by the rationalization that, for each 'excellent' binder, there will be many variants at one or two positions that will be poorer binders, but present in higher numbers, forcing some of their number to bind at equilibrium. The later selection/amplification cycles increase the representation of the excellent binders in the population, allowing them to compete more effectively with the poor binders. There are ways to influence this effect during the selection, which will be discussed later in this chapter. The practical consequence of this is that the selection/amplification process must be repeated until a satisfactory endpoint is reached. The best way to ascertain this endpoint is to characterize the binding behavior of the pool after successive rounds. *Figure 1b* shows how binding behavior changes during the course of a SELEX process. At a certain point (in the figure, between rounds 8 and 10), binding behavior no longer improves. At this point, individual members of the pool can be isolated and characterized by molecular biological methods, determining any prevalent sequences. Dominant sequences can be resynthesized for further characterization in terms of affinity, structure, and inhibitory activity.

The entire process can be roughly broken down into preparation (of the initial library of oligonucleotides), selection (binding, immobilization, and elution), amplification (through replication and transcription), and characterization of aptamers (binding for both pools and individual aptamer populations, sequencing and additional structural and functional characterization of individual aptamer populations). The aim of this chapter is to provide the basics for each of these, with the last item restricted primarily to binding, to allow the researcher enough technical information to perform his or her own SELEX.

3. Starting material: the library

The term 'library' is used to denote the collection of oligonucleotides that can be used as the starting material for SELEX experiments. The creation of the library requires three separate steps. First is the design, taking into account what sequences and structures are initially available for recognition of (or by) a target, as well as characteristics affecting its function as a replicon. The second step is the chemical synthesis, and third, this large collection of chemically synthesized oligodeoxynucleotides (ODNs) must be enzymatically amplified to provide a moderate representation of each individual. For those libraries with only a few up to about 15 positions randomized, this can be done using normal-scale PCR procedures. However, when the number of randomized positions exceeds this, the amplification must be done on a large scale in order to lose as little as possible of the complexity of the original synthesis.

3.1 Design

The library design is, in essence, a determination of constancy versus variability. For every position where a nucleotide monomer is to be added on to the growing chain, is a single base (constant), an equal mixture of all four bases (totally random), or a mixture where one or more of the bases are present in greater amount ('doped') in the coupling mix. A generic example is shown in *Figure 2a*. Two regions must be constant in all pools: the 5′-and 3′-terminal regions (shown in gray in the figure). These are the primer-binding sites necessary for replication, and all of the principles governing primer design apply to these regions (7–9). However, there are also unique considerations for pool design, given that they will be exposed to a dozen or more PCR amplifications, with 10–30 priming events in each (depending on the number of cycles). The occurrence of artefacts can be minimized by avoiding primers that form internal secondary structures or that pair with one another, and by making the 3′ termini of primers AT-rich (10). In addition, the 3′ (first synthesized) terminus will be subjected to the greatest number of chemical cycles. Although modern chemistry and machines minimize much of the problem, a certain amount of chemical damage accrues in this region, affecting replicability. This is primarily depurination, so making this priming region relatively poor in purines decreases the number of non-replicable molecules in the mix. Finally, although all care will surely be taken by any researcher to eliminate cross-contamination, it should go with saying that different pools should contain different priming sequences.

Between these two constant regions, the middle section of the oligonucleotide (shown in black in *Figure 2a*) can be completely random, partially randomized with a bias to a specific sequence, contain regions of constant interspersed with variable sequence (a few possibilities are illustrated in *Figure 2b*), or any combination of these. This decision is directed by the target being pursued. When the purpose of a selection experiment is to specify a target sequence for a nucleic acid-binding protein, several aspects of the design can be based on previously known recognition sequences. If the protein is known to bind to a loop at the end of a short stem, a random region

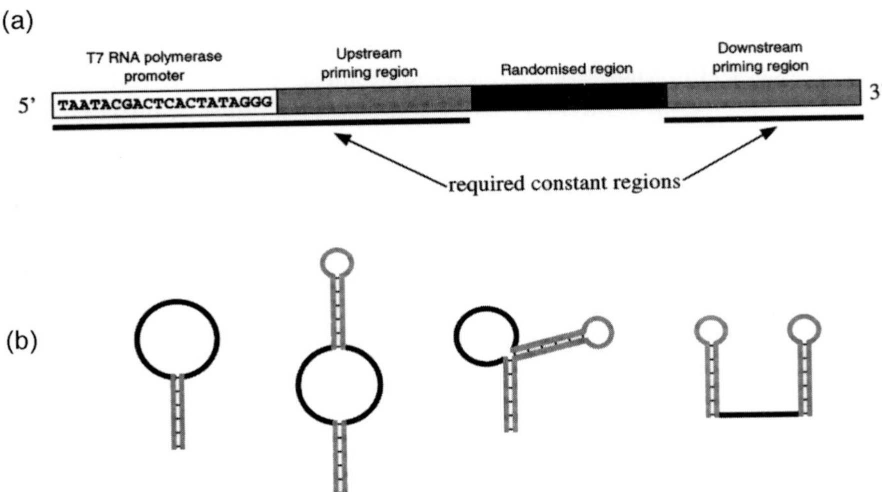

Figure 2. (a) Diagram of the design of an oligonucleotide pool, representing the 'sense' strand of the final dsDNA library. See the text for details. (b) Pictorial representations of the various formats that can be used in the randomized (black) region of the oligonucleotide design shown in panel (a). Thick gray lines represent constant sequence (with base-paired regions tied together with smaller black lines), while thick black lines represent partially or totally randomized sequence.

can be introduced between two fixed regions that form a base-paired stem, or it may be desired to dope the synthesis to correspond to a consensus recognition sequence, where the amount of the doped nucleotide phosphoramidite would be many times that of the other three. However, both these procedures are predicated on the assumption that the sequences discovered so far are representative of all that exist, and that the structure has been correctly predicted. To find a completely unbiased recognition site, use of a totally randomized region would be recommended. The same approach should be taken in those cases where a natural nucleic acid ligand for a molecular target is not known. By using a highly degenerate random sequence core, researchers' preconceptions will not bias the eventual results of the selection. Here, the *size* of the random region is the choice that must be made. Because the number of possibilities is 4^l, where l is the length of the random sequence; the ability to cover them all is limited to about a 15 nt stretch. This being said, there are arguments to be made in favor of large randomized regions. First, the larger tracts contain within them smaller sequences, which can be extracted from the selected aptamer sequences. Secondly, for larger nucleic acid structures there are often different sequence 'solutions' that yield similar three-dimensional shapes. This is borne out by the fact that, in our experience, different pools with large random tracts have been found to give different results with the same target.

3.2 Chemical (solid-state) DNA synthesis

Every new library that is generated requires three syntheses: the synthesis of the pool itself and the synthesis of the two primers for its amplification. If the synthetic ODN will be used only as a DNA pool (single- or double-stranded), then the primers need only match the terminal sections of the constant regions. However, if the synthetic ODN will eventually be transcribed into RNA, the upstream primer must also carry a promoter sequence, which will be lost during the transcription process. A popular choice is the strong promoter for bacteriophage T7 RNA polymerase, because this enzyme works efficiently with templates of all sizes. This sequence is shown in *Figure 2a*. The addition of a 4 nt 'clamp' upstream (any sequence) of the actual promoter sequence is recommended to increase the stability of the polymerase-binding site.

The procedures for pool synthesis have been described in detail elsewhere (11). In general, the synthesis is standard as described in the instructions for the individual synthesizer, with the unusual features being in the synthesis of the random region. Many DNA synthesizers include protocols for on-line mixing of phosphoramidites, and more sophisticated machines offer a more than adequate level of control for generation of doped and totally randomized regions. For simpler machines, this can be accomplished by manually mixing the four phosphoramidites off-line and then introducing this mixture on to a defined port of the synthesizer. It has been found that incorporation efficiency for all four bases is not equal (12). This skewing can be alleviated if the random sequence regions are synthesized using a 3:3:2:2 molar ratio of A:C:G:T. Sequence length as well as composition can be randomized, by performing several syntheses of differing lengths, then mixing them. This mixing can even be done with the still-active resin, followed by repackaging into a column and reattaching to the machine. This allows additional constant and random regions to be added in unison (13). Following synthesis, oligonucleotides are cleaved from their supports (and protecting groups removed) by prolonged incubation (16 h) with reagent ammonium hydroxide at 75 °C. Oligonucleotides are removed from the ammonium hydroxide solution by addition of ten volumes of isobutanol (absorbing all water) and centrifugation.

Shorter syntheses (primers) may be purified by precipitation alone. However, the chemical damage mentioned above for longer syntheses can result in significant strand cleavage during deprotection. Most of these products will not exponentially amplify in the PCR, but will still use up primers, nucleotides, and enzyme at each cycle, decreasing the overall yield of the desired full-length product. For this reason, long (>80 nt), random sequence oligonucleotides should be purified by gel electrophoresis before proceeding to the initial amplification. Some internal deletions may occur that do not interfere with amplification. Since these are still useful members of the population, it is advisable to cut out gel containing some slightly smaller products (10 nt less than full-length) along with the major band.

The procedure outlined in *Protocol 1* is applicable to all gel purifications mentioned in this chapter.

Protocol 1. Purification of an oligonucleotide using denaturing polyacrylamide gel electrophoresis (PAGE)

Equipment and reagents

- Formamide containing 0.01% bromophenol blue
- Acrylamide stock solution, 40% (19:1 monomer:bis)
- 10x TBE (890 mM Tris base, 890 mM boric acid, 20 mM Na_2-EDTA, pH 7.8)
- Urea (solid)
- TE solution (10 mM Tris–HCl (pH 7.5), 1 mM EDTA)
- 10% ammonium persulfate (APS)
- TEMED
- Vertical slab gel electrophoresis apparatus (e.g., from Hoefer Scientific Instruments or Gibco-BRL)

Method

1. Determine the appropriate gel percentage for the size of the oligonucleotide to be purified.[a]
2. Make enough gel solution to fill the apparatus (see manufacturer's instructions). Add an appropriate amount of acrylamide solution (e.g., 1/4 volume for a 10% gel), 1/10 volume of 10× TBE, 0.42 g/ml urea, and enough water to bring the gel solution to the final desired volume.
3. Gently heat the gel solution (using a hot water bath) to aid in dissolving the urea.
4. Add 1/100 volume of 10% APS and 1/1000 volume of TEMED, mix, and pour the gel solution into pre-cast gel plates. When choosing a comb, use the widest sample slots possible.
5. Once the gel has set (*ca.* 30–60 min), set up the apparatus and pour buffer into the upper and lower chambers.
6. Add an equal volume of the formamide solution to the synthetic oligonucleotide dissolved in water.
7. Heat the sample at 90 °C for 5 min. Using a syringe, rinse out urea that has diffused into the wells. Load the sample into the wells.[b]
8. Run the gel at about 0.1 W/cm^2 of surface area. The gel should be warm but not too hot to touch during the run (*ca.* 55 °C).
9. After the bromophenol blue tracking dye has run far enough to indicate that full-length oligonucleotides will be separated from truncated oligonucleotides, stop the run and remove the gel from the apparatus.

10. The position of the samples can be determined by shadowing the gel with short wavelength UV (254 nm) over a large TLC plate containing a fluorescent indicator. Excise the band and chop it into small pieces. Ease the pieces into an appropriately sized centrifuge tube.

11. Elute the oligonucleotide from the polyacrylamide gel into water or into 0.3 M sodium acetate at 37 °C with tumbling overnight. Elution works best if the volume of solvent used for elution exceeds gel volume by at least a factor of two.

12. Remove the eluate from the gel fragments. Precipitate the oligonucleotide from the eluate by bringing the concentration of sodium acetate to 0.3 M (if eluted into water) and adding 2.5 volumes of absolute ethanol. Incubate on dry ice for 30 min or at –20 °C overnight.

13. Spin down the precipitate at 10 000–15 000***g*** for 30 min. Wash pellet with 70% ethanol (95% for oligonucleotides of ≤30 nt) before drying. Dissolve the pellet in TE or water.

14. Determine the concentration of the oligonucleotide by reading the OD_{260} of an appropriate dilution.[c]

[a] Roughly: 20% for 10–20mers, 15% for 30–40mers, 10% for 50–100mers, 6% for 150–300mers.
[b] For a 15 cm wide, 1.5 mm thick gel, a total of 300 μg of crude oligonucleotide can be loaded over the entire gel.
[c] The concentration of single-stranded DNA can be estimated from the formula [ssDNA] = OD_{260} (of a 1 ml solution in a 1 cm path length) × dilution factor × 37 μg/ml.

3.3 Amplification to generate a dsDNA library

The chemical synthesis and purification provide a collection of unique single-stranded ODNs. These are without a transcription promoter and are not 100% replicable, due to the damage suffered by some molecules during chemical synthesis. By modestly amplifying the entire population (only about seven cycles of PCR), these attributes are all changed. Each replicable ODN is copied into several double-stranded DNA (dsDNA) molecules with a transcriptional promoter in place. Those molecules that are not replicable are now in the minority in this population. For libraries with relatively small random regions, there are many representatives of each sequence present in the initial synthesis, so amplifying the entire library together and for only a few cycles is not important. The cut-off point is around 15 random positions. The reasoning is that the maximum amount of DNA obtainable from a 100 μl PCR is about 2 μg, so for a 10-fold amplification, at most 0.1 μg of single-stranded template should be used. For a 20 nt random tract double-stranded oligonucleotide with two 20 nt priming regions, this represents 1.5×10^{12} molecules, which is about equal to the possibilities for a 20 nt stretch. Obviously, the chance of containing all sequences is negligible. By using a random region of 15 nt, the ratio of total molecules present to total sequence possibilities becomes about 1000. This is deemed a reasonable compromise between versatility (of structures) and probability (of containing a particular sequence).

In pools with larger random regions (≥27 nt), the initial synthesis cannot cover the entire sequence space, and virtually all members are unique. The emphasis here shifts to trying not to lose any of the complexity of the existent population. This means that the all or a substantial fraction of the original synthesis should be amplified 10- to 20-fold in the same mix, so that removal of an aliquot does not eliminate a particular species from the parent mix. This requires a huge (often >100 ml) PCR volume, with the thermal cycling done by hand in 15 ml tubes using separate water baths. The large volumes mandate longer times for each incubation step to ensure complete thermal equilibration. Where 0.1 μg is used for a 100 μl reaction, 100 μg is used as input for this 100 ml reaction volume. Remember that it is critical to re-mix the divided reaction volumes afterwards for the reasons mentioned above.

Protocol 2. Large-scale amplification of a synthetic oligonucleotide population

Equipment and reagents

- 10× PCR buffer: 100 mM Tris–HCl (pH 8.3), 500 mM KCl, 15 mM $MgCl_2$, 1% Nonidet P-40
- 50% acetamide
- 100 mM each dNTP, neutralized (Pharmacia PL Biochemicals, Milwaukee, WI, USA)
- TE: 10 mM Tris–HCl (pH 7.5), 1 mM EDTA
- Thermostable DNA polymerase from *Thermus aquaticus* (Perkin Elmer), 5 units/μl
- 15 ml screw-capped conical polypropylene tubes
- Upstream and downstream primers, 50 μM stock solutions (~1.6 ml each)

Method

1. Make up the PCR cocktail:
   - 10 ml of 10× PCR buffer
   - 10 ml of 50% acetamide
   - 0.2 ml of each 100 mM dNTP solution
   - 1.6 ml of each 50 μM primer solution
   - 77.5 ml deionized, distilled water
   - 0.5 ml of *Taq* polymerase stock (2500 U)
2. Add 2–4 nmol (in <1 ml) of the gel-purified, synthetic oligonucleotide to the PCR cocktail.
3. Distribute the mix between twelve 15 ml conical screw-capped tubes (*ca.* 8.3 ml per tube).
4. Using fixed-temperature water baths with lids, incubate the tubes for seven cycles according to the following schedule:
   - 94°C for 5 min for the first cycle or 3.5 min for each subsequent cycle

- 45 °C for 5 min[a]
- 72 °C for 7 min, 20 min total for the final cycle.

For ease of manipulation, a floating rack for the tubes can be fashioned out of polystyrene foam. The extent of amplification can be monitored by taking small samples at each cycle and comparing them with the original amplification reaction mix on an agarose gel, as described in *Protocol 4*.

5. Precipitate the entire amplification reaction. This can be carried out in large centrifuge bottles or in multiple centrifuge tubes:
   (a) add 100 ml of 4 M ammonium acetate and 400 ml of absolute ethanol;[b]
   (b) incubate at –80 °C for 1 h or –20 °C for 16 h;
   (c) centrifuge at 10 000–15 000*g* for 30 min;[c]
   (d) wash pellet(s) with 70% ethanol and vacuum dry.
6. Dissolve the pellet(s) and combine in a total volume of 1 ml TE.
7. Extract with an equal volume of phenol–chloroform (1:1), then with chloroform.
8. Precipitate as in step 5 (but decrease additions to 1 ml of 4 M ammonium acetate and 4 ml of ethanol).[d]
9. Dissolve the pellet in 500 μl of TE.
10. Determine the concentration of the DNA library by reading the OD_{260} of an appropriate dilution.[e]

[a] This temperature may have to adjusted depending on the melting temperature of the primer.
[b] Ammonium acetate minimizes the level of mononucleotide precipitation.
[c] Two 500 ml centrifuge bottles are convenient for this step.
[d] Clean Oakridge tubes are convenient for this step.
[e] The concentration of the dsDNA can be estimated using the formula [dsDNA] = OD_{260} × dilution factor × 50 μg/ml.

3.4 Conversion of the initial dsDNA library to an RNA pool

SELEX experiments routinely use an RNA pool. For this, the dsDNA library must first be transcribed *in vitro*, usually using bacteriophage T7 RNA polymerase. There are published procedures for this (14), but unless you can produce your own RNA polymerase, the use of commercially available kits (e.g., the Ampliscribe kit from Epicentre Technologies) presents an easy and very reliable means for performing this task. Such kits typically provide very consistent results using as little as 0.1 μg of PCR product as the initial template. Typically 5–10 μg dsDNA is used to make 50–100 μg RNA for the first round, and about 0.1 μg for subsequent rounds. After removing the DNA by DNase treatment, the RNA is gel-purified and quantified by measuring its OD_{260} (a solution with an OD_{260} of 1 contains 40 μg/ml RNA).

Other selections can rely on modified RNA or single-stranded DNA (ssDNA) pools. The production of modified nucleic acid pools uses modified nucleotides in place of their unmodified counterparts in RNA transcription reactions. Although they are incorporated by T7 RNA polymerase (15,16), the yield of the reaction is reduced. This loss of efficiency can be minimized when the first 12 bases of the transcription template contain no purines (17). An ssDNA pool can be generated directly from a dsDNA library. In this case a particular strand should be purified or at least in a majority in the pool. There are several protocols for accomplishing this end, including asymmetric PCR (3), the use of a mixed backbone primer (18), and incorporation of biotin into one primer (19).

4. Selection

SELEX experiments seek to provide a of pool of high-affinity binding species with minimal representation of low-affinity and non-specific binding species. Because of this, conditions need to be found for binding that favor this event. Because there are many ways to influence this, it is useful to speak in the general concept of stringency. Selections that are not stringent enough will not encourage competition between different aptamers, and will return a diverse population of mediocre as well as strong binding species. However, selections that are too stringent, especially at the start, will remove even the best aptamers from the selected population, leaving behind only non-specific binding species. We tend to carry out the first one to three cycles at low stringency, in order to firmly establish multiple copies of aptamers in a selected population, then increase the stringency of the selection to eliminate non-specific binders and weakly binding aptamers.

4.1 Binding

There are several considerations in determining the conditions under which the target and pool are mixed which affect stringency. These include solution composition, the presence of competitors, the temperature and length of the reaction, and the concentrations of pool and target.

The 'binding solution' is usually dictated by the target itself. Most proteins have known buffer and salt conditions which are used to assay activity. Since this is presumably the solution in which the aptamer will be asked to act, the selections should be made in it, or at least a modified version of it. The buffers themselves are forgiving: Tris (the majority of published selections), phosphate (20), and HEPES (21, 22) have all been successfully used. The ionic strength of the reaction has a large impact on the stringency of the selection. It should be high enough to buffer the repulsion of backbone phosphate groups, allowing formation of nucleic acid structure, but not so high that it interferes with ionic interactions between the target and nucleic acid—somewhere in the range of 50–150 mM. Divalent cations provide a much greater effect per molar amount than monovalents. In fact, at least one selection has been performed with Mg^{2+} as the sole cation (22). In general, selections with protein targets should include Mg^{2+} and/or Ca^{2+} at concentrations of 1–10 mM. Often the best course of action is to choose binding reaction conditions, presumably consistent with the end use of the aptamer, and test for the ability to bind a small fraction of the pool, as discussed in Section 6.1 below. Once a binding solution has been decided upon, the nucleic acid pool should be thermally equilibrated in this buffer prior to mixing with target. By heating in the buffer of choice to 75–90 °C, then cooling to the temperature of the binding reaction, individual members of the pool are scrambled and allowed to refold. A little-manipulated but potentially significant condition for binding is the final temperature. Although most selections are carried out at room temperature, selections carried out at higher temperatures may return fewer aptamers that form tighter structures. This must be balanced against the potential for target protein denaturation.

The concentrations of the pool and target affect the binding reaction in an obvious manner: the higher their concentration, the more complexes will form, and the lower the stringency of the selection. Performing the selection at higher dilution (lower concentrations of both target and pool) in later rounds is a simple and highly effective way to increase stringency. Again, the best strategy to determine initial selection conditions is to perform binding studies with various input amounts to find conditions that allow about 4% of the pool to be bound (23). In the absence of such knowledge, the initial selection should use relatively high (micromolar) concentrations of target, which can be reduced progressively with each round as shown in *Protocol 3*.

A final component that is readily applicable to increase stringency is the use of competitors, either specific or non-specific. Specific competitors would be used with nucleic acid-binding proteins, and would mimic known natural sequences. These lack priming regions and are therefore lost after the amplification step. When present, specific competitors should generally be included in at least a four-fold molar excess over the pool. Non-specific competitors would be polyanions like heparin or nucleic acids of indeterminate sequence (e.g. tRNA), again unamplifiable. These can be present in any concentration to displace low- or non-specifically-binding members of the amplifiable pool.

The length of the binding reaction can theoretically affect the kinetic characteristics of the aptamers selected, with faster-binding aptamers presumably the more desirable. In practice, this is affected by concentration as well. In general, incubation times should be within the range of several seconds to 30 min. Target protein stability or RNase activity of the protein preparation also play a role in this choice.

4.2 Isolation of bound nucleic acids

The critical step in the selection process is the specific isolation of nucleic acid complexed to the target. All procedures rely on a technique to immobilize the target. In certain cases the binding can be performed on a pre-immobilized target. These often involve covalent attachment of target on a chromatographic resin. Usually protein targets are immobilized after the binding reaction, trapping bound nucleic acids with them. This can be a specific retrieval from a protein mix or a general immobilization of all protein from a purified target preparation. In the first group of procedures would be immunoprecipitation or other affinity methods, which could use immobilized substrate, immobilized lectin to bind glycoproteins, or engineered protein sites (e.g. GST or streptavidin to bind to glutathione or biotin columns). The latter method can use panning on microtiter trays or the nitrocellulose filter procedure given in the following protocol. For any of these procedures, the bound nucleic acid aptamers are then eluted by competition with affinity elution or by denaturation. The selected nucleic acids can finally be concentrated by ethanol precipitation and amplified for the next cycle.

4.2.1 Nitrocellulose filter immobilization

The following protocol is a general procedure for isolating aptamers that bind to protein targets. Although the precise nature of the nitrocellulose membrane–protein interaction is not known, most proteins bind tightly to nitrocellulose. The word 'most' is stressed here, as some proteins, especially those under 30 kDa, are not retained by the nitrocellulose matrix. Therefore, before initiating a filter-binding selection, the ability of a protein target to bind to nitrocellulose should be checked. The easiest method is to check levels of target protein in a sample after passage through a nitrocellulose filter (versus control) by either Bradford assay or PAGE and R250 staining. During the selection procedure, passage of the entire binding mixture over a nitrocellulose filter under low vacuum traps the target and any associated nucleic acids. Aptamers are eluted by denaturation of the target. The following generic protocol should be customized to your own target, altering factors such as the binding buffer and the competitors according to the guidelines provided above. While the volume of wash should theoretically have a profound effect on the stringency of the aptamers selected, in practice this does not appear to be the case, making a 0.5–1 ml wash completely adequate. A final note on the procedure is the necessity to at least occasionally include a target-minus pass through nitrocellulose (a negative selection) to remove filter-binding species. For some selections, multiple negative selection steps (i.e. three filtrations prior to addition of target) may be necessary in every round to keep the population from being overrun.

Protocol 3. Selection procedure using nitrocellulose immobilization

Equipment and reagents

- Binding buffer (1× BB):[a] 20 mM Tris–HCl (pH 7.5), 150 mM NaCl, 1 mM $MgCl_2$, 0.5 mM dithiothreitol (DTT)
- 10× binding buffer (10x BB): 200 mM Tris–HCl (pH 7.5), 1.5 M NaCl, 10 mM $MgCl_2$, 5 mM DTT
- Target protein in storage buffer, at a known concentration
- HAWP filters, 1.3 mm diameter (Millipore)
- Thermally equilibrated RNA pool in binding buffer, at a known concentration
- 100 μM tRNA in water (from *Escherichia coli*, Boehringer Mannheim)
- Plastic holders for 1.3 mm diameter filters (Costar)
- Filter elution solution (FES): 20 mM Tris–HCl (pH 8.2), 4 M guanidinium thiocyanate

Method

1. Dilute the RNA pool to the concentration shown in the first line under the appropriate cycle in step 18, using 1× BB as diluent.
2. Pass the RNA through a HAWP filter. Collect flow-through.[b]
3. Mix this RNA with other components appropriate to the cycle as indicated in step 18.
4. Incubate the binding reaction at room temperature for 15 min.
5. Pass the binding mixture through a fresh HAWP filter, pre-wetted with 1× BB.[c]
6. After the entire 100 μl of binding mixture has cleared, pass 500 μl of 1× BB through the filter to wash it.
7. After the wash has cleared, with the vacuum still on and holder in place, dismantle the holder and remove the filter to a 1.5 ml microcentrifuge tube.
8. Cover the filter with 400 μl of FES.
9. Incubate the filter in FES at 75 °C for 15 min to elute the bound RNA.
10. Remove the eluate and transfer to a 1.5 ml microcentrifuge tube.
11. Add 1 μg of glycogen and mix thoroughly.[d]
12. Add 1 ml of absolute ethanol and mix.
13. Incubate at –80 °C for 30 min or at –20 °C overnight.
14. Precipitate the RNA by centrifuging at 15 000*g* for 30 min.
15. Wash the pellet with 1 ml of 70% ethanol.
16. Vacuum dry the pellet.
17. Dissolve the barely visible RNA pellet in 12 μl of double-distilled H_2O.

Protocol 3. *Continued*

18. Proceed to amplification (*Protocol 4*) under the following conditions:

Cycle 1:

- 50 μl of 10 μM RNA pool
- 5 μl 10× BB
- double-distilled H_2O to 100 μl
- 100 pmol of target (e.g. 10 μl of a 10 μM solution)

Cycle 2:

- 50 μl of 2 μM RNA pool[e]
- 5 μl of 10× BB
- double-distilled H_2O to 100 μl
- 100 pmol of target (e.g. 10 μl of a 10 μM solution)

Cycles 3–5:

- 10 μl of 1 μM RNA pool
- 9 μl of 10× BB
- 1 μl of 100 μM tRNA
- double-distilled H_2O to 100 μl
- 10 pmol of target (e.g. 10 μl of a 1 μM solution)

Cycles 6–8:

- 10 μl of 1 μM RNA pool
- 9 μl of 10× BB
- 1 μl of 100 μM tRNA
- double-distilled H_2O to 100 μl
- 1 pmol of target (e.g. 1 μl of a 1 μM solution)

The final concentrations are shown in the following table:

	Concentration (μM)		
Cycle	**RNA**	**target**	**tRNA**
1	5	1	0
2	1	1	0
3–5	0.1	0.1	1
6–8	0.1	0.01	1

[a] This is a generic recipe. See comments in Section 4.2.1.

[b] This can be accomplished by using positive pressure from an air-filled syringe loaded into the top of the filter holder. Some flow-through will remain in the Luer fitting below the filter. This can be removed with a micropipette. Handle filter only with forceps.

[c] The filter holder fits into standard Luer fittings, and can be used with a standard vacuum manifold or placed in a syringe needle inserted through a rubber stopper capping a vacuum flask. Either should be attached to a moderate vacuum source (~5 inches below atmospheric pressure). This corresponds to a standard faucet aspirator with a low water flow rate.

[d] Carrier for selected RNA; this is especially important with sub-nanogram amounts.

[e] Cycles 2 onwards will have less material for the RNA pool.

5. Amplification

To carry the selection forward, selected RNA must be reverse-transcribed into DNA, this cDNA amplified into double-stranded templates, and these templates transcribed into RNA. An essential part of these procedures is to retain significant amounts of the selected RNA and amplified DNA as an archive for 'going back' in case of a rethinking of experimental particulars or of experimental error. A reasonable fraction to archive is one-half of both the selected RNA population and the amplified DNA used to generate RNA. Also critical is the inclusion of controls in this process. Most crucial is a 'no reverse transcriptase (–RT)' control. If dsDNA products are prominent in this control, the amplification solutions should be checked for contamination or, more simply, all new fresh solutions used to see if the problem recurs. If so, that round's selection can be repeated using the archived sample. In the actual PCR, an additional step we have found useful is to monitor the production of products by withdrawing an aliquot every three or four cycles to examine using low-molecular weight agarose gel electrophoresis. Then the amplification can be stopped before the reaction has reached a plateau phase, resulting in population skewing. This also enables greater discrimination in using the '–RT' control, as appearance of a '–RT' band five cycles or more after the '+RT' band appears is usually not something to be overly concerned about (since *Taq* polymerase possesses some RT activity).

Protocol 4. *RT-PCR of selected RNA*

Equipment and reagents

- Selected RNA in 12 μl of double-distilled H_2O
- 10× RT buffer: 500 mM Tris–HCl (pH 8.0), 400 mM KCl, 60 mM $MgCl_2$
- 10× PCR buffer: 300 mM Tricine K (pH 8.4), 500 mM KCl, 10 mM $MgCl_2$, 50% acetamide, 0.5% Triton X-100, 2 mM DTT[a]
- Upstream (sense) and downstream (antisense) primers, 20 μM
- Solution of dNTPs, each at 4 mM
- AMV reverse transcriptase
- *Taq* DNA polymerase
- Thermocycling incubator
- 4% NuSieve agarose (FMC) gel in 1× TBE, prestained with ethidium bromide (5 μg/ml)
- 0.05% bromophenol blue in 40% glycerol

Method

1. Set up the '+RT' reaction mixture:
   - 4 μl of the selected RNA
   - 2 μl of 10× RT buffer
   - 10 μl of downstream primer, 20 μM
   - 4 μl of 4 mM dNTPs
   - 0.3 μl of AMV reverse transcriptase

Protocol 4. *Continued*

2. Set up the '–RT' reaction mixture:
   - 2 μl of RNA
   - 1 μl of 10× RT buffer
   - 5 μl of downstream primer, 20 μM
   - 2 μl of 4 mM dNTPs
3. Incubate both reactions at 42 °C for 30 min.
4. Set up the PCR reactions:[b]
   - 5 μl (– or +) RT reaction
   - 10 μl of 10x PCR buffer
   - 4 μl of 4 mM dNTPs
   - 2.5 μl of upstream primer, 20 μm
   - 0.5 μl (2.5 units) of *Taq* DNA polymerase
   - 78 μl of water
5. Overlay the PCR solutions with ~100 μl of mineral oil.
6. Program the thermocycling incubator with the following schedule:
   - 94 °C for 50 s;
   - 50 °C for 1 min;
   - 72 °C for 1.5 min.

   Finish the last cycle with an additional 1.5 min at 72 °C.[c]
7. Place the reaction tubes in the thermocycler and react for 12 cycles.
8. Remove 8–10 μl of the lower phase and deposit on Parafilm to remove oil.
9. Add 3 μl of 0.05% bromophenol blue in 40% glycerol.
10. Load each sample on the 4% NuSieve gel and electrophorese at 90 V for 15 min.
11. Observe the gel over a UV transluminator.
12. If no bands are present, replace the tubes in the thermocycler and perform three more cycles.
13. Repeat steps 8–12 until product is clearly visible in '+RT' sample only.
14. Add 200 μl of chloroform, mix thoroughly, and centrifuge at 10 000***g*** for 5 min.
15. Remove upper phase to another microcentrifuge tube, add 10 μl of 3 M $NaOOCCH_3$ and 250 μl of ethanol.
16. Centrifuge at 10 000***g*** for 30 min.

[a] The use of 30 mM Tricine and 5% acetamide aids replication of highly structured templates (40). To make this solution, solid acetamide and KCl (not stock solutions) must be used. The DTT is optional.
[b] Two PCRs using the '+RT' reactions are advised due to losses from sampling during the amplification.
[c] This ensures that all products are full-length.

6. Termination

In order to understand (a) whether or not a selection is succeeding and (b) when a selection should be concluded, the binding ability of the selected pool should be assayed every few cycles, comparing it with the binding activity of the initial pool. Single-point binding assays can quickly reveal how a selection is progressing, and binding curves as a function of protein concentration can serve as more detailed diagnostics. By the fifth or sixth cycle of the selection, the pool should demonstrate a significant (though not necessarily huge) increase in binding over the unselected pool. If not, the SELEX should be restarted using modified selection conditions. Once through this stage, the process should be continued until the binding activity plateaus, as shown in *Figure 1a*. This is the point to conclude the selection, cloning the individuals for further analysis. The researcher should not be dismayed if the number of rounds exceeds 10—well over 15 have been reported in the literature (6,21,24).

6.1 Binding assays

The following protocol for obtaining binding data utilizes immobilization on a nitrocellulose filter in a commercial dot-blot manifold (Schleicher and Schuell), modified so that O-rings form a seal at both the upper and lower surface of the membrane(s) being supported (25). The nitrocellulose filter has an additional, positively charged membrane placed under it to catch all nucleic acid not retained by the nitrocellulose membrane. The fraction of pool or aptamer that is bound at a given protein concentration can therefore be simply obtained by dividing the number of counts immobilized on the nitrocellulose by the total counts immobilized on both membranes. This can be readily quantified with a phosphor-screen β-particle capture system such as the Phosphorimager (Molecular Dynamics). If such a system is unavailable, the filter material for each well can be cut out and the amount of captured radioactivity quantified using a standard scintillation counter. The binding data can be plotted conveniently and analyzed to yield dissociation constants with many of the graphing software packages available (e.g. Kaleidagraph from Synergy Software).

Protocol 5. Assaying binding using nitrocellulose filter immobilization

Reagents and equipment

- Target proteins, 10 μM,[a] in storage buffer
- Storage buffer (for target protein)
- ^{32}P-labeled RNA pool,[b] 100 nM in binding buffer
- Binding buffer (1× BB)
- 10× concentrated binding buffer (10× BB)
- tRNA, 1 mM[c]
- Dot-blot manifold (Schleicher and Schuell)[d]
- BA85 nitrocellulose membranes (Schleicher and Schuell), cut to fit dot-blot manifold
- Hybond N+ positively charged nylon filters (Amersham), cut to fit dot-blot manifold

Protocol 5. *Continued*

Method

1. Set up the RNA binding reactions, omitting protein:[e]
   - 70 μl of RNA solution, 100 nM
   - 0.7 μl of tRNA solution
   - 63 μl of 10× BB
   - 426 μl of H_2O.
2. Aliquot 0, 1, 2, 5, 10 and 20 μl of the protein solution into chilled 0.5 ml microcentrifuge tubes.
3. Add storage buffer to each protein aliquot for a final volume of 20 μl.
4. To each of the protein solutions, add 80 μl of the RNA mix from step 1.
5. Incubate all binding reactions at room temperature for 15 min.
6. Place a Hybond N+ membrane on the bottom support of the dot-blot manifold.
7. Wet the membrane with 1x BB and place nitrocellulose filter on top (nitrocellulose membrane should be completely moistened).
8. Finish assembling the manifold.
9. Apply vacuum to the manifold (~12 cm below atmospheric pressure).
10. Load each of the binding reactions successively in predetermined wells of the manifold. Allow all wells to drain completely.
11. Wash each well with 500 μl 1× BB.
12. Quantify the radioactivity from each dot on each membrane.[f]

[a] This is an example. It is most straightforward to use the volumes given here and determine the final concentrations in the binding mixes to estimate K_ds.
[b] This is easily accomplished by adding [α-^{32}P]UTP to the transcription mix. Alternatively, the RNA can be phosphatased and labeled at the 5′ end with [γ-^{32}P]ATP and T4 polynucleotide kinase.
[c] Optional. This provides a non-specific competitor as well as a competitive RNase inhibitor.
[d] Modified as described in text.
[e] This is enough for seven reactions, to ensure sufficient volume for six reactions.
[f] See text.

After the conclusion of the SELEX, individual aptamers must be characterized. Aptamers are cloned from the population and their sequences determined; this allows for further characterization of prominent members or consensus sequences. Further analyses are dictated by the interests of the researcher. For example, if the target molecule was an enzyme, then assays can be carried out to identify agonists and antagonists. Usually, though, a general characterization of structures and affinities of individuals reduces the aptamers of interest to a manageable number, which can then be subjected to more specific tests. Once characterized, the interesting aptamers become tools for the study of the target and its related functions.

6.2 Cloning, sequencing, and structure determination

Although the final, selected pool can be used as a direct sequence template, there are usually too many sequences present to yield an intelligible composite one. That is one reason the PCR products from a selection experiment are cloned into a plasmid. Another is that, once cloned, any individual is retrievable through the power of molecular biology. Cloning can be accomplished through restriction enzyme recognition sites incorporated into the constant regions of the original library. These allow the directional insertion of aptamer sequences into any of a variety of vectors. Also, kits are now available (e.g. from Invitrogen or Promega) that allow the direct ligation of PCR products into pretreated vectors. Ligation of the PCR products into vectors, and transformation of the ligated vectors into bacteria, allows preparation of plasmid DNA from single bacterial clones. Each clone represents a single aptamer molecule, and the plasmid DNA provides both a sequence for records as well as an archive that can used to re-transform or as a template for PCR to make specific aptamers. For sequence comparison of the population, usually plasmid DNA from around 50 colonies is prepared and sequenced using standard techniques.

By comparing their sequences, two different results are possible. One is that a particular sequence of moderate length will be contained over and over again, with slight variations, in the larger random sequence. This will yield a consensus sequence that can be used to generate a core aptamer for further analysis and study. Davis *et al.* (26) have written a comprehensive treatise on how even subtle sequence and structural motifs can be recognized by computer analysis. A second possibility is when a particular full-length sequence is present in many individuals (with minor variations) of the population. Sometimes several of the sequence 'families' will be present in the final pool. These families are the 'winners' in the selective process, and presumably represent the high-affinity binders (but checking the binding behavior of 'orphans' is still a wise choice). The multiple consensus sequences of these families are the subjects for further study.

A variety of procedures drawn from nucleic acid biochemistry and molecular biology can be used for further structural analysis. Procedures for determining the minimal binding domain (27), chemical and enzymatic studies to reveal secondary and tertiary structural features and what regions of an aptamer interact with its target (17,24,28–31), and cross-linking and proteolysis procedures (32) all have been published.

References

1. Conrad, R. C., Brück, F. M., Bell, S., and Ellington A. D. (1998) In: Smith, C. W. J. (Ed.), *Nucleic Acid–Protein Interactions: A Practical Approach*, p. 285. Oxford University Press, Oxford.

2. Fitzwater, T. and Polisky, B. (1996). In: Abelson, J. N. (Ed.), *Methods in Enzymology*, Vol. 267, p. 275. Academic Press, London.
3. Conrad, R. C., Giver, L., Tian, Y., and Ellington, A. D. (1996). In: Abelson, J. N. (Ed.), *Methods in Enzymology*, Vol. 267, p. 336. Academic Press, London.
4. Gold, L., Polisky, B., Uhlenbeck, O., and Yarus, M. (1995) *Annu. Rev. Biochem.*, **64**, 763.
5. Uphoff, K. W., Bell, S. D., and Ellington, A. D. (1996) *Curr. Opin. Struct. Biol.*, **6**, 281.
6. Nieuwlandt, D., Wecker, M., and Gold, L. (1995) *Biochemistry*, **34**, 5651.
7. Breslauer, K., Frank, R., Bl_cker, H., and Marky, L. (1986) *Proc. Natl Acad. Sci. USA*, **83**, 3746.
8. Rychlik, W. and Rhoads, R. A. (1989) *Nucleic Acids Res.*, **17**, 8543.
9. Freier, S. M., Kierzek, R., Jaeger, J. A., Sugimoto, N., Caruthers, M. H., Neilson, T., and Turner, D. H. (1986) *Proc. Natl Acad. Sci. USA*, **83**, 9373.
10. Crameri, A. and Stemmer, W. P. C. (1993) *Nucleic Acids Res.*, **21**, 4410.
11. Ellington, A. D. and Green, R. (1989). In: Ausubel, F. M., Brent, R., Kingston, R. E., Moore, D. D., Seidman, J. G., Smith, J. A.,and Struhl, K. (Eds), *Current Protocols in Molecular Biology*, pp. 2.11.1–2.11.18. John Wiley and Sons, Inc., New York.
12. Bartel, D. P. and Szostak, J. W. (1993) *Science*, **261**, 1411.
13. Giver, L., Bartel, D. P., Zapp, M. L., Green, M. R., and Ellington, A. D. (1993) *Gene*, **137**, 19.
14. Pokrovskaya, I. D. and Gurevich, V. V. (1994) *Ann. Biochem.*, **220**, 420.
15. Aurup, H., Williams, D. M., and Eckstein, F. (1992) *Biochemistry*, **31**, 9636.
16. Ueda, T., Tohda, H., Chikazumi, N., Eckstein, F., and Watanabe, K. (1991) *Nucleic Acids Res.*, **19**, 547.
17. Lin, Y., Qui, Q., Gill, S. C., and Jayasena, S. D. (1994) *Nucleic Acids Res.*, **22**, 5229.
18. Silveira, ?. and Orgel, L. E. (1995) *Nucleic Acids Res.*, **23**, 1083.
19. Stahl, ?., Hultman, T., Olsson, A., Moks, T., and Uhlen, M. (1988) *Nucleic Acids Res.*, **16**, 3025.
20. Jellinek, D., Lynott,C. K., Rifkin, D. B., and Janjic, N. (1993) *Proc. Natl Acad. Sci. USA*, **90**, 11227.
21. Chen, H., McBroom, D. G., Zhu, Y. Q., Gold, L., and North, T. W. (1996) *Biochemistry*, **35**, 6923.
22. Conrad, R., Keranen, L. M., Ellington, A. D., and Newton, A. C. (1994) *J. Biol. Chem.*, **269**, 32051.
23. Irvine, D., Tuerk, C., and Gold, L. (1991) *J. Mol. Biol.*, **222**, 739.
24. Chen, H. and Gold, L. (1994) *Biochemistry*, **33**, 8746.
25. Wong, I. and Lohman, T. (1993) *Proc. Natl Acad. Sci. USA*, **90**, 5428.
26. Davis, J. P., Janjic, N., Javornik, B. E., and Zichi, D. A. (1996). In: Abelson, J. N. (Ed.), *Methods in Enzymology*, Vol. 267, p. 302. Academic Press, London.
27. Ringquist, S., MacDonald, M., Gibson, T., and Gold, L. (1994) *Biochemistry*, **32**, 10254.
28. Kubik, M. F., Stephens, A. W., Schneider, D., Marlar, R. A., and Tasset, D. (1994) *Nucleic Acids Res.*, **22**, 2619.
29. Kjems, J., Calnan, B. J., Frankel, A. D., and Sharp, P. A. (1992) *EMBO Journal*, **11**, 1119.

30. Harris, M. E. and Pace, N. R. (1995) *RNA*, **1**, 210.
31. Ehresmann, C., Baudin, F., Mougel, M., Romby, P., Ebel, J.-P., and Ehresmann, B. (1987) *Nucleic Acids Res.*, **15**, 9109.
32. Mirfakhrai, M. and Weiner, A. M. (1993) *Nucleic Acids Res.*, **21**, 3591.

14

Ribozymes: oligonucleotides with enzymatic activity have potential as regulators of gene expression in the CNS

LEONIDAS A. PHYLACTOU, MARC B. LEE and MATTHEW J. A. WOOD

1. Introduction

The central nervous system (CNS) is the site of many neurological diseases; much of the total gene population of the body is expressed there. The complexity of the system provides a great puzzle in determining the function of its molecular components. It is essential to determine the role of these expressed genes both during normal and disease processes. The ability to down-regulate neuronal gene expression using antisense technology makes the above task possible since it is feasible to achieve this at the single-gene level. Moreover, genetic diseases, non-monogenetic diseases and malignant neoplasia could be challenged through the antisense-based gene knockdown approach.

Recently, a new class of genetic tools, called ribozymes (1,2) has been identified, capable of controlling gene expression through the manipulation of RNA. Ribozymes are catalytic RNA molecules which can be designed to bind RNA in an antisense-like specific manner. They also have catalytic properties which enable them to cleave or edit RNA molecules (3–5).

According to the 'RNA-world' view, there was a time when all biological reactions were catalysed by RNA. This theory first received support with the identification of natural ribozymes. RNA catalysis was first described by Altman and Cech with the discovery of RNase P and the group I intron respectively (1,2). This makes RNA the only known molecule with information-carrying capacity and inherent catalytic activity.

Several natural ribozyme motifs have been identified; their physical structure, biological and biochemical properties have been the subject of reviews (6,7). In general, natural ribozymes are categorized according to their specialized catalytic properties:

- The hammerhead, hairpin and hepatitis delta virus (HDV) ribozyme motifs can be characterized by their ability for self-cleavage of a particular phosphodiester bond. These motifs are typically found in viral or viroid RNAs.
- Group I and group II intron ribozymes, which are found in lower eukaryotes and also in some bacteria, can self-splice, and can cleave and ligate phosphodiester bonds.
- The ribonuclease P ribozyme was first identified in *Escherichia coli*; in conjunction with a protein cofactor, it cleaves a phosphodiester bond in a variety of cellular tRNA precursors.

There has been considerable effort to study the structure and function of natural ribozymes and convert them into tools for manipulation of RNA. The hammerhead ribozyme, the smallest ribozyme identified, is composed of approximately 30 nucleotides and is capable of site-specific cleavage of a phosphodiester bond (7). The demonstration that the self-cleaving hammerhead ribozyme can be resolved into a substrate strand and a catalytic strand (ribozyme) (see reference 8 and *Figure 1a*), led to much attention being paid to the application of antisense hammerhead ribozymes to biological systems (3,9–13). The hammerhead ribozyme has been extensively studied in order to understand the relation between structure and function, since it may be a very valuable tool for gene therapy through its RNA-mediated inhibition of gene expression. Many hammerhead ribozymes have been synthesized against RNA targets, some of which have medical relevance. However, in the case of the CNS, very few attempts have been made to use ribozymes to regulate neuronal gene expression and most of these have been at the cell culture level. In a particular case, hammerhead ribozymes have been synthesized against the amyloid peptide precursor (β-APP) which is involved in the pathogenesis of Alzheimer's disease (14). Problems like this one, where the product of a neuronal gene may be toxic or unwanted in the cell, could be challenged with ribozyme-mediated down-regulation of gene expression.

Another ribozyme, the group I intron ribozyme, has recently emerged as a potential regulator of gene expression. The *Tetrahymena* group I intron catalyzes a two-step trans-esterification reaction resulting in joining of the two rRNA exons and release of the intron (2,15). The ligase activity of the group I intron ribozyme has recently been applied to *trans*-splicing of RNA molecules. It can *trans*-splice an exon joined to its 3′ end on to a separate 5′ exon (target RNA) (references 16–18 and *Figure 1b*).

The establishment of ribozyme-mediated *trans*-splicing of RNA target molecules has tremendous implications for gene therapy. The main advantage of this system is the repair of genetically defective messages. Many of the genetic defects underlying inherited neurological disorders have recently been characterized. It may therefore be feasible to design therapeutic group I intron ribozymes to repair mutations responsible for neurodegenerative and

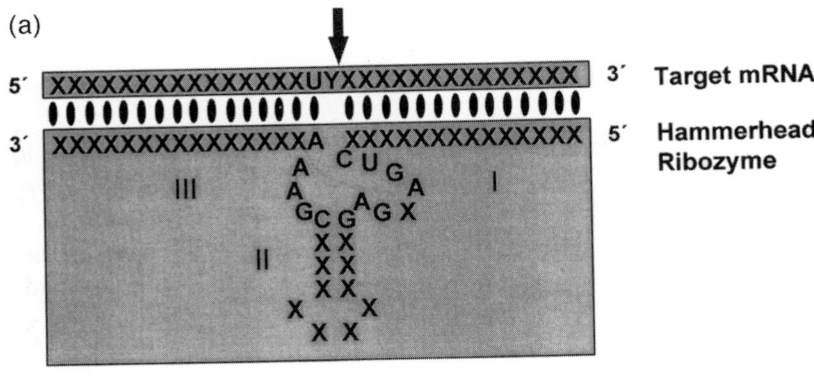

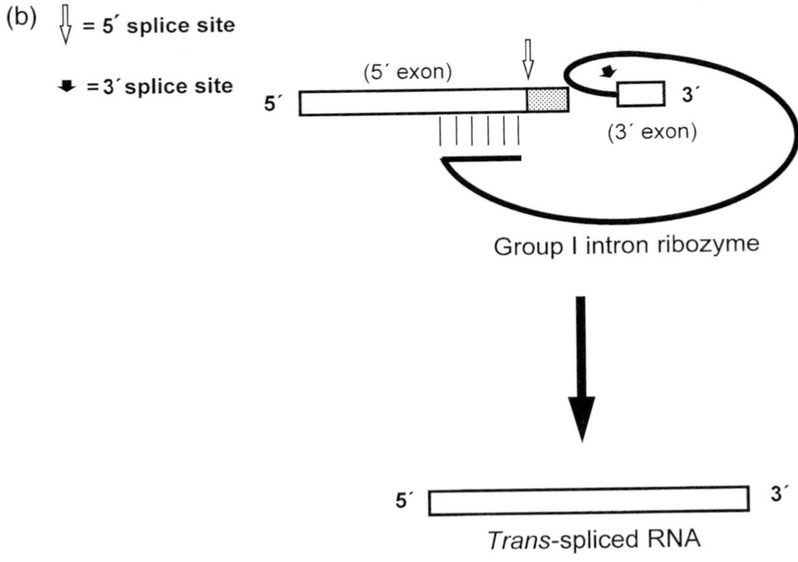

Figure 1. (a) Design of a hammerhead ribozyme against an RNA molecule. The hammerhead ribozyme (shown as the bottom strand), bound to its target RNA (shown as the top strand), forms a typical three-stemmed structure (numbered I–III) which leads to the cleavage of the target RNA at the site indicated with an arrow. The absence of conserved bases in arms I and III of the ribozyme strand provides great flexibility for the selection of appropriate targeted sequence. The only sequence requirement for target RNA selection is the presence of an XUY cleavage site, where X is any base, and Y is any base but G. The rest of the conserved bases, necessary for cleavage, are situated in the ribozyme strand. (b) Group I intron ribozyme-mediated *trans*-splicing of RNA molecules. Following binding via Watson–Crick base pairing, the ribozyme cleaves its target RNA (5′ exon) at a specific site (5′ splice site). A second cleavage then occurs at the 3′ end of the ribozyme strand (3′ splice site) which releases the 3′ exon. This results in the replacement of part of the 5′ exon (shown as a gray rectangle).

neuromuscular disorders as well as CNS tumours (16,19). In addition to the repair of defective RNA molecules, some other possible uses of RNA *trans*-splicing are the creation of toxic proteins, for example to inhibit viral replication, or proteins with completely novel functions.

2. Targeted down-regulation of gene expression in the CNS using hammerhead ribozymes

Since the discovery that some RNAs can act as biological catalysts, much effort has been devoted to exploiting their catalytic activities as regulators of gene expression. Of the ribozymes identified to date, the hammerhead ribozyme has attracted substantial interest, as it can induce site-specific endonucleolytic cleavage. Hammerhead ribozymes may be designed to down-regulate the expression of, theoretically, any gene. It should therefore be possible to down-regulate neuronal gene expression involved in CNS diseases, using the RNA-cleaving abilities of hammerhead ribozymes. Moreover, reduction in the expression of a specific gene product may reveal clues about neuronal protein function.

2.1 Design considerations

In order to design and synthesize a functional hammerhead ribozyme against a CNS RNA target, a series of design steps must be followed. The nucleotide sequence of the neuronal target RNA to be cleaved by a hammerhead ribozyme must be known. This is necessary in order to design the part of the hammerhead ribozyme that will have affinity for the target RNA. The only real sequence requirement in the neuronal target RNA is the presence of a putative hammerhead ribozyme cleavage site. There has been extensive investigation about the choice of a functional cleavage site in the target RNA (20). In the naturally occurring hammerhead ribozyme the most common cleavage site is GUC; however, GUA and AUA have also been identified. The general rule for choosing a triplet cleavage site in a target RNA is that it must be of the type XUY (where X is any nucleotide and Y any nucleotide but G) (*Figure 1a*).

Arms I and III on the hammerhead ribozyme comprise the recognition signal responsible for holding the target and ribozyme structures together (*Figure 1a*). The nucleotide sequences in these two arms have not been found to be conserved and thus can be designed to be complementary to the RNA sequence to be cleaved. However, certain sequences—in either the target RNA or the ribozyme—may prove to be problematic since they can be inaccessible to each other. This problem can be overcome by using specialized computer software to analyse the secondary structure of ribozyme and target RNA and to predict the efficiency of ribozyme cleavage. Alternatively, a trial-and-error approach can be used to determine ribozyme cleavage efficiency, since the nucleotide sequences in arms I and III vary in each design. The length of ribozyme arms I and III is critical for ribozyme efficiency and specificity. Binding of the ribozyme to the target RNA through arms I and III should be stable, and therefore last long enough for cleavage to occur. Different arm lengths have been found to be optimal in different experiments: some studies showed that arms comprising 7 or 8 nucleotides each gave optimal cleavage (21) whereas others showed optimal RNA cleavage with 30 nucleotides (22,23). This variability could be due to the different RNA target sequences. Although stable formation of stems I and III should be achieved to ensure efficient target RNA cleavage, the hammerhead ribozyme must be able to dissociate from its target. Hybridizing arms containing 7 or 8 nucleotides can achieve catalytic turnover.

Arms I and III should be joined by a series of conserved nucleotides (catalytic core) necessary for catalysis (*Figure 1a*). For a more detailed review on experiments carried out to identify the conserved nucleotides and the nucleotide interactions, see references 24 and 25. Stem II contains two conserved nucleotides adjacent to the catalytic core (26,27) and ribozyme activity can be dramatically reduced if the stem II length drops below two base pairs (28). Finally, the loop that terminates stem II has very little effect on ribozyme activity and can be replaced by non-nucleotide linkers (29).

2.2 Construction and cell-free functional assays

Ribozymes can be cloned into vectors as synthetic double-stranded oligonucleotides. They can then be synthesized by run-off *in vitro* transcription from the linearized vectors. Alternatively, ribozymes can be directly synthesized chemically, although this approach can be quite costly.

An easy and fast way to screen for functional hammerhead ribozymes is to check their ability to cleave a small part of the cellular target RNA. Similar to the construction of ribozymes, target RNA molecules can be cloned into vectors in the form of cDNA. This can be in the form of synthetic double-stranded DNA or PCR product. The PCR product, which would contain the DNA sequence of the target RNA, can be made as follows:

(1) Total RNA is extracted from cells expressing the gene of interest, then reverse transcribed using either an oligo(dT) or a target RNA-specific primer.
(2) The cDNA template is amplified by PCR using target cDNA-specific primers.
(3) The PCR product is then cloned into a vector; target RNA can be made by *in vitro* transcription from the linearized vector.

Ribozyme and target RNA can then be incubated in the presence of magnesium ions or other divalent metal ions at a physiological pH and temperature. Cleavage products can be identified by denaturing gel electrophoresis (*Figure 2*).

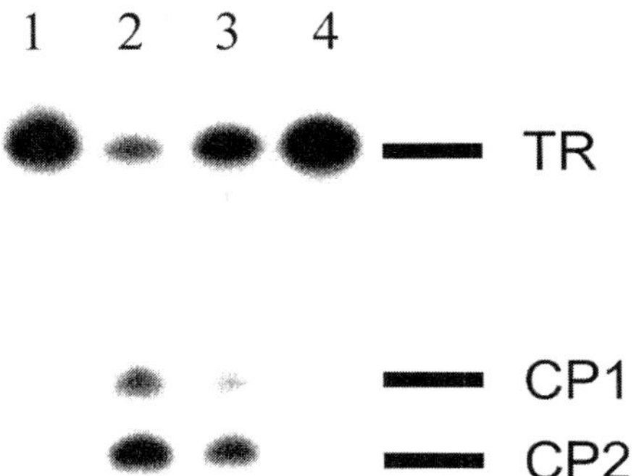

Figure 2. Cleavage of dopamine transporter (*DAT*) RNA by a hammerhead ribozyme. Lanes 2 and 3 show incubation of the ribozyme with its labeled *DAT* RNA target (TR) at different concentration ratios and at physiological temperature. Cleavage products (CP1 and CP2) can be detected by denaturing gel electrophoresis. Lane 4 shows incubation of the *DAT* target RNA in the presence of a catalytically inactive ribozyme and lane 1 shows incubation of the target in the absence of a ribozyme.

Following the identification of functional hammerhead ribozymes and prior to cell culture experiments, ribozyme activity can be tested in the presence of total RNA extracted from cells expressing the target RNA of interest.

2.3 *In vivo* applications

Hammerhead ribozymes have to face a completely different environment *in vivo* compared with the cell-free situation. There has been considerable progress in the area of ribozyme delivery and expression. Ribozymes can be delivered into cells in two ways: exogenously or endogenously. The latter is based on the expression of the DNA equivalent of ribozymes inside cells, whereas the former is based on the delivery of presynthesized ribozymes.

2.3.1 Endogenous delivery

Tissue-specific (5,30) or strong viral promoters (5,31) can be used for selective or constitutive ribozyme expression, respectively. Additionally, Pol II and Pol III promoters (32,33) have been extensively used for ribozyme transcription. For example the Pol III promoter, a natural tRNA- and snRNA-driving promoter, can achieve a very high level of ribozyme expression. Sometimes an unavoidable outcome of cloning a ribozyme into a vector is the presence of extraneous sequence in the transcript, originating from the parental vector. While this may provide extra resistance against cellular nucleases, it may adversely affect the structure of the ribozyme and therefore reduce its ability to cleave the target RNA. One way to overcome this potential problem would be to clone *cis*-acting ribozymes (ribozymes that can cleave themselves) adjacent to the ribozyme to order to induce, by cleavage, release of the ribozyme from the unnecessary RNA sequence (34,35). Another important requirement for enhanced ribozyme efficiency is that it is brought into close proximity with the target RNA. For example, it might be useful to clone the ribozyme into a tRNA gene with its regulatory elements which can deliver the ribozyme close to the translational machinery where mRNA is localized.

A potential way to increase ribozyme delivery and efficiency in the CNS would be the use of viral vectors (36,37; see Chapter 11). Other alternative methods to deliver nucleic acids, such as the use of cationic lipids and transferrin polylysine conjugates (5,38,39), have also been used in the CNS and other systems.

2.3.2 Exogenous delivery

As mentioned above, presynthesized ribozymes can be delivered to the CNS. These are chemically modified ribozymes designed to confer resistance to cellular nucleases. Modifications such as fluoro-, allyl-, amino- or *O*-allyl-groups can be introduced into the 2′ position and such methods have been successful in providing increased ribozyme survival with no decrease in ribozyme efficiency (11,40,41,42). Synthesis of this type of modified ribozyme can, unfortunately, be quite costly.

In summary, the use of hammerhead ribozymes in the CNS looks very promising, but delivery of ribozymes to the relevant tissue and cell compartments remains a critical issue. Specific delivery of ribozymes to the CNS will be beneficial for the understanding of complex neuronal functions and for the design of therapeutic strategies aimed at treatment of some neurological diseases. For example, in Parkinson's disease, where it is known that a certain population of neuronal cells degenerates, it might be possible to specifically deliver therapeutic ribozymes to the affected area of the brain with the help of viral vectors. Moreover, ribozymes might target messages such as tyrosine hydroxylase or the dopamine transporter which are essential for the synthesis and regulation of dopamine, to aid in the understanding of the pathogenesis of the disease.

3. Targeted RNA repair using group I intron ribozymes

Recently, another ribozyme has emerged as a potential regulator of gene expression. Group I intron ribozyme, one of the first to be discovered in nature, may prove to be an important tool for RNA-directed therapy. It can be specifically designed to repair abnormal mRNA molecules (16–18). In its naturally occurring form, the *Tetrahymena* group I intron ribozyme catalyzes its own splicing (15). The reaction proceeds by two consecutive trans-esterification reactions in the presence of a divalent cation. The first of these is initiated by an endogenous guanosine that attacks the 5′ splice site. The 5′

exon, terminating in a 3′-hydroxyl group, then attacks the 3′ splice site; this results in ligation of exons and excision of the intron. Recently, it has been demonstrated that a group I intron can *trans*-splice RNA both *in vitro* and in cultured cells (16–18), where the intron to be spliced out is part of a different RNA molecule that shares complementarity with the ribozyme.

3.1 Design considerations

The construction of group I intron ribozymes is similar to that of hammerhead ribozymes. The group I intron ribozyme can *trans*-splice an exon joined to its 3′ end ('new' part RNA) on to a separate 5′ exon (target RNA) (*Figure 3a*). For *trans*-splicing to occur, the group I intron ribozyme must possess a target RNA binding site in its 5′ end, which will allow binding of the ribozyme to its target RNA via base pairing. The only sequence requirement in the binding site is the formation of a U:G base pair (15) (*Figure 3a*). The catalytic nucleotides in the ribozyme are all present between the binding site and the 3′ exon (15), so the presence of a uridine is the only sequence requirement for choosing the RNA target to be *trans*-spliced. Binding of the ribozyme to its target causes cleavage of the latter at the 3′ end of the uridine, followed by the release of the 3′ exon ('new' part RNA) and the ligation of the two exons. It is thus possible to design a group I intron ribozyme to repair a mutant RNA by replacing the faulty genetic information with the wild type, engineered to be attached to the ribozyme. Moreover, repair of RNA can be widely applied since the only sequence requirement in the two exons is a uridine preceding the 5′ splice site in the target RNA. A target RNA splice site, containing the conserved uridine residue, can be selected upstream of the mutation area. The splice site can be in the form 5′-NNNNNU-3′, where N is any nucleotide.

The precautions taken regarding the secondary structure of the target RNA (5′ exon) should be similar to those for hammerhead ribozyme structure. The structure of either or both ribozyme and target RNA may be such that access to each other is inhibited. A group I intron ribozyme should contain the conserved nucleotides necessary for catalysis, and these should be flanked by the target RNA binding site (based on the splice site and the 3′ exon, i.e. the normal allele sequence which will replace the mutation). The uridine preceding the 5′ splice site must be base paired with a guanosine residue.

3.2 Construction and cell-free functional assays

The whole group I intron ribozyme can be cloned, in its DNA form, into a vector and synthesized by *in vitro* transcription. Similar to hammerhead ribozymes, the ability of group I intron ribozymes to *trans*-splice their target RNA can be tested in a cell-free environment. Small RNA targets, synthesized by *in vitro* transcription, or whole target RNAs from total RNA extracts can be used as substrates for the group I intron ribozyme. *Trans*-splicing assays can be performed in the presence of divalent metal ions such as

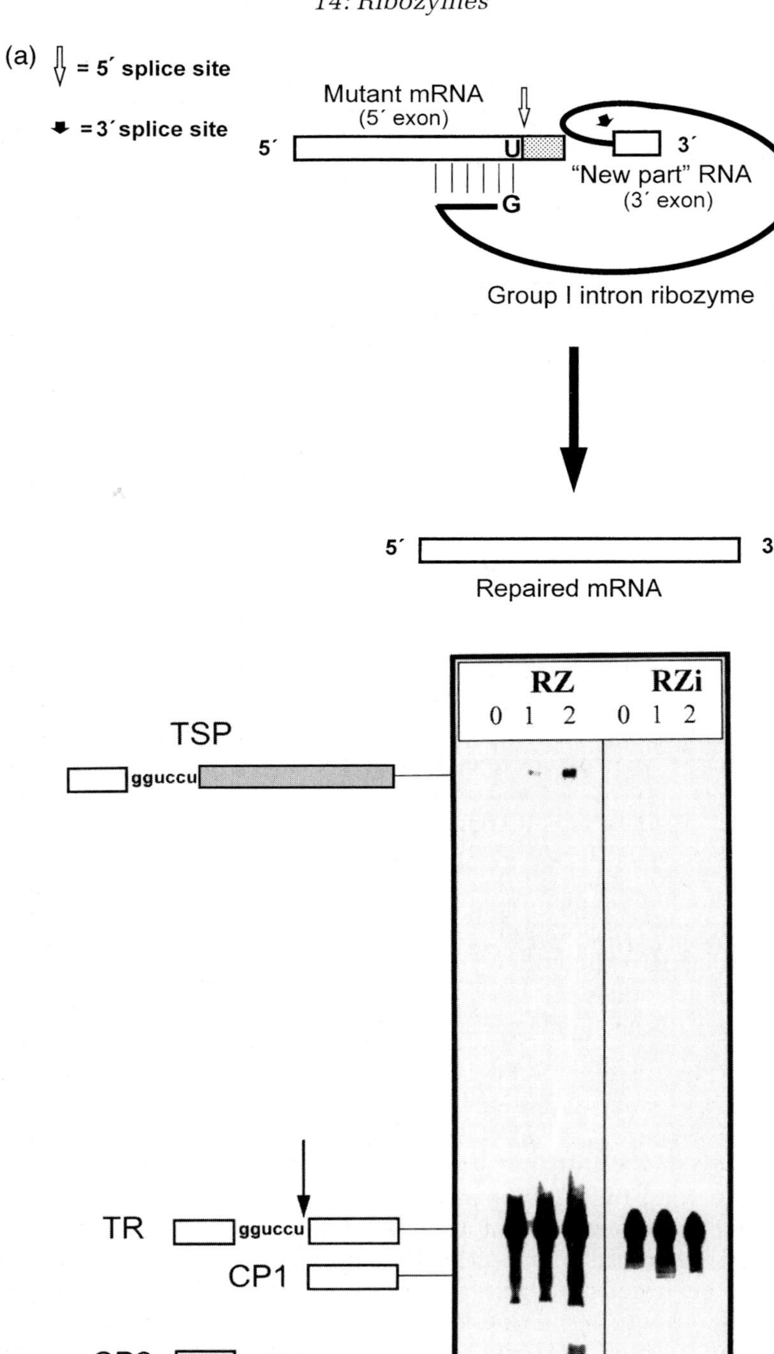
(a)
= 5´ splice site
= 3´ splice site
Mutant mRNA
(5´ exon)
5´
U
G
3´
"New part" RNA
(3´ exon)
Group I intron ribozyme
5´
3´
Repaired mRNA
RZ
RZi
0 1 2
0 1 2
TSP
gguccu
TR
gguccu
CP1
CP2
gguccu

Figure 3. (a) Group I intron ribozyme-mediated repair of mutant RNA molecules by *trans*-splicing. Following binding via Watson–Crick base pairing, the ribozyme cleaves its target RNA at a specific site (5′ splice site). A second cleavage then occurs at the 3′ end of the ribozyme strand (3′ splice site) which releases the 'new' RNA. This results in the replacement of the mutation (shown as a gray rectangle) in the mutant RNA, with the wild type sequence contained in the 'new' part RNA. The only sequence requirement for the selection of appropriate target sites is a uridine preceding the 5′ splice site. (b) Ribozyme-mediated *trans*-splicing of *DMPK* RNA. The labeled *DMPK* target RNA (TR) was incubated in the presence of a group I intron ribozyme (lanes RZ) or in the presence of an inactive version of the ribozyme (lanes RZi) at 37 °C. Reactions were stopped immediately (0), after 1 h (1) or 2 h (2). Target RNA (TR), cleavage products (CP1 and CP2) and *trans*-splicing product (TSP) are indicated schematically; 5′-gguccu-3′ indicates the ribozyme-binding site and the arrow shows the predicted 5′ splice site.

Mg^{2+} and guanosine triphosphate at physiological pH and temperature. *Trans*-splicing and cleavage products can be detected by denaturing gel electrophoresis (*Figure 3b*).

3.3 *In vivo* applications

Although the group I intron ribozyme was one of the first natural ribozymes to be discovered, very few attempts have been made to use such molecules as *trans*-splicing agents. Therefore, the *trans*-splicing system is in its infancy and current reports describe their effects only in cell culture systems. The principle, however, is similar to that of the *trans*-cleaving system: the ribozyme gene needs to be delivered efficiently and specifically to the place where the target RNA is located, and expressed under the appropriate promoter and regulatory elements. A potential drawback in using group I intron ribozymes for RNA repair is the small RNA target recognition site in the ribozyme which limits its specificity. However, derivatives of the *Tetrahymena* ribozyme have been synthesized with increased specificity for their target *in vitro* (43).

The potential of the ribozyme-mediated *trans*-splicing system for therapy in the nervous system is enormous. A number of inherited diseases affect the nervous system. Gene mutations are responsible for many types of neurological disorders including some neurodegenerative and neuromuscular diseases. Any type of mutation involved in such disease could theoretically be targeted by ribozyme-mediated *trans*-splicing, which could repair the mutation by replacing it with the wild-type sequence. For example, recently it has been demonstrated that a group I intron ribozyme can be used to correct the genetic defect underlying myotonic dystrophy (DM). DM has an autosomal dominant genetic trait and is the most common inherited neuromuscular disease in adults (44,45). The DM mutation is an amplification of a CTG repeat that lies in the 3′ untranslated region of the *DMPK* gene on chromosome 19 (46–49). The CTG repeat is highly polymorphic in the normal population (5–35 repeat units) and alleles responsible for DM have >50 repeat units, rising to 2000 in patients with the classical or congenital form of the disease (50). The pathogenesis of DM is thought to be complicated, but some good evidence suggests that the mutant *DMPK* mRNA is trapped in the nucleus and that, at this site, the CUG expansion alters binding of RNA-binding proteins to the molecule (51,52).

4. Conclusion

Ribozymes are RNA molecules which, when designed properly, can be used to manipulate endogenous RNA molecules and therefore control cellular gene expression. The CNS is the site of expression of many genes, and some of those expressed genes are involved in neurological diseases. The use of the catalytic abilities of ribozymes may make it possible to down-regulate or edit neuronal gene expression in specific cases and intervene in such disease processes. Although the rationale is very simple, in practice there still are problems that need to be tackled before application of ribozymes in the CNS can become an established protocol for therapy of neurological diseases as well as for the study of neuronal gene function.

References

1. Guerrier Takada, C. and Altman, S. (1984) *Science* **223**, 285.
2. Cech, T. R., Zaug, A. J. and Grabowski, P. J. (1981) *Cell* **27**, 487.
3. James, W. and al Shamkhani, A. (1995) *Curr. Opin. Biotechnol.* **6**, 44.
4. Kiehntopf, M., Esquivel, E. L., Brach, M. A. and Herrmann, F. (1995) *Lancet* **345**, 1027.
5. Rossi, J. J. (1994) *Curr. Biol.* **4**, 469.
6. Cech, T. R. (1987) *Science* **236**, 1532.
7. Symons, R. H. (1989) *Trends Biochem. Sci.* **14**, 445.
8. Haseloff, J. and Gerlach, W. L. (1988) *Nature* **334**, 585.
9. Sarver, N., Cantin, E. M., Chang, P. S. Zaia, J. A., Ladne, P. A., Stephens, D. A. and Rossi, J. J. (1990) *Science* **247**, 1222.
10. Steinecke, P., Herget, T. and Schreier, P. H. (1992) *EMBO J.* **11**, 1525.
11. Rossi, J. J. (1995) *Trends Biotechnol.* **13**, 301.
12. Thompson, J. D., Macejak, D., Couture, L. and Stinchcomb, D. T. (1995) *Nature Med.* **1**, 277.
13. Gibson, S. A. and Shillitoe, E. J. (1997) *Mol. Biotechnol.* **7**, 125.
14. Denman, R. B., Smedman, M., Ju, W., Rubenstein, R., Potempska, A. and Miller, D. L. (1994) *Nucleic Acids Res.* **22**, 2375.
15. Cech, T. R. (1990) *Annu. Rev. Biochem.* **59**, 543.
16. Phylactou, L. A., Darrah, C. and Wood, M. J. A. (1998) *Nature Genet.* **18**, 378.
17. Jones, J. T., Lee, S. W. and Sullenger, B. A. (1996) *Nature Med.* **2**, 643.
18. Sullenger, B. A. and Cech, T. R. (1994) *Nature* **371**, 619.
19. Karpati, G., Lochmuller, H., Nalbantoglu, J. and Durham, H. (1996) *Trends Neurosci.* **19**, 49.
20. Shimayama, T., Nishikawa, S. and Taira, K. (1995) *Biochemistry* **34**, 3649.

21. Lieber, A. and Strauss, M. (1995) *Mol. Cell. Biol.* **15**, 540.
22. Beck, J. and Nassal, M. (1995) *Nucleic Acids Res.* **23**, 4954.
23. Crisell, P., Thompson, S. and James, W. (1993) *Nucleic Acids Res.* **21**, 5251.
24. Scott, W. G., Finch, J. T. and Klug, A. (1995) *Cell* **81**, 991.
25. Pley, H. W., Flaherty, K. M. and McKay, D. B. (1994) *Nature* **372**, 111.
26. Nakamaye, K. L. and Eckstein, F. (1994) *Biochemistry* **33**, 1271.
27. Symons, R. H. (1992) *Annu. Rev. Biochem.* **61**, 641.
28. Tuschl, T. and Eckstein, F. (1993) *Proc. Natl Acad. Sci. USA* **90**, 6991.
29. Thomson, J. B., Tuschl, T. and Eckstein, F. (1993) *Nucleic Acids Res.* **21**, 5600.
30. Ohta, Y., Kijima, H., Kashani Sabet, M. and Scanlon, K. J. (1996) *J. Invest. Dermatol.* **106**, 275.
31. Couture, L. A. and Stinchcomb, D. T. (1996) *Trends Genet.* **12**, 510.
32. Kawasaki, H., Ohkawa, J., Tanishige, N., Yoshinari, K., Murata, T., Yokoyama, K. K. and Taira, K. (1996) *Nucleic Acids Res.* **24**, 3010.
33. Thompson, J. D., Ayers, D. F., Malmstrom, T. A., McKenzie, T. L., Ganousis, L., Chowrira, B. M., Couture, L. and Stinchcomb, D. T. (1995) *Nucleic Acids Res.* **23**, 2259.
34. Yuyama, N., Ohkawa, J., Koguma, T., Shirai, M. and Taira, K. (1994) *Nucleic Acids Res.* **22**, 5060.
35. Liu, Z., Batt, D. B. and Carmichael, G. G. (1994) *Proc. Natl Acad. Sci. USA* **91**, 4258.
36. Morgan, R. A. and Anderson, W. F. (1993) *Annu. Rev. Biochem.* **62**, 191.
37. Lieber, A. and Kay, M. A. (1996) *J. Virol.* **70**, 3153.
38. Kilpatrick, M. W., Phylactou, L. A. Godfrey, M., Wu, C. H., Wu, G. Y. and Tsipouras, P. (1996) *Human Mol. Genet.* **5**, 1939.
39. Sakamoto, N., Wu, C. H. and Wu, G. Y. (1996) *J. Clin. Invest.* **98**, 2720.
40. Heidenreich, O., Benseler, F., Fahrenholz, A. and Eckstein, F. (1994) *J. Biol. Chem.* **269**, 2131.
41. Pieken, W. A., Olsen, D. B., Benseler, F., Aurup, H. and Eckstein, F. (1991) *Science* **253**, 314.
42. Sproat, B. S. (1995) *J. Biotechnol.* **41**, 221.
43. Young, B., Herschlag, D. and Cech, T. R. (1991) *Cell* **67**, 1007.
44. Harper, P. S. (1989) *Myotonic Dystrophy.* W. B. Saunders, Philadelphia.
45. Shelbourne, P. and Johnson, K. (1992) *Human Mutat.* **1**, 183.
46. Davies, K. E., Jackson, J., Williamson, R., Harper, P. S., Ball, S., Sarfarazi, M., Meredith, L. and Fey, G. (1983) *J. Med. Genet.* **20**, 259.
47. Buxton, J. *et al.* (1992) *Nature* **355**, 547.
48. Brook, J. D. *et al.* (1992) *Cell* **68**, 799.
49. Mahadevan, M. *et al.* (1992) *Science* **255**, 1253.
50. Tsilfidis, C., MacKenzie, A. E., Mettler, G., Barcelo, J. and Korneluk, R. G. (1992) *Nature Genet.* **1**, 192.
51. Hamshere, M. G. and Brook, J. D. (1996) *Trends Genet.* **12**, 332.
52. Davis, B. M., McCurrach, M. E., Taneja, K. L., Singer, R. H. and Housman, D. E. (1997) *Proc. Natl Acad. Sci. USA* **94**, 7388.

15

Antisense gene knockdown technology in the nematode *Caenorhabditis elegans*: applications to cholinergic synaptic transmission

EMMANUEL CULETTO and DAVID B. SATTELLE

1. Introduction

One of the most important challenges of the post-genome era will be to determine the functions of sequenced genes and their relevance to human disease. Functional genetics is a multidisciplinary approach to determining the roles of genes, gene products, their interactions and regulatory mechanisms; it encompasses genomics, genetics, proteomics and molecular physiology and can be directed towards central questions in physiology, including neural signalling. The first metazoan genome for which genome sequencing has been completed is that of the small invertebrate *Caenorhabditis elegans*, a model organism that is ideally suited to exploration of functional genetics using a wide range of experimental methods (1,2). The relatively small genome (97 megabases) of this nematode not only provides a useful vehicle for pilot functional genetics investigations in the period while sequencing of the human genome is incomplete, but also offers experimental access to genes which are homologous to those implicated in human genetic disorders (3). For example, it is estimated that following completion of the *C. elegans* genome project, at least 70% of positionally cloned human disease genes will have identifiable orthologues in the worm. The use of *C. elegans* facilitates analysis of mutant and wild-type genes *in vivo*. The analysis of a gene's function begins by isolation of worms possessing the mutated gene of interest.

Several attempts have been made to find a good strategy for specifically (and reliably) shutting down the actions of selected genes in *C. elegans*. A major impetus for this effort has been the wealth of new information emerging from the *C. elegans* genome sequencing project (4,5). Another major step forward will be the development of a method for routinely knocking down the activity of predicted genes by the *C. elegans* Genome Consortium. Recently, A. R. Coulson and colleagues at The Sanger Centre have initiated a new project, a systematic (chemical) knockdown approach, which will throw light on the biological roles of gene products. Here we shall endeavor to summarize the various experimental approaches in current use in many laboratories and outline recent progress. For readers not familiar with the biology of *C. elegans*, we examine first the experimental advantages of using this organism for functional genetics. There follows a brief section showing how reverse genetics can be applied in *C. elegans* (see also reference 6). This is an essential prerequisite to a detailed evaluation of antisense approaches to neural signalling in *C. elegans*, with particular emphasis on its potential for enhancing our understanding of cholinergic synaptic transmission.

2. Experimental advantages of using *C. elegans* for analysis of gene function

2.1 A model organism for neurogenetics

C. elegans is a free-living soil nematode, 1 mm long with a transparent body (*Figure 1*). It is easily cultured on Petri dishes on a simple agar medium where it is fed with the bacterium *Escherichia coli*. Its organization is very simple, with only 959 somatic cells of which 302 are neurons in the hermaphodite (381 in the male). This simple organization, and a development that is essentially invariant, has allowed a complete description of cell lineage in

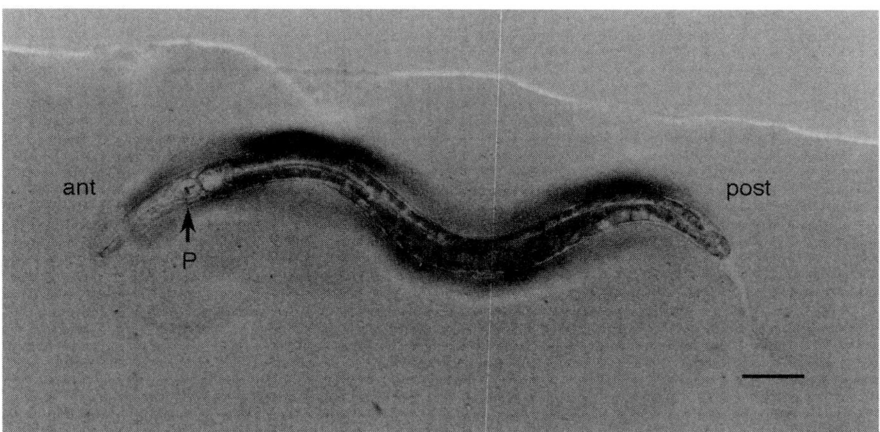

Figure 1. Bright-field illumination photomicrograph of a young adult hermaphrodite *C. elegans* (wild type (N2)) . This adult worm is about 1 mm long and is moving on a layer of bacteria on the surface on an agar plate. Anterior is to the left, posterior to the right. P = pharynx. Bar represents 100 μm.

C. elegans (7). Moreover, the synaptic connections of most neurons have been reconstructed by means of serial section electron micrographs (8). The rapid generation time of *C. elegans* (one embryo becomes an adult in 3 days at 25°C and gives birth to 300 progeny) and its reproduction by self-fertilization make *C. elegans* amenable to genetic analysis (9). Mutagenesis, mutant screening, genetic mapping, complementation and mosaic analysis, as well as studies of gene interaction through suppressor selection and epistatic analysis, are experimental approaches that can be adopted (reviewed in reference 2). Also, transgenic worms are easily produced by injection of DNA into the syncitial part of the gonad of an adult hermaphrodite *C. elegans* (10,11; see *Figure 2*).

2.2 Genetic and physical maps

The *C. elegans* genome is relatively small and compact (20 times the size of the *Escherichia coli* genome, one thirtieth the size of the human genome). Its content is distributed on five autosomes and one sexual chromosome (hermaphrodites are XX and males are X0).

The relative ease with which mutants can be obtained (9) has permitted the construction of a detailed genetic map (with about 2000 loci). This genetic map has been completed by the generation of a physical map (13–15) in which almost the complete genome has been subcloned into overlapping cosmids and yeast artificial chromosomes (YACs). The physical and genetic maps have been aligned (*Figure 3*). In addition to many other advantages, *C. elegans* offers an unparalleled resource for cloning genes by rescue transformation, since it is possible to select DNA clones from the physical map to inject into a selected mutant.

2.3 Genome sequence

The physical map provided the starting point for the Genome Sequencing Project, which is spearheaded by the laboratories of J. E. Sulston (MRC Laboratory of Molecular Biology and The Sanger Centre, Cambridge, UK) and R. Waterston (Department of Genetics and Genome Sequencing Center, Washington University School of Medicine). Together they form the *C. elegans* Genome Consortium and the DNA sequence is now complete. A total of 97 Mb have been sequenced (December 1998). Current estimates indicate a total of about 19 100 *C. elegans* protein coding genes (2). The *C. elegans* genome resource is now the subject of intense analysis by reverse genetics including antisense approaches.

Publicly available *C. elegans* sequences can be located at the following websites: http://www.sanger.ac.uk/Projects/C_elegans and http://genome.wustl.edu/gsc/gschmpg.html. To obtain more information on *C. elegans* see http://elegans.swmed.edu/

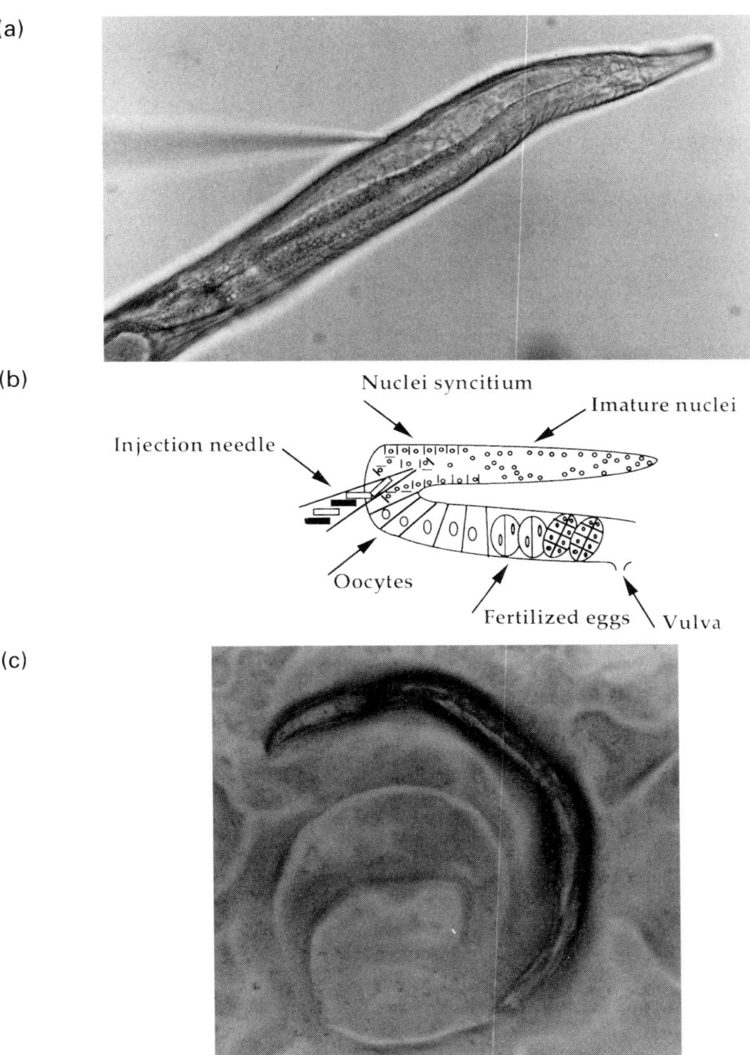

Figure 2. (a) Photomicrograph showing the injection of DNA into the syncitial part of the gonad of an adult hermaphrodite. Bar represents 25 μm. (b) Schematic representation of the micro-injection technique. A suspension containing the DNA of interest (white bars) together with a marker DNA (*rol-6* gene in pRF4 plasmid, black bars) is injected into the syncitial cytoplasm of the gonad where mature syncitial nuclei are about to become oocytes. Injected DNAs undergo linear recombination to form a large DNA array; when the array is large enough it becomes heritable as an extrachromosomal element and is transmitted to the progeny. (c) Photomicrograph of a *C. elegans* expressing *rol-6* that is used as a co-marker for identifying successful transformants. Plasmid pRF4 codes for a dominant collagen mutation, *rol-6* (su 1006; reference 12) that confers a roller phenotype: transformed animals with the pRF4 plasmid roll distinctively, moving in circles, and so are easy to select from the plates. Bar represents 100 μm.

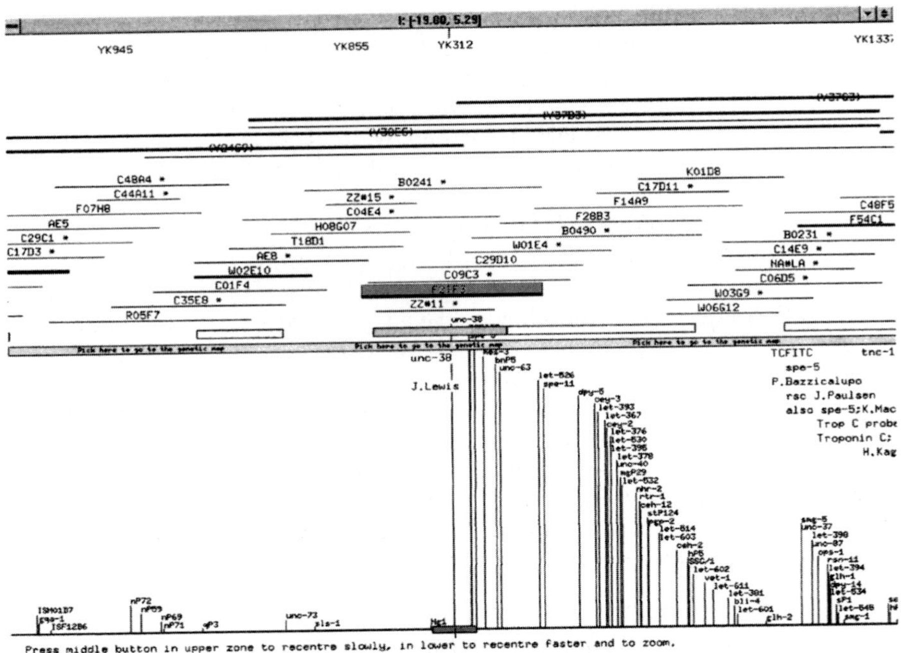

Figure 3. Localization of *unc-38* on the physical and genetic maps. This is a printout from a computer screen displaying ACeDB (a *Caenorhabditis elegans* database). It shows, from the top downwards: cDNA determined by hybridization with YACs; YACs determined by hybridization with selected cosmids; cosmids whose overlap was determined by fingerprinting; discontinuous bar beneath the cosmids indicating the extent of genomic sequence; continuous bar providing rapid access within ACeDB to some position on the genetic map; positions of defined genes (including the nAChR α subunit encoded by the *unc-38* gene along with comments relating to the assembly of the map). At the bottom is an overview of the region of the chromosome in which the above map lies. Cosmids marked with an asterisk indicate the presence of additional analyzed clones not shown on this particular screen.

3. Reverse genetics

3.1 Tc1 insertion mutants

One of the most widely adopted strategies in current use has been developed by the laboratories of R. H. A. Plasterk and colleagues. This involves the use of the Tc1 insertion mutant. Tc1 is one of the mobile genetic elements in *C. elegans* and its insertion into a gene can inactivate it (16,17). A very precise protocol has been designed by the laboratory of Plasterk (18) which is based on PCR screening of pools of DNA samples from a *C. elegans* strain active for Tc1 transposition (*Figure 4*). Once a pool that is positive for the Tc1 insertion has been identified, it is divided and retested until the isolation of a single homozygous Tc1 insertion worm is achieved. Since Tc1 elements are often inserted into intronsor removed from pre-mRNA by the *cis*-splicing machinery, difficulties might well have been anticipated for mutant generation. However this problem can be overcome by rescreening the pools for a random excision of the Tc1 motif from the gene of interest. This leads to deletions (of several kilobases) in the gene which can be detected by PCR screening. Under optimal conditions it requires 2 months to obtain a null Tc1 insertion mutant (3).

3.2 Chemically induced deletion mutants

A new protocol has been devised by R. Barstead and colleagues working at the Oklahoma Medical Research Foundation (Oklahoma City, OK, USA). First deletion mutants are obtained using trimethylpsoralen–ultraviolet light (TMP-UV), diepoxybutane (DEB) or ethyl methanesulfonate (EMS) treatments. F1 generation worms are then pooled in samples and used for nested PCR screening (*Figure 4*). This has been done successfully for more than 10 genes, including *unc-41*, the focal adhesion kinase gene.

Both Tc1 insertion mutants and chemically induced deletion mutants have proved to be useful, though some limitations still exist. For example, small genes may be entirely deleted and in this case mutants escape detection when using primers derived from the gene sequence.

3.3 Homologous recombination

The homologous recombination approach to knock down genes is widely used in mammals (19). However this targeted gene replacement approach has not been so fruitful in the nematode. Only one example of such an experiment has been reported so far in *C. elegans* (20). A plasmid containing a synthetic fusion of two genes encoding *C elegans* yolk protein (*vit-2* and *vit-6* genes) has been injected into a wild-type animal using the micro-injection transformation technique (see *Figure 2*). Generally, injected DNA recombines into large extrachromosomal arrays, but this time the authors selected for smaller extrachromosomal arrays using a transformant marker deleterious at high copy numbers. The molecular analysis of transformed animals showed that in most cases plasmids were randomly integrated at non-homologous sites. However, two strains showed effective homologous recombination between plasmid genes and the endogenous *vit-2* locus. To date no other successful examples of homologous recombination have been reported in the *C. elegans* literature. This may be due to differences in the nature of enzymes (e.g. lack of proteins that catalyze recombination) and/or competition with enzymes involved in the production of the large recombinant array.

4. Use of antisense technology for knockdown

4.1 The demonstration of antisense knockdown in *C. elegans*

Other recombination experiments have been attempted by A. Fire and colleagues (21) and several early results led them in the direction of antisense

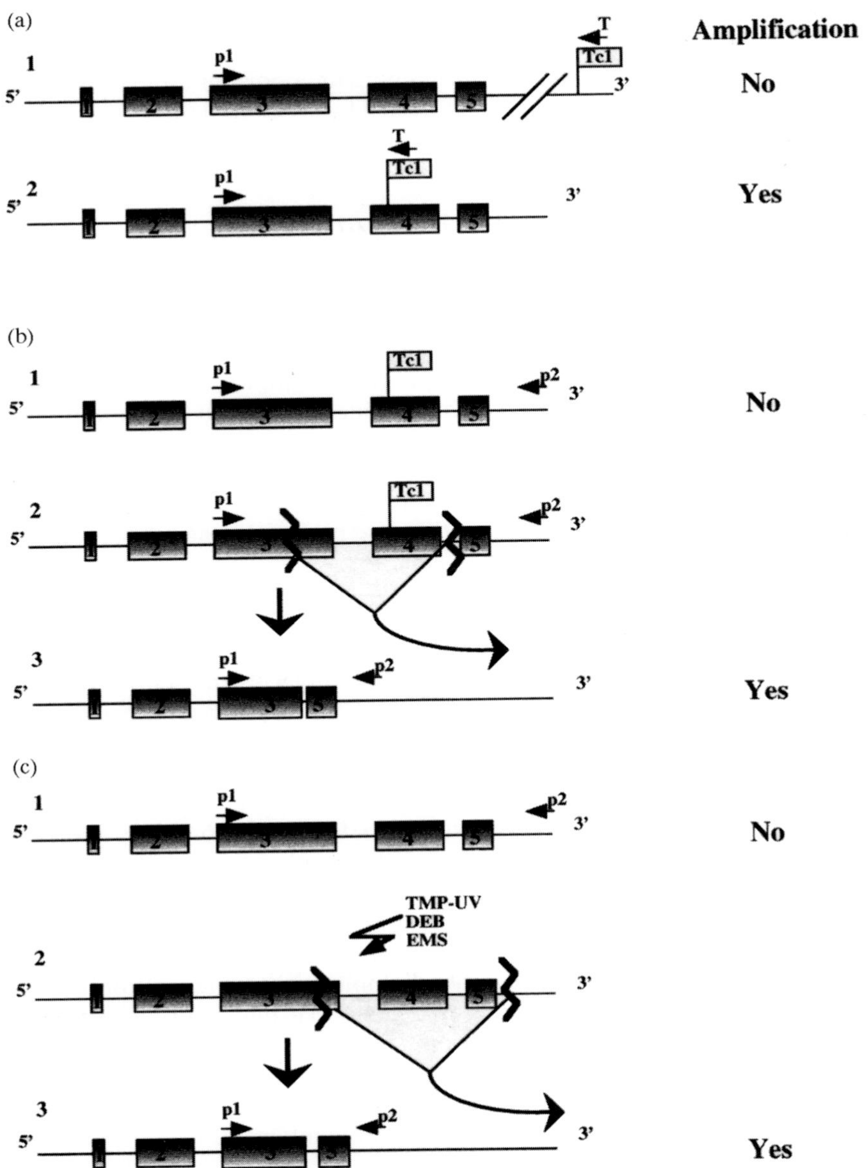

knockdown approaches. In these experiments they injected plasmid DNA, containing the *unc-22* gene, into wild-type *C. elegans*. The *unc-22* gene codes a muscle protein (twitchin) associated with the thick (myosin) filament. Twitching mutants were obtained, phenocopying the *unc-22* null mutant phenotype. Unexpectedly, the transformed worms did not contain a mis-recombination between the plasmid DNA and the chromosome (as described

Figure 4. Schematic representation of two reverse genetic methods for isolating specific mutants in *C. elegans*. (a) A method using the *C. elegans* strain MT3126, which has a high frequency of the Tc1 mobile genetic element. The presence of Tc1 is detected by PCR. Several DNA sample pools from the MT3126 strain are screened by PCR using one primer deduced from the gene of interest (p1) in combination with one primer complementary to the Tc1 sequence (T). There will only be one amplification if the Tc1 element is sufficiently close to the p1 primer (a2). Once the pool containing the gene of interest with the Tc1 insertion has been identified, PCR screening is performed on diluted samples until the mutant is located. The final goal is to identify a single worm homozygous for the Tc1 insertion. (b) Sometimes Tc1 is excised from the pre-mRNA by the *cis*-splicing machinery of the cell leaving the mRNA unaffected. In this case, a second round of PCR must be performed on the same strain looking for animals with imprecise excision of the mobile element. Imprecise excision of Tc1 results in genomic deletion, since varying lengths of DNA flanking the Tc1 element could be removed (b2), which are in turn detected by PCR using a set of well spaced primers (b3). There will not be amplification on intact DNA (fragment to amplify is too large, (b1)) but one amplification can be obtained on the deleted sequence (b2). (c) Genomic deletion can be induced with TMP-UV, DEB and EMS treatments (c2). Pools of DNA samples from mutagenized worms are screened by PCR using one set of primers deduced from the gene of interest. PCR is performed on divided pools until isolation of the pure mutant is achieved. In this case pools giving one amplification are selected (c3). Filled boxes are exons and arrows indicate primers.

in Section 3.3), but only extrachromosomal arrays. Moreover, these results have been reproduced by injecting plasmid DNA containing the *unc-22* cDNA in antisense orientation. One possible conclusion is that antisense RNA is produced from extrachromosomal arrays by a cryptic promoter. The explanation for phenocopying of the null mutant has been sought in terms of interference by antisense RNA produced from the extrachromosomal array with endogenous mRNA. This rationale has been utilized subsequently by several groups to examine the phenotypes of animals in which maternal RNA is interfered with by antisense RNA injections. Guo and Kemphues (22) injected antisense RNA directly into the gonad of wild-type *C. elegans*. Animals injected with antisense *par-1* RNA showed the typical *par-1* mutant phenotype: arrested development, no morphogenesis, and no intestinal cells. Surprisingly, the same results can be obtained by injecting sense RNA (22, 23). A contrasting example comes from the study of atypical protein kinase C (encoded by the *pkc-3* gene). In this case, the injection of antisense RNA resulted in embyonic lethality, but the injection of sense RNA did not result in a distinct phenotype (24).

4.2 Mechanism underlying antisense knockdown action involves double-stranded RNA interference

In order to enhance understanding of the mechanism underlying the effects of injected sense and antisense RNA, two laboratories have further investigated this phenomenon. Fire and colleagues (25) worked on very pure sense and antisense RNA synthesised from the *unc-22* gene. Separate injections of each single-strand RNA (sense and antisense) did not lead to any phenotypic abnormality in F1 animals, but injection of a mix of the two strands resulted in a strong twitcher phenotype phenocopying the *unc-22* null mutant. The same result has been obtained for other genes whose functions and expression patterns are very different. This result demonstrates that the RNA injection knockdown effect following micro-injection is not mediated directly by either antisense or sense RNA, but rather by a double-stranded RNA structure. This phenomenon has been designated double-strand RNA interference (dsRNAi). Previous single-strand RNA injection results (21,22,23) can also be explained in these terms (see reference 26). For example, if contaminated DNA is injected into the worm (n.b. linear plasmids are used for the RNA transcription), it can form an extrachromosomal array and so antisense and sense RNA may be synthesized from this structure (as shown by Fire *et al.* (21)). Another explanation is that contaminant sense RNA is formed when antisense RNA is prepared, and vice versa, due to the non-specific action of the bacterial polymerase resulting in double-stranded RNA formation.

Protocol 1. Outline of double-stranded RNA preparation, based on Fire *et al.* (25)

1. Prepare microgram quantities of DNA template using, for example, a Qiagen preparation kit.
2. Linearize DNA sample using blunt end restriction site or restriction enzyme leaving 5′ overhanging end at the 3′ end of the template.
3. Extract the linearized plasmid with phenol-chloroform, precipitate in ethanol and resuspend in water to a final concentration of 1 μg/μl.
4. Synthethize single-stranded RNA from the linearized template using T3 or T7 polymerase.
5. Remove the DNA template by DNase treatment.
6. Extract reaction products with phenol–chloroform, precipitate in ethanol and resuspend in water.
7. Anneal the two complementary RNA strands at 37 °C for 10–30 min; either inject them directly or store at –20 °C.

4.3 Possible mechanisms invoked to explain dsRNAi

The mechanism underlying dsRNAi is not known. It is possible to summarize some characteristics of dsRNAi from the work of Fire and colleagues (25). There is no clear stable heritable effect, despite the observation that effects of dsRNAi are observed in F1 but not in subsequent generations. The effect of RNA interference is concentration dependent and genes may have different degrees of susceptibility, depending on the developmental stage at which they are expressed. Injections into the body cavity, the head region, or the gonad give quite similar results. The fact that the effect can occur in parts of the body remote from the injection suggests the presence of an active transport of dsRNA. This implies the existence of an, as yet unknown, biological process involving dsRNA, possibly functioning as a whole organism defense mechanism against dsRNA viruses. A similar process seems to operate in plants (reviewed in reference 26). On the other hand, it has been suggested that a dsRNA adenosine deaminase activity could make edited RNA into the dsRNA. Then a recombination of this RNA with the genomic copy will integrate the mutation caused by the editing (27). The fact that RNA interference is not heritable argues against this hypothesis. The mechanism is still under investigation in the laboratory of A. Fire. One of the approaches is to isolate *C. elegans* mutants resistant to dsRNAi.

5. Applications to neural signalling

Classical forward genetics has allowed the identification of more than 35 genes involved in synaptic transmission in *C. elegans* (*Figure 5*) based on screening for mutants resistant to either the anthelmintic drug levamisole (*lev* genes) or the anticholinesterase aldicarb (*ric* genes) and on characterization of mutants defective in well defined enzymatic activities involved respectively in the synthesis (*cha-1*) and breakdown (*ace* genes) of the neurotransmitter acetylcholine (ACh). Some genes have been used to clone their mammalian counterparts (*unc-18*, *unc-13*) or to understand further their functional roles (*snt-1*, *rab-3*). All these examples show that it is the disruption of a given gene that yields the most information. This type of approach will only detect obvious mutant phenotypes. If the gene belongs to a multiple gene family whose activity is redundant, no mutant will be detected (28).

In this section we will consider strategies for the use of the dsRNAi technology in addressing central questions in cholinergic synaptic transmission.

5.1 Functional roles of nicotinic acetylcholine receptor gene family members

Fast actions of ACh are mediated by nicotinic acetylcholine receptors (nAChRs). These are pentameric receptors transiently permeable to cations composed of various combinations of α and non-α subunits. The α subunits are defined by the presence of adjacent cysteines in one extracellular loop involved in the ACh binding site. A number of nAChR subunits have been characterized at the molecular level by classical forward genetics (9,30,31). Taking advantage of the *C. elegans* genome resource, our group has provided evidence for the transcription of more than 20 previously unknown nAChR subunits. Sequence analysis has identified four distinct families of α subunits

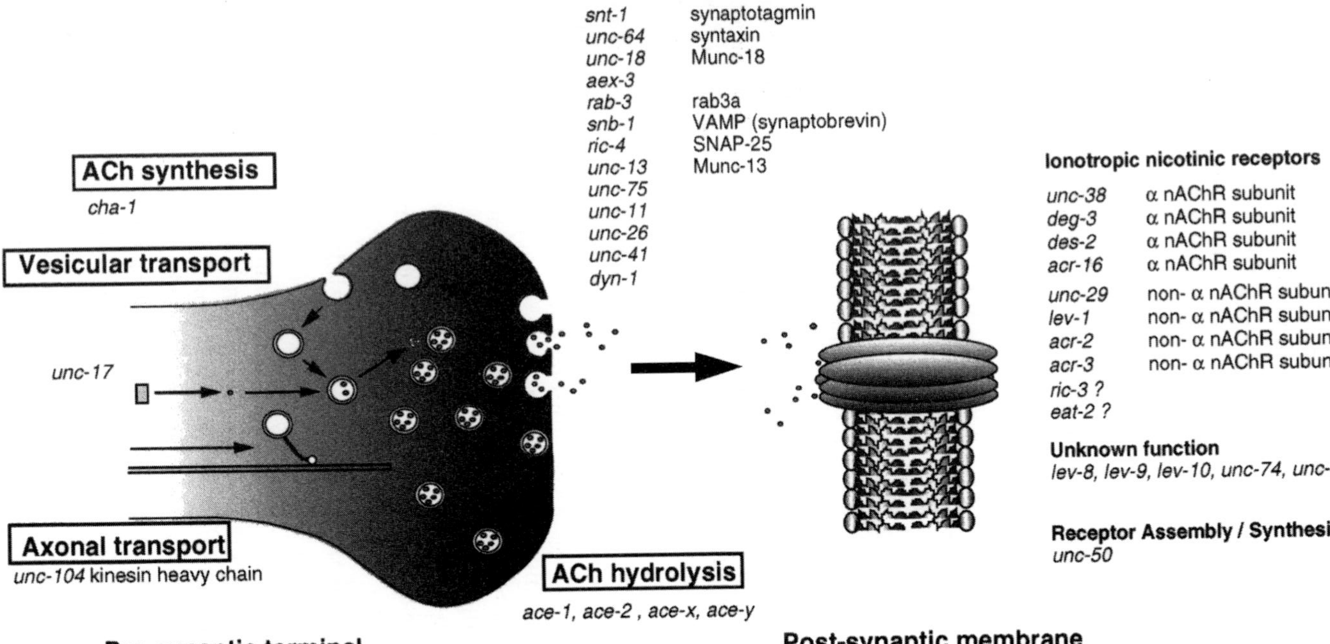

Figure 5. *C. elegans* mutants involved in cholinergic transmission. Genes known to act on axonal transport, acetylcholine synthesis and transport are shown; genes involved in exocytosis, endocytosis and the regulation of both mechanisms are also depicted. In the synaptic cleft genes (*ace*) encoding the hydrolytic enzyme acetylcholinesterase (AChE) are shown. On the postsynaptic element genes encoding nicotinic receptors and other proteins involved in receptor function, assembly and/or synthesis are indicated. Several synaptic mutants have been isolated based on their resistance to the anthelmintic drug levamisole (*lev*), uncoordinated locomotion (*unc*), resistance to inhibitors of acetylcholinesterases (*ric*) or defects in pharyngeal pumping (*eat*). Other three-letter abreviations are as follows: *deg*, degeneration; *dyn*, dynein; *acr*, acetylcholine receptor. Based on Jorgensen and Nonet (29).

(32). Although defects in single nAChR genes can produce striking phenotypes (30), there may be gene redundancy between members of such a large family, i.e. knocking down one gene may not necessarily affect the phenotype, especially in the laboratory context where worms have unlimited access to food, and no predators. We are using dsRNAi to investigate the role(s) of each nAChR α subunit, injecting at the same time multiple dsRNAs derived from genes belonging to the same family of nAChR subunits. This could circumvent the potential problem of redundancy (28).

5.2 Functional roles of the four acetylcholinesterase genes in *C. elegans*

Acetylcholinesterase (AChE) is a key enzyme at cholinergic synapses, where it hydrolyses ACh terminating its synaptic actions. It was reported previously that three genes, *ace-1*, *ace-2* and *ace-3*, encode three pharmacological classes of AChE in the nematode *C. elegans* (reviewed in reference 33). The triple mutant *ace-1*, *ace-2*, *ace-3* is lethal at developmental stage L1. To make such a mutant it is necessary to combine the double mutant *ace-1;ace-2* with the *ace-3* mutant producing the triple mutant with some maternal *ace-1* and *ace-2* RNA furnished by the *ace-3* mutant. The question arises as to whether there is any contribution of these RNAs in development. It is hard in other systems to address experimentally the early role of AChE genes. However, this can be investigated in *C. elegans*. It has been shown that maternal *mex-3* mRNA is no longer observed in *C. elegans* early embryos present within animals injected with dsRNA from the *mex-3* gene (25). Using dsRNAi techniques one can perhaps address the early role of maternal AChE RNAs in *C. elegans*. It has been shown in vertebrates that AChE could play an unconventional role in neurite outgrowth (34).

Recently a fourth AChE gene has been cloned in *C. elegans*; it is responsible for 0.1% of the total AChE activity (35). It will be impossible to obtain a mutant by the method adopted for the three other genes (brute-force screening using a class-specific enzymatic AChE assay) and dsRNAi will be necessary here to address the mutant phenotype.

6. Conclusions

The dsRNAi technique is a very fast approach to generating transient gene knockdown in *C. elegans*. Moreover, as suggested by A. Fire, the biological process on which it relies is likely to be present in nematodes other than *C. elegans*. This technique could thus provide a way to knock down genes in pest species of nematodes which are not themselves amenable to gonad DNA micro-injection. It would then be possible to test the effects of the knockdown of a given gene in animal- and plant-parasitic nematodes, on the efficacy of host infection. This may help identify new targets for drug and crop

Onchocerca volvulus UNC-38	RTKN**Y**LTSFSDEAFIDIIFYLELRR
C. elegans UNC-38	RAKN**Y**PS**CC**PQSAYIDVTYYLQLRR
C. elegans DEG-3	HEYK.**Y**A**CC**.AEPWVILQASLVIQR

Figure 6. Alignment of loop C of three nematode nicotinic acetylcholine receptor α subunits: UNC-38 from the free-living nematode *C. elegans* (30); orthologue of *C. elegans* UNC-38 from the human parasitic nematode *O. volvulus* (36); DEG-3 from *C. elegans* (37).

protection agents (*Figure 6*). The dsRNAi technique also provides a way to help identify which members of a complex receptor gene family (32,38) are targetted by a particular drug/chemical.

Acknowledgements

The authors thank the BBSRC and the MRC for financial support, and Dr Marta Grauso for comments on the manuscript.

References

1. Hodgkin, J., Plasterk, R. H. A., and Waterston, R. H. (1995) *Science* **270**, 410.
2. Hodgkin, J., and Herman, R. K. (1998) *Trends Genet.* **14**, 352.
3. Ahringer, J. (1996) *Curr. Opin. Genet. Dev.* **7**, 410.
4. Sulston, J. E. *et al.* (1992) *Nature* **335**, 37.
5. Wilson, R. *et al.* (1994) *Nature* **368**, 32.
6. Kuwabara, P. E. (1997) *Trends Genet.* **13**, 455.
7. Sulston, J. (1988) In: Wood, W. B. (Ed.), *The Nematode Caenorhabditis elegans*, pp 123–155. Cold Spring Harbor Laboratory Press, Cold Spring Harbor, NY.
8. White, J. G., Southgate, E., Thomson, J. N., and Brenner, S. (1986) *Phil. Trans. Roy. Soc. London, B: Biol. Sci.* **314**, 1.
9. Brenner, S. (1974) *Genetics* **77**, 71.
10. Fire, A. (1986) *EMBO J.* **5**, 2673.
11. Mello, C. C., Kramer, J. M., Stinchcomb, D., and Ambros, V. (1991) *EMBO J.* **10**, 3959.
12. Kramer, J. M., French, R. P., Park, E. C., and Johnson, J. J. (1990) *Mol. Cell. Biol.* **10**, 2081.
13. Coulson, A. R., Sulston, J., Brenner, S., and Karn, J. (1986) *Proc. Natl Acad. Sci. USA* **83**, 7821.
14. Coulson, A. R., Waterston, R. H., Kiff, J. E., Sulston, J., and Kohara, Y. (1988) *Nature* **335**, 184.
15. Coulson, A. R., Kozono, Y., Lutterbach, B., Shownkeen, R., Sulston, J., and Waterston, R. (1991) *BioEssays* **13**, 413.
16. Zwaal, R. R., Broeks, A., van Meurs, J., Groenen, J. T., and Plasterk, R. H. (1993) *Proc. Natl Acad. Sci. USA* **90**, 7431.

17. Rushforth, A. M., Saari, B., and Anderson, P. (1993) *Mol. Cell. Biol.* **13**, 902.
18. Plasterk, R. H. (1995) *Methods Cell Biol.* **48**, 59.
19. Capecchi, M. R. (1989) *Science* **224**, 1288.
20. Broverman, S., MacMorris, M., and Blumenthal, T. (1993) *Proc. Natl Acad. Sci. USA* **90**, 4359.
21. Fire, A., Albertson, D., Harrison, S. W., and Moerman, D. G. (1991) *Development* **113**, 503.
22. Guo, S. and Kemphues, K. (1995) *Cell* **81**, 611.
23. Rocheleau, C. E., Downs, W. D., Lin, R., Wittman, C., Bei, Y., Cha, Y. H., Ali, M., Priess, J. R., and Mello, C. C. (1997) *Cell* **90**, 707.
24. Wu, S.-L., Staudinger, J., Olson, E. N., and Rubin, C. S. (1998) *J. Biol. Chem.* **273**, 1130.
25. Fire, A., Xue, S., Montgomery, M. K., Kostas, S. A., Driver, S. E., and Mello, C. C. (1998) *Nature* **391**, 806.
26. Montgomery, M. K. and Fire, A. (1998) *Trends Genet.* **14**, 255.
27. Wagner, R. W. and Sun, L. (1998) *Nature* **39**, 744.
28. Thomas, J. H. (1993) *Trends Genet.* **9**, 395.
29. Jorgensen, E. M. and Nonet, M. L. (1995) *Semin. Dev. Biol.* **6**, 207.
30. Fleming, J. T. *et al.* (1997) *J. Neurosci.* **17**, 5843.
31. Lewis, J. A. *et al.* (1980) *Neuroscience* **5**, 967.
32. Mongan, N. P., Baylis, H. A., Adcock, C., Smith, G. R., Sansom, M. S. P., and Sattelle, D. B. (1998) *Receptors and Channels* **6**, 218.
33. Arpagaus, M., Combes, D., Culetto, E., Grauso, M., Fedon, Y., Romani, R., and Toutant, J.-P. (1998) *J. Physiol. (Paris)* **92**, 363.
34. Sternfeld, M., Ming, G. C., Song, H. J., Sela, K., Timberg, R., Poo, M. M., and Soreq, H. (1998) *J. Neurosci.* **18**, 1240.
35. Grauso, M., Culetto, E., Combes, D., Fedon, Y., Toutant, J.-P., and Arpagaus, M. (1998) *FEBS Lett.* **424**, 279.
36. Ajuh, P. and Egwang, T. (1994) *Gene* **144**, 127.
37. Treinin, M and Chalfie, M. (1995) *Neuron* **14**, 871.
38. Sattelle, D. B. (1998) *J. Physiol.* 513P, 18S.

Index